To

Miss Anna Holt

Here it is. Hope you like it. Your aid & encouragement has been greatly appreciated

Jack Smellie

Oct 4 - 1955

PUBLIC HEALTH
Its Promise for the Future

The roads you travel so briskly lead out of dim antiquity, and you study the past chiefly because of its bearing on the living present and its promise for the future.

LIEUTENANT GENERAL JAMES G. HARBORD
K.C.M.G., D.S.M., L.L.D., U.S. Army (ret.)
1866-1947

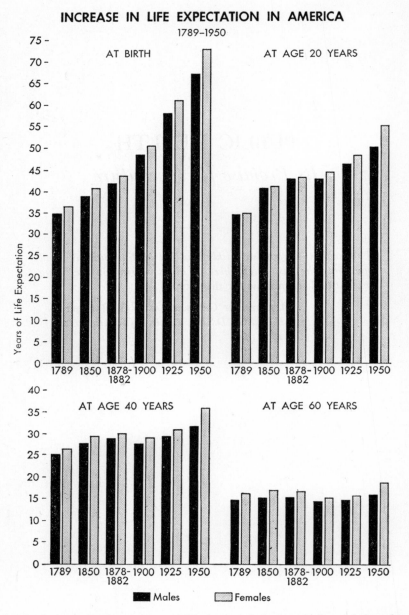

INCREASE IN LIFE EXPECTATION IN AMERICA
1789–1950

AT BIRTH

AT AGE 20 YEARS

AT AGE 40 YEARS

AT AGE 60 YEARS

Years of Life Expectation

■ Males ☐ Females

The increase in expectation of life is one of the best indices of the advancement of the public health of a people. In America there has been a great increase in life expectancy at birth. At 20 years the gain has been considerable, and at 40 some gain has been made although there was an actual loss during the early industrial years. But our great-grandfathers who reached the age of 60 had as good a life expectation as we have ourselves.

PUBLIC HEALTH
Its Promise for the Future

*A Chronicle of the Development of Public Health
in the United States, 1607-1914*

WILSON G. SMILLIE

A.B., M.D., D.P.H., SC.D. (Hon.)

PROFESSOR OF PUBLIC HEALTH AND PREVENTIVE MEDICINE
CORNELL UNIVERSITY MEDICAL COLLEGE
NEW YORK, NEW YORK

The Macmillan Company   New York   1955

PREFACE

This book is a chronicle of the development of public health in the United States during the period of 1607-1914. The reader may ask just why a book of this sort was written. It is not a history. A historian is a person who is quite objective. He collects and then systematizes the mass of data that he has assembled and, in a completely detached manner, either holds it at full arm's length or places it under a microscope for analysis and interpretation. The essential quality of his work is that his subject must be viewed dispassionately and quite objectively.

But this cannot be an impersonal book. When a man has devoted his entire professional career to a single phase of human advancement, he cannot present the subject objectively. For public health is a service to mankind to which one dedicates his life. Whatever talents he may possess are poured unstintingly into his work. His activities and his ideas are blended with those of his co-workers, and public health becomes to him almost a religious fervor, a form of devotion and a spiritual ideal. Thus, a book of this type cannot be written dispassionately, for it is, in truth, a justification of one's way of life.

A great inspiration comes from a review of the achievements of our forefathers. We gain understanding and courage from their foresight, their strength, and their fortitude. An analysis of past events provides us with a more complete knowledge of the philosophy which gave birth to new social concepts and to the application of advances in science.

But the consummate value that is derived from a study of the past is "its bearing on the living present and its *promise for the future.*" For this reason we have chosen the inspiring quotation from Harbord which is to be found on the first page and from which we have selected the title for this book—*Public Health: Its Promise for the Future.*

If we can observe the actual birth of a new social concept, if we learn and understand how these ideas were conceived, and follow

their growth through the long years, we are placed in an informed
position to make sound judgments for the present and to formulate
wise plans for the future. This is the great value of the chronological
approach in gaining understanding of social growth and development. Thus our title is not a whimsy, but is based on a fundamental
truth.

The circumstances that led to the compiling of this text were
quite fortuitous. Nearly twenty years ago I was asked by a pub-
lisher to select a list of twenty-five names of men who had contributed
most to the field of public health in America. It seemed a simple
task, one that would require perhaps a few hours of contemplation
and some routine library abstracting. I have now completed that
task. In the Appendix will be found a list of names of twenty-five
great men who have been pioneers in the development of the concepts and principles of public health in America during the years
1610-1925. They have been chosen with the assistance of my colleagues in this field and represent our present considered judgment.
A century from now, this list of the names of men that we believe
have contributed most effectively to public health during the first
315 years of our history will be entirely rewritten. But to us, at
this time, these men are the most outstanding. In selecting the names
of those who have contributed to the many different fields of public
health, a study of their deeds became essential. I soon learned that
the man himself is not too important. Often it was not the man who
developed a new principle—or point of view. Rather, a social
situation arose that required a solution. New social concepts are
born out of an impelling need of the people. The very press of
circumstances develops the leaders of the people and opens new
avenues of progress.

I learned that, although an outstanding leader may be important
in bringing about a social change, any given individual is not essential to the development of a new social procedure. The man who
is selected by circumstances to be the leader may hasten the process
of social growth or the promotion of community service, but he is
not unique. If he did not step forward as a leader, someone else
would, for the situation demands it. In other words, social development of a people is a mass phenomenon, and does not result simply
because of the emergence of outstanding personalities.

The truly great man is the originator of ideas—the person who
develops his theoretical concepts out of his inner being and forces

his mind to penetrate the true causes of social maladjustment. These men are inspired. They are encountered rarely. Seldom are they great leaders. Often they are born years before their time and live very lonely existences, misunderstood and often despised. Many times they die before a single one of their dreams is realized. Only the dusty document or the lowly disciple keeps the flame alight. But out of the minds of these men come our real understanding and interpretation of human needs. This results eventually in an evolution of methods for the prevention of human suffering and sorrow, and the promotion of human happiness.

For the most part, historians have paid little or no attention to the impact of disease upon our civilization. Public health is not even mentioned as a social phenomenon. It is true that Zinsser in his *Rats, Lice and History* drove home the important fact that plagues and pestilences have had a profound influence on human progress, and the greatest history of all—The Old Testament of the *Bible*—is replete with examples of the influence of epidemics and disease processes in changing the current of history. But one may scan the pages of modern American histories with care and find no reference at all to public health. We encounter full discussions of the vagaries of petty politicians, and read detailed descriptions of unimportant skirmishes that are called battles, but no mention is made of the influence on the people of tuberculosis, of smallpox, of a high infant death rate, or the disastrous consequences of a pandemic of influenza. Even the great triumph of yellow fever control is barely mentioned.

Oliver Wendell Holmes once said: "The state of medicine is an index of civilization of an age and country, and one of the best perhaps by which it can be judged." A century later Kendall Emerson said the same thing in a different way: "The health standard of a nation is a fair gauge of its intelligence and its degree of social development." Thus this text is, to some degree, a measure of the development of American culture.

In 1937 the medical historian Shryock stated that "no one to this day has attempted to write a general history of public health in the United States." Although, as I have previously explained, this book cannot be considered a history text, it is, however, an attempt to meet this obvious need. We believe that, as the chronicle unfolds, we shall witness and understand the slow, steady, painful march of the social development of a people. Some other social index might have been chosen by another author, such as public education of children, the development of transportation, the interchange of information, the growth of urbanization, or some other measure of social evolution. I have chosen the development of the field of public health because it is the subject that I know best. Furthermore, I believe that it is one of the best indices of the march of civilization, since it is a true measure of the growing consciousness in the minds of the whole people that the community itself has a direct and vital responsibility for the promotion of individual and family welfare.

I have chosen, arbitrarily, to bring this book to its close with the year 1914. It is quite true that this was the end of an era for America and the beginning of a new world. But the termination date I have selected is again fortuitous. For this is a personal book and it so happens that 1914 was the year that I entered the field of public health. No one who has been active in a given social or scientific field is in a position to judge and evaluate the historical worth of the work of his contemporaries, nor to appraise the results of their efforts. His eyes are too close to the pages and his heart often affects his judgments. Thus the story of public health in America after 1914 should be written by my successors.

I take this opportunity to thank all those who have aided me in the compilation of this material. To the librarians of medical colleges and schools of public health in various parts of America, I send due appreciation, particularly to Miss Anna Holt, librarian of Harvard Medical School. To all those who have read critically and helpfully certain sections of this text, I give sincere thanks. Particularly to Mrs. Dorothy Rhoades Duerschner, who has borne the heavy burden of editorial assistance and criticism, I extend sincere gratitude and full appreciation.

W. G. S.

CONTENTS

CHAPTER 1. *Introduction*

> *The legitimate object of government is to do for the people what needs to be done, but which they cannot by individual effort do at all, or do so well, for themselves.*
>
> ABRAHAM LINCOLN QUOTING JEFFERSON, *1854*

Medicine is a social science. In the full comprehension of the term, medicine is not simply the care of the sick by a physician, but encompasses all those activities in the community that relate to the prevention of illness and suffering, as well as the promotion of health, and to the improvement of the physical and emotional welfare of the people. Medicine includes hospital care, physician care, nursing service, medical social service, and preventive medicine. It includes also the rehabilitation of those who have met with physical or mental disaster. One of the most important aspects of medicine is the division of activity that is called *public health*.

What is *public health?* It is that responsibility which rests upon the community for the protection of life and the promotion of the health of its people. It is one of the basic community functions, comparable to public education of children, police protection, construction and maintenance of highways, and other public services. It is not a constant, but a changing concept. This change is due to a gradual increase in understanding by the people of the social structure of self-government and a growing recognition of the necessity for community action in promotion of individual and community health and welfare.

The broad general principle upon which public health rests is that every member of the community is entitled to protection in regard to his health, just as in regard to his liberty and property. But his liberty and the control of his property are guaranteed to him on condition that they not be injurious to the health or welfare of the community at large. "Health is not merely analogous to capital, *it is*

1

capital, the value of which to a certain extent may be expressed in coin."[1]

Has the state the right to interfere with the liberty of the individual for the purpose of securing the health of the next generation? May the community invade a man's home and remove him forcibly to an isolated spot as a measure of community protection? These were the questions our forefathers asked themselves. John Stuart Mill denied that the state should attempt directly to improve the physical welfare of its citizens on the ground that such interference would do more harm than good. On the contrary, Sir James F. Stephens stated, "If the object aimed at is good and if the good obtained overbalances the inconvenience of the compulsion, then the compulsion is good."

One important objective in compiling this book is that it may give a historical perspective to those who are interested in community service, particularly as it is related to the field of public health. The knowledge acquired should help us to understand what our job really is. What is the philosophy upon which our community-wide public health structure rests? What is the logic which determines the things that we now do? What does the future have in store? When did the local community first assume responsibility for the health protection of its citizens? What circumstance brought about this event? Why were there no health officers nor departments of health during the Colonial period? Why, at about the beginning of the nineteenth century, did so many towns begin to establish local health services? Why were there no state departments of health until after the Civil War? How could it be that the brilliant and farsighted men who wrote our national Constitution completely ignored the establishment of public health as an essential function of federal government? Only by understanding these matters is it possible to see public health in its proper perspective and to understand its relationships to other community services. Only thus can one plan adequately for the future.

The historical perspective gives a student of this field a very firm foundation on which to stand. He learns from the mistakes that others have made. He becomes more tolerant and more patient. He is less insistent on getting things done—at once. All social development is a very slow and gradual process. Each new concept must be carefully nurtured, and time must be regarded as one of the most important of all elements in its growth. Overstimulation may be

[1] See Billings, J. S.: "Jurisprudence of Hygiene," *Treatise on Hygiene and Public Health,* edited by A. H. Buck, Vol. I, p. 34, 1879.

disastrous. The trunk and branches may seem vigorous, but a poor root system will result in luxuriant foliage without fruit.

During the Colonial period the government assumed little responsibility for promotion of individual or community health. The care of the poor, the unfortunate, the orphans, and the mentally ill was assumed by the community. But this was a private philanthropy, and a good Samaritan act of charity. The local community aided in care of the sick and burial of the dead. Each community cared for its own. In the larger seaports the government took aggressive steps to quarantine incoming ships in the face of impending disastrous epidemics, but this was almost the sole responsibility that was assumed by the Colonial government in the field of public health.

A new concept arose, at about the end of the Revolutionary War, that disease—all disease—was due to bad air, contaminations of the ambient environment by floating miasmata which arose from a great variety of sources. Some of these bad odors were a result of community uncleanliness. Thus the public health became a matter of cleanliness and sanitation of the environment. This required organized community action, but it was obviously not a federal nor a state responsibility. It was purely a local function. Therefore, community sanitation was added to quarantine as a local public health procedure.

The humanistic aspect of public health was initiated at the beginning of our industrial revolution, early in the nineteenth century. The community began to realize that it had a direct responsibility for, and an enlightened self-interest in, promotion of the health of the individual and of the family. This concept was not directly allied to disease prevention; rather it was concerned with the long hours of labor by children in the textile mills, the malnutrition of the factory workers, and the terrible housing conditions of the poor who lived in the industrial slums. These matters became the concern of the entire community. This concept is as distinctly a creation of recent civilization as is the factory system. Galdston has emphasized that "the relationship between the two is causal and organic. It is rooted in the humanism of the Eighteenth Century."[2] It was a protest against the degrading conditions which were a direct result of industrial expansion. There arose spontaneously an awakening desire of the people for social betterment, which resulted in an accepted conviction of group responsibility for health promotion.

[2] Galdston, Iago: "Humanism and Public Health," *Annals of Medical History,* Third Series, Vol. III, No. 6, p. 518. Paul B. Hoeber, Inc., New York, 1941.

As we advanced through the nineteenth century, public health lost most of its humanistic qualities. It became less concerned with the habitations of the poor, with the filth, dirt, and misery of the slums. The development of the science of bacteriology completely absorbed the scientific world. Medical scientists became immersed in the study of the etiological factors in disease production, and, quite logically, public health turned to the epidemiological approach in control of disease. This resulted in a narrowing of the horizon of public health. Public health, according to Galdston, became "microbistic," with the resultant "elimination of its human affinities, and consequent loss of its social effectiveness." Another development occurred at about this period (1870-1875). For the first time the states and, to a limited degree, the federal government began to assume some responsibility for protection of the health of the people. Not until the end of the century, however, did the pendulum swing back to its humanistic concepts, and public health again acquire some interest in the promotion of the health of the individual. Thus the very concept of public health is changing constantly. It is quite different now from what it was 100 years ago. It seems probable that 100 years hence this subject will have advanced, as a social concept, to a much more effective degree than prevails at the present time.

A study of the historical development of those concepts which relate to the public health and to human welfare gives one a feeling of great humility. All our fresh and original ideas that we promote as our own with so much enthusiasm have been proposed many years ago—sometimes almost in our own words. Many of the modern principles of public health practice that are today considered progressive or even revolutionary were clearly formulated at the initial meeting of the American Public Health Association in 1872. Our present teachers of public health administration feel quite complacent about their advanced ideas and modern concepts, but a few quotations from J. S. Billings,[3] written in 1879, illustrate that our predecessors were fully abreast of modern thinking. Following are certain excerpts from Billings on "Jurisprudence of Hygiene." They have a very modern sound.

A. County lines are not natural boundaries and have no relation to causes of disease.
B. Administrative health areas should be large enough and populous enough to require full time of sanitary and executive forces.

[3] Billings, J. S.: *op. cit.*

C. There should be non-practicing full-time health officers with medical education.
D. The Health Officer should be specially trained for his job.
E. If a municipal board of health be properly constituted so that its relationships to the medical profession are harmonious, it should be charged with the supervision of *all medical charities such as hospitals and dispensaries.*

Billings proposed these principles seventy-five years ago. We have not yet carried them to fulfillment.

Another important purpose of this text is that it demonstrates so clearly that public health is an integral part of social development. Each step in advance is interrelated to other social changes in the community. New scientific discoveries may evolve, but make no impact upon community life. One important reason for this phenomenon is that these new discoveries cannot be applied effectively to social betterment until they are well understood and fully accepted by the great majority of the people. Furthermore, old measures that have been applied for years may be quite outmoded. Because of scientific advances, they may no longer be of public health benefit. But they will be retained in community law and custom for many years after their usefulness has disappeared. They are firmly imbedded in the social structure and cannot be dislodged. Through a study of the past we can understand just why some of the public health measures that now seem to us so foolish were once quite logical and well adapted to existing needs. This frame of mind makes it possible to view critically the things we ourselves are now doing and to rationalize as to their true worth both for the present and for the future.

The most important lesson that we have learned in compiling this book is the growing realization that social development is a slow, continuous, onflowing process, very gradual, but irresistible. It follows certain well-defined trends, and flows at a fairly constant rate of speed. Thus the chief value of the historical perspective in public health, as in any other social field, is that by looking at the past and extending it through the present, we can predict the future with a reasonable degree of certainty. Furthermore, we can foresee not only the future but can participate, each in his own way, in bringing about these changes which will result inevitably in benefit to generations yet unborn. We shall never live to see these changes, we cannot greatly speed their flow, but we can channel them in the right directions, break down the impeding barriers, check the deviations from the central stream, and thus make our efforts an integral part of all the ideals of those men, great and small, who have devoted their lives to these matters throughout the past. To these efforts of ours and theirs will be added the efforts of those who, in future time, will continue to contribute to the development of this great public service.

In outlining our text, we have tried, as the systematic historians do, to divide the epochs into certain chronological periods. This classification has been attempted before with considerable success.

Bowditch in 1876 stated that "Public Hygiene in the United States has been woefully neglected except under the stimulus of great epidemics. It may be divided into unequal periods:

1776-1832 Period of theory and dogmatism.
1832-1869 Period of strict observation and bold, even reckless scepticism.
1869-1876 Development of State Medicine."[4]

Chapin[5] has divided American public health development very succinctly. His grouping is as follows:

1. Earliest days to 1790   Quarantine, isolation, fumigation.
2. 1790-1870   Environmental cleanliness. Exceptions are smallpox and maritime quarantine.
3. 1870-1900   Almost purely the control of infectious diseases.
4. 1900-   Promotion of the health of the individual.

At the outset we attempted to divide the development of public health in America into seven periods, but eventually we realized that our divisions were quite arbitrary and inconvenient. Each period merged into the other. It was a continuous development rather than a compilation of a series of volumes in which one book was written and closed, and another volume started. We also attempted to divide our text into subjects, but here again we were unsuccessful. One subject may develop more rapidly than another; there is no true chronology. One must carry one subject through a period of time, then set it down to rest and go back and pick up another subject to bring it abreast of its fellows. But this results in overlapping

[4] Bowditch, Henry I.: "Hygiene and Preventive Medicine." Address to the International Congress of Medicine. Philadelphia, 1876.
[5] Chapin, Charles: "History of State and Municipal Control of Disease," *A Half Century of Public Health.* American Public Health Association, New York, 1921, pp. 133-37.

and repetition. In the end three natural divisions emerged as well-defined epochs. The first period began with the establishment of the North American colonies and lasted until the establishment of the new Republic. This we have termed the *Colonial period.* The second epoch we have called the *pioneer period,* which began about 1790 and lasted to the beginning of the Civil War. This great national catastrophe influenced all social development of our nation and was, in fact, a very natural ending of old concepts and beginning of new ones.

The third period we have called the *developmental period* of public health in America. This period began with the initiation of the Civil War and extended to the beginning of World War I. This war was our next great national catastrophe, and its end was the beginning of a new era in America. It also so happens that 1914 is the year that the author entered the field of public health, and here our chronicle ends.

Thus we have elected to close the pages of this book when the most interesting and by far the most important and fruitful developments were just getting under way. There has been a great upsurge in public health in America during the past forty years. Perhaps more concrete results have been achieved during these years than during the previous 100 years of our history. Some believe that public health has moved ahead more rapidly than other elements in our social structure, although this statement is perhaps debatable. But we are convinced that some other author who is more detached and objective than we can be must record the deeds of this present generation. He will evaluate the achievements and the errors of the first half of the twentieth century and place everything in its proper order, fitting the entire picture into the flowing panorama of time and of social growth.

As an excellent exercise in the evaluation of public health procedure, we shall close this chapter with Benjamin Rush's concepts of a physician's place in health protection—160 years ago—and shall measure his concepts against our present knowledge. This will give a clear illustration of the influence of time upon public health concepts.

We are sincere when we say so proudly that greater advances have been made in public health during the past forty years than during the entire previous period of our American history. What will be the judgment of the historian who writes *our* story? Benjamin Rush

also stated with equal certainty at the beginning of the nineteenth
century that greater advances had been made in medicine during
the past forty odd years—1766-1809—than during the entire previous
history of the country. He wrote as follows:

From a review of what has been effected within the last nine and thirty
years, in lessening the mortality of many diseases, we are led to look
forward with confidence and pleasure to the future achievements of our
science.

Could we lift the curtain of time which separates the year 1847 from
our view, we should see cancers, pulmonary consumptions, apoplexies,
palsies, epilepsy and hydrophobia struck out of the list of mortal diseases
and many others which still retain an occasional power over life, rendered
perfectly harmless, provided the same number of discoveries and improvements shall be made in medicine in the intermediate years, that have been
made since the year 1776.[6]

> We think our fathers fools, so wise we grow,
> Our wiser sons, *I hope,* will think us so.
> —POPE

With this quotation Benjamin Rush ends the chapter on "The
Phenomena of Fever,"[7] but there is little reason to think that he
really hoped or expected that his theories of disease and his favorite
methods of treatment would ever be superseded. For he was the
greatest physician in America in his time, and even today he is considered by many people to be the greatest physician that America
ever produced. In fact, in 1938, when it was suggested that the por-
trait of a distinguished physician be selected by the national government for a postage stamp issue, the first name suggested for this
honor was Benjamin Rush.

But if we analyze the life and activities of Dr. Rush, it becomes
quite clear that he did more to retard medical progress in the United
States than any other one man. He has been called "the man who
was always wrong," but this is hardly fair, for after all he did sign
the Declaration of Independence. He was so sure of himself that he
convinced others and overwhelmed those who refused to follow in
his steps. He had such a strong personality, spoke so well, and wrote
so eloquently that he influenced the medical philosophy and public

[6] Rush, Benjamin: "An Inquiry into the Comparative State of Medicine between the
Years 1760-1766 and the Year 1809," *Medical Inquiries and Observations,* Fourth Edition, Vol. IV, p. 248, 1815.
[7] Rush, Benjamin: "Outlines of the Phenomena of Fever," *Medical Inquiries and
Observations,* Fourth Edition, Vol. III, p. 36, 1815.

health practice of America for seventy years after his death. But if we have gained any wisdom in medical science, then we can be sure of one thing, namely, that Benjamin Rush was a fool of the highest order.

This fact is well illustrated by his conduct during the terrible yellow fever epidemic in Philadelphia in 1793.[8] In the period from August 1 to November 9, over 4,000 people died of this disease in Philadelphia, the next largest and most prosperous city of America and its national capital. Dr. Rush himself had the disease, as did every person in his household. He saw his sister die, and lost three of the five young assistants who lived and worked with him. He was the first to make the diagnosis of the disease and the first to inform the authorities of the presence of yellow fever in the city.

He believed that there was and could be but one fever, and that all its varieties, e.g., typhus fever, pleurisy, consumption, measles, intermittent fever (malaria), yellow fever, and all the rest, were symptoms of a "primary disease in the sanguiferous system." All kinds of fever were preceded by general debility, and this debility was brought about in various ways, from miasmata to violent emotion. On this extraordinary and preposterous foundation he built his complicated structure of the phenomenon of fever through thirty-three pages of confused thinking and completely erroneous conclusions.[9]

Thus, when yellow fever struck Philadelphia in August, Dr. Rush was sure that it was not contagious, nor had it been introduced from the West Indies. It was due to a pile of spoiled coffee that had been "thrown on Mr. Ball's wharf . . . on the 24th of July . . . which had putrefied there." He traced the early cases to this source of infection, communicated his information to Dr. Hutchinson, "inspector of sickly vessels," and, having expressed himself forcefully on this matter of the cause of the outbreak, he set about his deadly rounds of treatment.

Fifteen grains of jalap and 10 grains of calomel was the dose for a single treatment. Three doses were given six hours apart. "The effects of this powder not only answered, but far exceeded my expectations," says Rush, "but I did not rely upon purging alone to cure the

[8] Rush, Benjamin: "An Account of the Bilious Remitting Yellow Fever as It Appeared in Philadelphia in the Year 1793." *Medical Inquiries and Observations,* Fourth Edition, Vol. III, pp. 37-193, 1815.

[9] Rush, Benjamin: "Outlines of the Phenomena of Fever," *Medical Inquiries and Observations,* Fourth Edition, Vol. III, pp. 3-36, 1815.

disease. The theory of it which I had adopted led me to use other remedies to abstract excess of stimulus from the system. These were *blood-letting, cool air, cold drinks, low diet,* and *applications of cold water* to the body." This last technique consisted in "buckets full of cold water to be thrown frequently" upon the patient, but later was modified to application "by means of napkins to the head," and to injection "into the bowels by way of clyster," after "three out of four of my patients died, to whom the cold bath was administered." "A gentle vomit of ipecacuanha" was resorted to on the first day of the fever and, of course, infusion, powder, and tincture of cinchona bark were given freely, with blisters "to the limbs, neck, and head." "The quantity of blood drawn was proportioned to the violence of the fever. Sometimes the loss of a hundred ounces was required for a cure."

Dr. Rush consulted with patients until he became so exhausted that he was in a complete daze. He went to bed, but got no rest; he saw a hundred patients a day at their bedsides; thirty or more distressed fathers talked to him in quick succession while he ate his dinner. He became so steeped in the dreadful miasmata that when he rubbed his hands they gave off a sulphurous odor, and his night perspiration became so offensive that he had to draw his bedclothes close about the neck to defend himself from the smell.

He saw his best friends die in quick succession, and lost all sense of sorrow and grief. With dogged courage he fought his way from home to home to administer to the sick, yet all this time his active mind was casting about for the causes of this epidemic. He notes, "The weather was hot and dry, with very little wind. *Moschetoes, the usual attendants of a sickly autumn, were uncommonly numerous.* Here and there a dead cat added to the impurity of the air. A meteor was seen at 2 o'clock in the morning about the 12th of September."

In his review of the epidemic he devoted twenty-seven pages to a discussion of the noncontagious nature of yellow fever, and then went on to prove that it arose from putrefying animal and vegetable matter. His enumeration of the substances that may produce the summer and autumnal fevers encompassed most of the bad smells of the day. Among others may be mentioned exhalations from marshes, rotten cabbage (which was particularly dangerous), rotten potatoes, onions, peppers, Indian meal, coffee, wet cotton, hemp and flax, musty old books and paper money, the timber of an old house, green timber in a new ship, bilge water, stagnating rain water, hog-sties, duck ponds, locusts, spoiled salt beef and salt pork, raw hides, fish entrails, and privies. Putrid vegetable matter was worse than putrid animal matter. He was able to cite instance after instance in which exposure to each and every one of these various effluvia had resulted in sudden illness and death of individuals, sometimes wiping out whole families, in the destruction of the entire crew of a ship, and even in the development of widespread epidemics.

These views of Dr. Rush as to the cause and mode of spread of many of the common communicable diseases were so strongly entrenched in the minds of physicians, and of the laymen as well, that they persisted right down through the nineteenth century and well beyond the period of the development of the science of bacteriology.

Dr. Rush apparently borrowed most of his etiology from Boerhaave and his epidemiology from Noah Webster. His fearful and devastating therapy was his own, built on the absurdities of his theories and the complete, unreasoning blindness of his conclusions. He observed and described the symptoms of the disease accurately. But if a patient of his got well, his method of therapy cured the man; if death occurred, then the patient had not observed carefully the regimen to which he had been subjected, or was perverse of nature or a weakling.

The extraordinary reasoning that he employed in proving that yellow fever cannot be contagious can only be duplicated by his reasoning in advocacy of the great dangers of putrid air. The disappearance of the disease with the first frost was easily explained. "The miasmata were annihilated from the atmosphere." But to be consistent, one must reason that, since smallpox and measles are only varieties of fever, they should logically be destroyed by frost also. Not at all. Yellow fever miasmata exist in the *outside air* and must come in through the windows. (As indeed the disease did, on the wings of a mosquito.) Smallpox is directly contagious by emanation from person to person, and thus since the frost makes it necessary to exclude air from sickrooms, these diseases naturally spread more widely.

As we review the naive absurdities of Dr. Rush's reasoning, we find only a few grains of sound wheat in all the chaff. He made an exact early diagnosis of the disease and warned the authorities of an approaching epidemic. His clinical description of his cases was precise, and many of his epidemiological observations were exact. For example, he determined the fact that the disease began at Ball's Wharf, that white refugees from the recent revolution in the French West Indies were immune, and that Negroes were less afflicted than the whites. The universally hot, dry weather, with stagnation of streams and springs, and particularly the stagnant water in the rain barrels and cisterns were noted, but their true relationship to the epidemic was not understood. Finally, we find this sentence: "Moschetoes, the usual attendants of a sickly autumn, were uncommonly numerous."

It is all so simple to us, for we now know the secret. Things are so plain to us that, like children playing the game of "hunt the thimble" when everyone in the room knows just where the thimble is except the seeker, we cannot understand why Dr. Rush could have been so stupid when the evidence was all at his finger tips. The true solution was that the disease came from the West Indies by ship during the hottest part of July. The mosquitoes on board the ship transmitted the infection. Because of the hot, dry season, conditions were unusually favorable for development of the household mosquito responsible for transmission of yellow fever. If someone had only overturned the rain barrels and checked mosquito breeding, the whole chain of tragic events would have been broken. The tremendous efforts that Rush expended in his treatment of patients did more harm than good, for the disease, once established, runs its course. Stephen Girard, the financier who had volunteered to organize and run the emergency hospital at Bush Hill, really accomplished something, for he gave the patients rest, food, and nursing care and organized a home for the children made orphans by the epidemic.

When frost finally came, and infected "moschetoes" were destroyed, the epidemic ceased.

We know now, of course, that the whole population might have been injected with a simple yellow fever vaccine, which would have prevented the epidemic from gaining any headway.

"We have grown so wise, we think our fathers fools." Can it be possible that 150 years from now our sons will read our medical texts, this text perhaps, and find that all our naive satisfaction with ourselves and the intricate methods that we have developed for the control of disease are a mass of blundering folly, and that only a few grains of truth are hidden in the chaff of our immense conceit? Our present-day leaders are just as courageous as Benjamin Rush, as honorable, as energetic, and as fine in character. Perhaps a few of them may have as much influence upon the future thought and actions of our nation. But are they more wise?

SECTION I. *The Colonial Period*

1600 TO 1790

CHAPTER 2. *Colonial Unawareness of*

Public Health

Local self-government seems to many [to be] a great obstacle to sanitary progress, but an attempt should be made to secure both rather than sacrifice either for the sake of the other.

J. S. BILLINGS
Jurisprudence of Hygiene
1879

The Colonial era that we have covered in this text lasted about 200 years—from 1607 almost to the end of the eighteenth century. During this entire period we find little evidence that the authorities realized that they had a direct and continuing responsibility for promotion of the health of the people. Certainly there was an almost complete lack of community organization for health services.

The outstanding health crises that had to be faced were recurring epidemics which sometimes developed to disaster proportions. These epidemics were met as emergencies and, as in all disasters, the universal pattern of human reaction was followed.

At the outset, in any human disaster, chaos prevails, every man searching madly for a resolution of his own situation. The major motive is self-preservation. Out of this turmoil certain natural community leadership emerges, usually from the most unexpected sources and almost never from the vested authorities. Often the community drunkard or wastrel is the momentary hero. Eventually a temporary, highly autocratic organization is set up to meet the most pressing needs; sometimes this organization has an official basis, sometimes an entirely unofficial one. Through superhuman effort, the holocaust is stayed; or more often, simply burns itself out. As the disaster recedes there occurs a gradual disintegration of the organization. The heroes have no further titanic deeds to perform. The emergency fades away and ends. A normal situation is regained and no organization is formed in preparation for further emergencies, nor for prevention of similar disasters.

These five steps were followed in every disaster that occurred in the Colonial period. They were followed in three disasters in which this author was an active participant during the first half of the twentieth century, and will probably be followed in the next great disaster that occurs in this nation.

Nevertheless, some lessons are always learned from disasters. During the first 200 years of Colonial life, seeds were sown in the community consciousness for each of the present facilities that are now established as suitable measures for health protection and for promotion of public welfare. They germinated slowly and did not always develop in direct ratio to existing community needs. For example, child health protection, although greatly needed, was undeveloped as a community function until the end of the nineteenth century.

Colonial Health Service Was Fragmentary

Our Colonial forefathers must have been men of iron. It is true that they lived in desperate times, and hard conditions always breed a race of hardy men. Life in Europe was bitter and treacherous, driving the people to any desperate resource. The actual reasons for the establishment of the separate settlements on the North American coast were varied: one group of people left England because of religious persecution, another because of the pressure of economic circumstances. Life at home in Europe was cheap enough. The punishment for a petty thief, if caught, was hanging, and many of the early adventurers to the various colonies had taken the choice between death on the gallows and, what some considered as worse, expulsion to the colonies.

A few scattered points of settlement lay along an enormous seacoast, with little contact between settlements and with no cohesion, no bond of sympathy, not even the wildest dream that all these colonies would be fused eventually into a unified, powerful, populous nation.

The forbidding forests reached to the water's edge, the hostile savages impeded every effort toward permanent settlement. The hardships of wresting a living from the barren soil of New England, the uncompromising winter, the discouragement, privation, and actual starvation, destroyed almost one-half of the first contingent of settlers from the "Mayflower" before a single year had passed.

Sir Walter Raleigh's first colony on Roanoke Island, North Carolina, was completely wiped out. Where they went, how they were destroyed, no one has ever known.

Savage conditions, bitter struggles for life itself, left little time for consideration of community protection against disease. The colonists were so concerned with the construction of stockades about their settlements that they gave little thought to repelling the less obvious, but no less malignant enemy, epidemic illness. Physicians came with the first settlers, of course. No leader of such an enterprise could hope to be successful without some medical and surgical assistance. The first settlers at Jamestown, Virginia, brought a surgeon with them, Dr. Walter Russel, but apparently he did not stay. In one of John Smith's chronicles he noted that Dr. Russel "accompanied him from Jamestown to Chesapeake Bay, up the Potomac to the Falls." Russel was succeeded by another and another. Dr. Anthony Bagnal is mentioned also by Captain Smith as accompanying him on an expedition. These doctors were under contract with the Company, but apparently the rough life of the new world was not to their liking, for they promptly returned home. When John Smith was wounded by a gunpowder explosion the very next year, 1609, there was no surgeon at the colony, and Captain Smith had to return all the way to England for treatment.

Dr. Samuel Fuller was our first American doctor who came to stay. He accompanied the settlers on the "Mayflower" in 1620. He was "zealous in the cause of religion and eminently useful as a physician and surgeon." In 1633 an epidemic of infectious fever occurred at Salem. Dr. Fuller went over the Bay to help the newly settled colony, developed the disease himself, and died from it shortly thereafter. We do not know the nature of this outbreak, but presumably it was smallpox.

Epidemics frequently invaded the colonies with disastrous results. The worst of all were the virulent outbreaks of smallpox. There was no method of protection or evasion when these visitations came. The very isolation of the colonists built up a large nonimmune population, which produced favorable conditions for an overwhelming epidemic. When smallpox arrived, the Indians suffered much more seriously than the colonists. Epidemic after epidemic of various diseases which the Indians contracted from the whites decimated their numbers; doubtless this situation was an important factor in saving the colonies from complete and overwhelming destruction by the savages in the early Colonial days.

As always happens among isolated peoples, the colonists enjoyed long periods of freedom from pestilence. But when an infection did arrive with a ship from Europe, it found a fertile soil and struck with great violence. These epidemics always began at the center of the colony, spreading gradually to the most remote homes. Simple "child-hood diseases" such as measles seem to have caused havoc, and there is some reason to believe that the great Indian epidemic about 1618 that destroyed so many of the savages was measles and not smallpox. (See page 39.)

Influenza, scarlet fever, diphtheria, and epidemic lobar pneumonia as well as meningococcus meningitis added their toll in the winter, while typhoid fever and dysentery were a constant scourge during the summer months.

The old records give us a very imperfect idea of the exact diagnosis of these various epidemic diseases. We do not know what many of them were, for their clinical description is so incomplete. Scarlet fever was not differentiated from diphtheria—both were called "angina maligna." Malaria was not differentiated from yellow fever. Typhus and typhoid fever were not separated until the early part of the nineteenth century. The terrible "spotted fever" epidemic which began in the Connecticut River Valley in 1806 may have been typhus fever, but more probably it was epidemic cerebrospinal meningitis.

Medical science in the early seventeenth century was just emerging from the morass of the Middle Ages. The whole of current medical knowledge could be encompassed within the pages of a few books. These books were written in Latin and Greek; thus only the highly educated few could read them.

The educated men of the day were, in great part, clergymen. Many of them were trained in medicine as well. It was not uncommon that a clergyman, as part of his general education, would study Hippocrates, Galen, Aesculapius, and Celsus, thus obtaining the medical knowledge of the day while gaining the accomplishments of the finished scholar.

In the New England colonies particularly, many of the clergymen also practiced medicine, and the Puritans enjoyed a religious confidence in the skill of these clerical physicians which carried them through many a severe crisis.

The early colonists knew that epidemic diseases were contagious and were spread from one community to another by human contacts, but apparently it never occurred to them to take any direct community-wide action in an endeavor to check the spread of these outbreaks within their own communities. They preserved the spirit of submission to privations that were incident to a new pioneer settlement, and assumed a fatalistic philosophy in the presence of disaster.

Over 100 years elapsed after the founding of the original colonies before we find any of the communities making a definite, continuous, and positive effort to protect themselves from the spread of epidemic disease.

When a disastrous outbreak of disease occurred, a commission was appointed by the governor of the colony to investigate the situation and make recommendations. Some physicians were appointed to these committees, but the chief effort of the committee was amelioration of suffering, care of the sick, provision for orphans, and burial of the dead.

The major public health activities that developed gradually during the Colonial period were related to control of contagion. The most effective weapons of defense were isolation of the sick and quarantine of their contacts. This included not only household quarantine but community quarantine as well. Since epidemic disease usually entered through the ports, ships' quarantine was frequently invoked, although it always was a most disturbing procedure.

As the seventeenth century advanced, we encounter some early ideas concerning the role of environmental sanitation as a means of controlling disease, but any measures that were planned were primarily for community tidiness rather than for health protection. As the eighteenth century progressed, occupational hygiene, health education, infant hygiene, and mental hygiene, as well as the recording of vital statistics, began to emerge as measures for promotion of community health. These early concepts are most fragmentary, but they were important indices of things to come.

We shall present some data concerning the development, during the Colonial period, of hospitals, dispensaries, pesthouses, quarantine stations, medical colleges, and auxiliary community health facilities. Most of these facilities were organized as private philanthropic undertakings rather than as official health services.

In our discussion of contagious disease, we shall not cover the historical period of the Spanish conquest which began in 1492, but shall start our story with the establishment of the Jamestown colony in Virginia in 1607. We shall attempt to glean, from the sparse and confused records, a consecutive account of the trials and disasters of our forefathers during the long period that was required to establish a nation, and to learn of the measures that were employed in the prevention of illness and death from infection. Much of the data is fragmentary and equivocal. We are quite certain that many of our statements can be only guesses, and often our conclusions will be based on fallacy. But the general over-all picture is as true and accurate as we can interpret it.

The presentation will have some chronological order, though there will be a great deal of overlapping of time and topic. Some of our data are not subject to documentation and thus must be taken as probable rather than certain evidence of the facts. We have done the best we could. We shall begin with smallpox.

CHAPTER 3. *Communicable Disease during the Colonial Period*

The best index to public health may be deduced from the proportion in which epidemic diseases prevail.

LEMUEL SHATTUCK
Census of the City of Boston
1845

SMALLPOX

Smallpox was the outstanding epidemic disease of the colonies during the *seventeenth century. Yellow fever* exceeded it in interest and importance during the *eighteenth century,* whereas the dread disease of the first half of the *nineteenth century* was *cholera.*

Smallpox spared no community, but seems to have been more troublesome in the northern colonies (particularly in New England) than elsewhere. Perhaps the New Englanders wrote more about it than the other colonists. In any case, all the colonies had good reason to hold this terrible epidemic disease in greatest dread.

Rhazes,[1] in the early part of the tenth century, described smallpox as a clinical entity, although he confused it with measles. The disease was distinguished from the Great Pox (syphilis) in 1518. Smallpox was introduced into Mexico by the Spaniards as early as 1520 and killed "over one half the native population."[2] Repeated outbreaks occurred among the Indians throughout North America and South America. Thus it was no new disease to the Indians at the time of the settlement of Jamestown in 1607 when our story begins.

An epidemic which occurred among the Indians during the years

[1] Rhazes: *Treatise on the Small Pox and Measles,* translated by W. A. Greenhill. Sydenham Society, London, 1848.
[2] Rolleston, J. D.: *The History of the Acute Exanthemata.* The Fitzpatrick Lectures for 1935 and 1936 delivered before the Royal College of Physicians, London. William Heinemann, Ltd., London, 1937.

1616 to 1619, just before the arrival of the Plymouth colony, killed "nine out of ten of the savages," according to Cotton Mather. We do not know what caused this epidemic. Oliver Wendell Holmes[3] thought it was smallpox, but there is considerable evidence that it was some other type of infection. The Indians themselves were sure that it was not smallpox. This outbreak did not spread to the few explorers who were in America that winter (1618) and who were exposed to it. (See pages 39-43.)

In 1633, however, an epidemic of smallpox did strike the Massachusetts Bay colony. It was worst in the settlement of Salem. The disease spread to the Indians and killed "whole plantations" of them. The disease struck again and again during the seventeenth century, decimating the new colonies. In Europe it was a disease of childhood, as was measles; but in the colonies, where isolation prevented continuous or frequent exposure, the infection might be postponed for almost a generation, then it would attack the whole nonimmune population with terrible force. The disease broke out in New Netherlands (New York) in 1663, and struck the Virginia colony in 1667.

The year 1677 is notable, since it was then that an epidemic of smallpox called forth the first medical publication in America. This was Thacher's *A Brief Rule to guide the Common-People of New-England, How to order themselves and theirs in the Small Pocks, or Measels.*[4] Thomas Thacher was a minister at the Old South Meeting House. Beloved by his parish, he ministered to physical as well as to spiritual needs. The disease was epidemic in Boston at the time. Thacher obtained the information that is contained in the broadside from Sydenham's works. His *Brief Rule,* which gave great comfort to the people, was republished at least twice—in 1702 and in 1721.

Two years after Thacher's broadside (1679), Sydenham pointed out the distinguishing characteristics of smallpox as differentiated from measles, and emphasized that both are primarily diseases of childhood.

Cotton Mather has given us an account of the smallpox epidemic of 1689-1690 in New England. "In about a twelvemonth, one thousand of our neighbours have been carried to their long home." It must be remembered that the total population of the town of Boston

---

[3] Holmes, O. W.: *Medical Essays,* Second Edition. Houghton Mifflin Co., Boston, 1883, p. 314.

[4] See description of this broadside by Dr. Henry Viets, Johns Hopkins University Press, Baltimore, 1937.

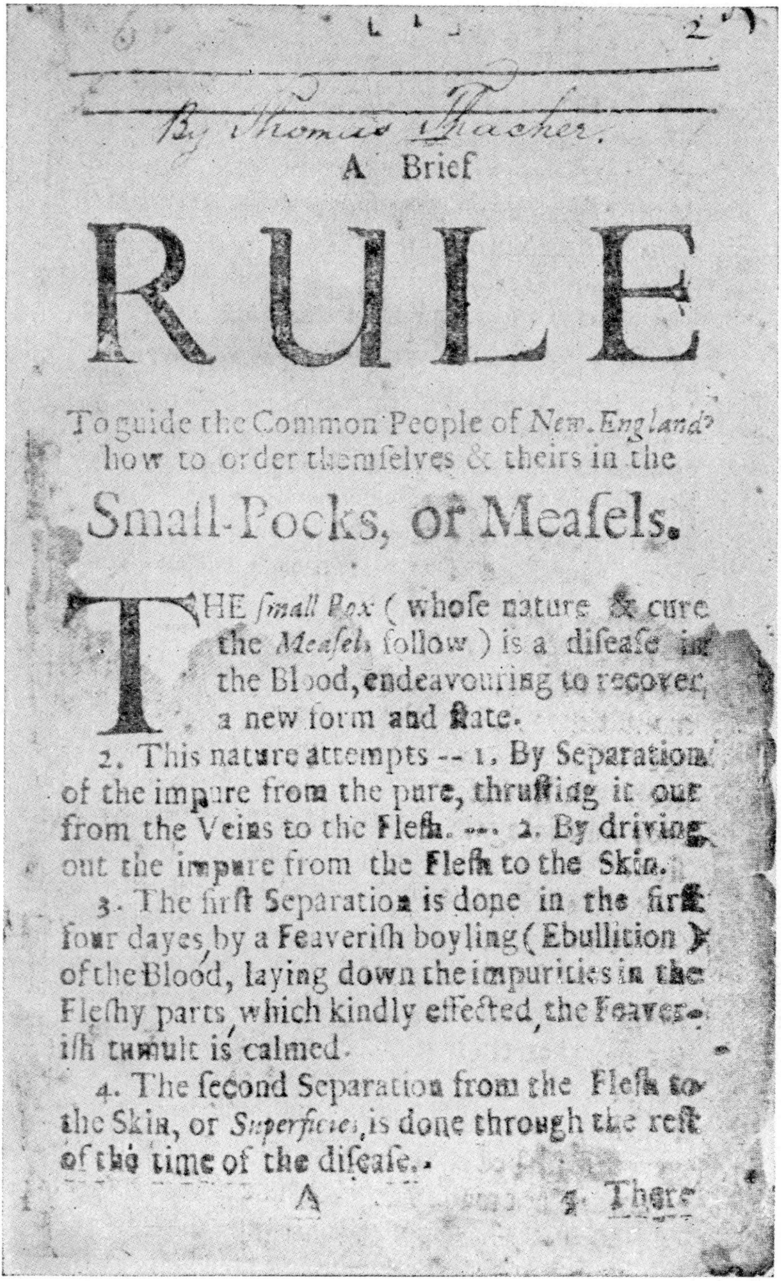

By Thomas Thacher

A Brief

RULE

To guide the Common People of *New.England*
how to order themselves & theirs in the

Small-Pocks, or Meafels.

THE *small Pox* (whofe nature & cure
the *Meafels* follow) is a difeafe in
the Blood, endeavouring to recover
a new form and ftate.

2. This nature attempts -- 1. By Separation
of the impure from the pure, thruffing it out
from the Veins to the Flefh. --- 2. By driving
out the impure from the Flefh to the Skin.

3. The firft Separation is done in the firft
four dayes by a Feaverifh boyling (Ebullition)
of the Blood, laying down the impurities in the
Flefhy parts, which kindly effected, the Feaverifh tumult is calmed.

4. The fecond Separation from the Flefh to
the Skin, or *Superficies*, is done through the reft
of the time of the difeafe.

A   5. There

Fig. 1. The first medical publication in America, 1677, Thacher's *Brief Rule,* as republished in 1702.

at that time was only 7,000. Another epidemic occurred in New England in 1702.

The year 1721 was an historical one, for active immunization procedures were first employed in America during the smallpox epidemic of that year. In 1714 Timonius, a Greek physician, had written in *Philosophical Transactions* an article on smallpox inoculation as practiced in Constantinople. This account was read by Cotton Mather, who determined to try the method at the first opportunity.

Some years before (1706) Mather had been given a Negro slave, who stated that he would never have smallpox. Mather, in a letter to Dr. Woodward, writes:

I had from a Servant of my own, an Account of its being practiced in *Africa.* Enquiring of my Negro-man *Onesimus,* who is a pretty Intelligent Fellow, Whether he ever had ye *Small-Pox;* he answered both, *Yes,* and, *No;* and then told me, that he had undergone an *Operation,* which had given him something of ye *Small-Pox,* and would forever Praeserve him from it; adding, That it was often used among ye *Guramantese,* and whoever had ye Courage to use it, was forever free from ye fear of the Contagion. He described ye Operation to me, and shew'd me in his Arm ye Scar, which it had left upon him; and his Description of it, made it the same, that afterwards I found it related unto you by *Timonius.*

. . . .

How does it come to pass, that no more is done to bring this Operation, into experiment and into Fashion—in *England?* When there are so many Thousands of People, that would give many Thousands of Pounds, to have ye Danger and Horror of this frightful Disease well over with ym. I beseech you, syr, to move it, and save more Lives than Dr. *Sydenham.* For my own part, if I should live to see ye *Small-pox* again enter into our City, I would immediately procure a Consult of our Physicians, to Introduce a Practice, which may be of so very happy a Tendency. But could we hear, that you have done it before us, how much would That embolden us![5]

Cotton Mather's opportunity came with the smallpox epidemic that occurred in Boston in 1721, as we shall see by the following excerpts from his diary of that year.

May 26. The grievous Calamity of the Small-Pox has now entered this Town. The practice of conveying and suffering Small-Pox by Inoculation has never been used in America. But how many lives might be saved by it,

[5] Leikind, Morris C.: "Colonial Epidemic Diseases," *Ciba Symposia,* 1:374. (March) 1940. Reproduced by permission.

if it were practiced? I will procure a Consult of our physicians and lay the matter before them.

June 22. I prepare a little Treatise on the Small-Pox first awakening the Sentiments of Piety which it calls for: then exhibiting the best Medicines and Methods which the world has yett had for the managing of it: and finally adding the new Discovery to prevent it in the way of Inoculation. It is possible this Essay may save many Lives, yes and the Souls of many people.

Mather was in great distress about his son Sammy, who was begging his father "to have his Life saved by receiving Small-Pox in the way of Inoculation." The father feared that if the boy should die, "our People who have Satan remarkably filling their Hearts and Tongues will go on with infinite Prejudices against me and my ministry." Finally, very privately, the boy was inoculated, with excellent outcome.

The minister of Roxbury parish, a kinsman, came to Mather's house on November 14 to undergo smallpox inoculation. About three in the morning, a homemade grenade was thrown into the room where his kinsman lay, but it did not explode, for the burning fuse shook out upon the floor. Attached to the grenade was a message.

"Cotton Mather: you Dog, Damn you, I'll inoculate you with this, and a Pox to you."

The 1721 episode has been graphically described by Oliver Wendell Holmes:

The Reverend Mather,—I use a mode of expression he often employed when speaking of his honored brethren,—the Reverend Mather was right this time, and the irreverent doctors who laughed at him were wrong. One only of their number disputes his claim to giving the first impulse to the practice in Boston. This is what that person says:
"The Small-Pox spread in *Boston, New England,* A. 1721, and the Reverend Dr. *Cotton Mather,* having had the use of these Communications from Dr. *William Douglass* (that is, the writer of these words); surreptitiously, without the knowledge of his Informer, that he might have the honour of a New fangled notion, sets an Undaunted Operator to work, and in this Country about 290 were inoculated."
All this has not deprived Cotton Mather of the credit of suggesting and a bold and intelligent physician of the honor of carrying out, the new practice. On the twenty-seventh day of June, 1721, Zabdiel Boylston of Boston inoculated his only son for smallpox,—the first person ever submitted to the operation in the New World. The story of the fierce resistance to the introduction of the practice; of how Boylston was mobbed,

Several REASONS

Proving that Inoculating or Tranfplanting the *Small Pox,* is a Lawful Practice, and that it has been Bleffed by GOD for the Saving of many a Life.

By *Increafe Mather,* D. D.

Exod. XX. 13. *Thou fhalt not kill.*
Gal. I. 10. *Do I feek to pleafe Men? if I pleafe Men, I fhould not be a Servant of* CHRIST.

It has been Queftioned, Whether *Inoculating* the Small Pox be a Lawful Practice. I incline to the Affirmative, for thefe Reafons.

I.   **B**Ecaufe I have read, that in *Smyrna, Conftantinople,* and other Places, Thoufands of Lives have been faved by Inoculation, and not one of Thoufands has mifcarried by it. This is related by Wife & Learned Men who would not have impofed on theWorld a falfe Narrative. Which alfo has been publifhed by the *Royal Society* ; therefore a great Regard is due to it.

II. WE hear that feveral *Phyficians,* have Recommended the Practice hereof to His *Majefty,* as a Means to preferve the Lives of his Subjects, and that His Wife and Excellent *Majefty King* GEORGE, as alfo his *Royal Highnefs* the *Prince* have approved hereof, and that it is now coming into practice in the Nation. In one of the Publick Prints are thefe Words, " *Inoculating the Small Pox is a fafe and* " *univerfally Ufeful Experiment.* Several Worthy Perfons lately arrived from *England* inform us, that it is a fuccefsful Practice there : If Wife & Learned Men in *England,* declare their Approbation of this *Practice,* for us to declare our Difapprobation will not be for our Honour.

III. GOD has gracioufly owned the *Practice of Inoculation,* among us in *Bofton,* where fome Scores, yea above an hundred have been *Inoculated,*& not one mifcarried ; but they Blefs GOD, for His difcovering this Experiment to them. It has been objected, that one that was Inoculated, died, viz. Mrs. D——*ll :* but fhe had the *Small Pox,* in the common way before, & her Friends and neareft Relations declare that fhe received no hurt by *Inoculation,* but was by a fright put into Fits that caufed her Death. It is then a wonderful Providence of GOD, that all that were *Inoculated* fhould have their Lives preferved· ; fo that the Safety and Ufefulnefs of this Experiment is confirmed to us by Ocular Demonftration : I confefs I am afraid, that the Difcouraging of this Practice, may caufe many a Life to be loft, which for my own part, I fhould be loth to have any hand in, *becaufe of the Sixth Commandment.*

IV. IT cannot be denied but that fome Wife and Judicious Perfons among us, approve of Inoculation, both *Magiftrates* and *Minifters* ; Among Minifters I am One, who have been a poor Preacher of the Gofpel in *Bofton* above Threefcore Years, and am the moft Aged, Weak and unworthy Minifter now in *New-England.* My Sentiments, and my Son's alfo, about this *Matter* are well known. Alfo we hear that the Reverend and Learned Mr. *Solomon Stoddard* of *Northampton* concurs with us ; fo doth the Reverend Mr. *Wife* of *Ipfwich,* and many other younger Divines, not only in *Bofton,* but in the Country, joyn with their Fathers. Furthermore, I have made fome Enquiry, Whether there are many Perfons of a Prophane Life and Converfation, that do Approve and Defend *Inoculation,* and I have been anfwered, that they know but of very few fuch. This is to me a weighty Confideration. But on the other hand, tho' there are fome Worthy Perfons, that are not clear about it ; neverthelefs, it cannot be denied, but that the known Children of the Wicked one, are generally fierce Enemies to Inoculation. It is a grave faying of Old *Seneca, Peffimi Argumentum Turba eft.* For my part I fhould be afhamed to joyn with fuch Perfons ; *O my Soul come not thou into their Secret, unto their Affembly be not thou United.* I am far from reflecting upon all that are againft *Inoculation.* I know there are very worthy Perfons (with whom I defire to Live and Die) that are not clear in their Judgments for it, and they are greatly to be commended and honoured in that they will not act againft a doubting Confcience ; yet it may be fome of them might change their minds, if they would advife with thofe who are beft able to afford them Scripture Light in this as well as in other Cafes of Confcience.

Novemb. 20. 1721.

That the Caufe may have Two Witneffes, here are fubjoyned the Sentiments of another, well known in our Churches, of which I declare my hearty Approbation.

Sentiments on the Small Pox Inoculated.

A *moft Succefsful, and Allowable Method of preventing* Death, *and many other grievous Miferies, by the* Small Pox, *is not only* Lawful *but a* Duty, *to be ufed by thofe who apprehend their Lives immediately endanger'd by the terrible Diftemper.*

But the *Method of managing and governing the* Small Pox *in the way of* Inoculation, *is a moft fuccefsful and allowable Method of preventing* Death, *and many other grievous Miferies by this dreadful Diftemper. Therefore,* 'tis not only Lawful, *but alfo*

Fig. 2. A defense of smallpox inoculation by Increase Mather (1721).

and Mather had a hand-grenade thrown in at his window; of how William Douglass, the Scotchman, "always positive, and sometimes accurate," as was neatly said of him, at once depreciated the practice and tried to get the credit of suggesting it, and how Lawrence Dalhonde, the Frenchman, testified to its destructive consequences; of how Edmund Massey, lecturer at St. Albans, preached against sinfully endeavoring to alter the course of

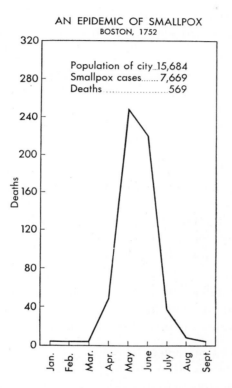

AN EPIDEMIC OF SMALLPOX
BOSTON, 1752

Population of city...15,684
Smallpox cases.......7,669
Deaths 569

Fig. 3. This epidemic of smallpox among a highly susceptible population produced a classic curve of the spread of infection in a community.

nature by presumptuous interposition, which he would leave to the atheist and the scoffer, the heathen and unbeliever, while in the face of his sermon, afterwards reprinted in Boston, many of our New England clergy stood up boldly in defence of the practice,—all this has been told so well and so often that I spare you its details. Set this good hint of Cotton Mather against that letter of his to John Richards, recommending the search after witch-marks, and the application of the water-ordeal, which means throw your grandmother into the water, if she has a mole on her arm;—if she swims, she is a witch and must be hanged; if she sinks, the Lord have mercy on her soul![6]

In 1726 Boylston published a report of this work. There were 5,759 cases of smallpox in the city of Boston in 1721, which represented more than half the total population, with a case fatality rate of 15 per cent. Among the 286 inoculated persons, there were only 6 deaths (fatality rate, 2 per cent).

In 1752 Boston had a population of 15,684 persons. That year smallpox struck again. The following vital data tell the story.[7]

> 5,998 had had the disease already
> 1,843 fled the city to escape the epidemic
> 5,545 developed smallpox in the natural way
> 2,124 were inoculated
>   174 escaped infection
> ————
> 15,684 — total

It seems incredible that of the nonimmune population only 174 persons escaped infection, but this is characteristic of the epidemiology of smallpox. The death rate in the uninoculated population was over 10 per cent, whereas only 1.5 per cent of the inoculated population succumbed to the disease.[8]

A fatal epidemic of smallpox invaded Charleston in 1738. Dr. Mowbray, an English surgeon, inoculated 450 persons and secured splendid results. The method did not gain much headway, however, in Carolina because of the following reasons:

1. Scruples of conscience.
2. Question of lawfulness of the procedure.
3. Fear of the inoculation, which had a mortality rate of 1 to 2 per cent.

Governor Clinton of New York issued a proclamation *against* inoculation in 1747. In 1764 inoculation was forbidden in Carolina without permission from the governor, and during the same year Massachusetts prohibited inoculation in each town unless the consent of the selectmen was obtained. Opposition to inoculation was also strong in the Virginia colony at this period.

Nevertheless, we find an advertisement in the *Connecticut Courant*, November 30, 1767, in which Dr. Uriah Rogers of Fairfield

---

[6] Holmes, O. W.: *op. cit.*, pp. 346-47.

[7] *Gentleman's Magazine*, June, 1753.

[8] Letter from Benjamin Franklin, written in London, 1759, at the request of Dr. William Heberden.

claims to be an inoculation specialist and agrees to carry the patient through the entire course of his infection, with medical and hospital care, for a flat charge of four pounds.

Smallpox again struck Boston at the beginning of the War of the Revolution in 1776. The whole nonimmune population—9,152 persons—was inoculated in three days, with a resultant 165 deaths. This

Table 1

Great Epidemics of Small Pox in Boston*†

1721-1792

YEAR	CASES	DTHS	RATIO PER 100 POPULATION		NATURAL			INOCULATED		
			SICK	DIED	CASES	DTHS	RATIO PER CENT	CASES	DTHS	RATIO PER CENT
1721	6,006	850	54.6	7.7	5,759	844	14.8	247	6	2.4
1730	4,000	500	26.6	3.3	3,600	488	13.5	400	12	3.0
1752	7,669	569	48.9	3.6	5,545	539	9.7	2,124	30	1.7
1764	5,646	170	36.4	1.1	669	124	18.5	4,977	46	.9
1776	5,292	57	44.1	1.0	304	29	9.5	4,988	18	.5
1778	2,243	61	16.6	.4	122	42	34.4	2,121	29	.9
1792	8,346	198	46.0	1.0	232	33	14.2	8,114	165	1.8

* NOTE: There were seven big epidemics during the century. In five of the epidemics nearly one-half the population was infected. A steady decline occurred during the century in the actual number of deaths from smallpox. The case fatality rate in persons inoculated remained remarkably constant.

† SOURCE: Shattuck, Lemuel: *Report of the Sanitary Commission of Massachusetts, 1849.* Dutton & Wentworth, Boston, 1850, p. 70.

heroic immunization campaign knows no parallel in vigor and effectiveness in all our national history. Washington required nonimmune soldiers to be inoculated promptly at Valley Forge, and the disease was kept in check during that year.

Smallpox returned to Massachusetts in 1792. Boston now had a population of over 18,000, of whom 10,655 had had smallpox. Of the remainder:

> 262 fled the city
> 221 remained unaffected
> 232 had smallpox in the natural way
> 8,114 were inoculated

The death rate in natural smallpox was 14 per cent, and in the inoculated group was 1.8 per cent.

Apparently smallpox inoculation had completely demonstrated its worth to the people. Four years later Jenner, a country doctor in England, introduced cowpox vaccine.

Many persons had observed, before the time of Jenner, the value of cowpox in producing an immunity against smallpox. A farmer,

Benjamin Jesty of Dorchestershire, as early as 1774 successfully vaccinated his wife and two sons. But it remained for Edward Jenner, an obscure country practitioner, to make the sound scientific observation that gave full proof of the value of the procedure. In May, 1796, Jenner began his studies by the selection of a dairy maid, Sarah Nelms, who had scratched her hand with a thorn and who became infected with cowpox while milking a cow that had the disease. This variolous matter, originally from the udder of the cow, was inserted into a scratch on the arm of a boy who had not had small-pox. A perfectly characteristic attack of vaccinia followed.

The following July, this same boy was inoculated with material from the pustules of a smallpox patient. He was found to be immune. This experiment was repeated several months later, with a confirmation of the first result. We can justify Dr. Jenner in making this human experiment, since it had been common practice for nearly a century to immunize persons against smallpox by actually inoculating them with the disease.

On the basis of his first experiment, Jenner now selected ten persons who had developed cowpox from nine months to fifty years previously and inoculated them with material from a case of small-pox. All proved to be immune. As Jenner wrote, "I placed it on a rock where I knew it would be immovable, before I invited the public to take a look at it." Nevertheless, his paper which reported these results, when presented to the Royal Society, was refused. In 1798 he published his classic monograph on *An Inquiry into the Causes and Effects of Variolae Vaccinae*. With this brief and modest report began the world-wide conquest of one of the greatest enemies of mankind.

Jenner's work was announced in America in 1799 in the current newspapers and in the *Medical Repository*. Jenner had already sent the virus and a copy of his manuscript to Dr. David Hosack—of New York—in 1798.

Dr. Benjamin Waterhouse, a professor at the Harvard Medical School, wrote to Jenner and obtained from him some dried vaccine impregnated on silk thread. On July 8, 1800, Dr. Waterhouse vaccinated his five-year-old son with this material, and thus the child became America's first vaccinated person. Two years later the Boston Board of Health conducted a carefully controlled vaccination experiment. John Warren, Josiah Bartlett, and Benjamin Waterhouse made the study on eleven boys at Noddles Island. The experiment was beautifully planned and completely proved the effectiveness of cowpox vaccine as a preventive against smallpox, since all eleven boys were subsequently immune to smallpox inoculation. In 1803 the junior physicians of the city formed a free vaccination clinic for the indigent.

A Vaccination Institute was formed in New York in 1802 to give free vaccination to the poor. Dr. Valentine Seaman volunteered to serve as its physician.

The town of Milton, Massachusetts, in 1809 was the first community to organize an official vaccination clinic. The selectmen arranged with Dr. Amos Holbrook of the town to vaccinate, at a cost of 25 cents each, all who would come to the schoolhouse beginning July 20. Within a few days 337 persons were vaccinated—or more than a fourth of the town's total population.

Thomas Jefferson, who later became President, greatly aided Waterhouse and his colleagues in promoting vaccination. In 1806 Jefferson wrote a letter to Jenner in which he said, "Future nations will know, by history only, that the loathsome smallpox had existed, and by you has been exterminated." One hundred and fifty years have passed, and although Jefferson's prophecy will eventually be realized, it is still far from fulfillment.

Nevertheless, a great page in history had been turned. Those of us who have lived in the period after vaccine was discovered by Jenner can only faintly conceive of the dread and despair that formerly fell upon a community when the first case of smallpox appeared. There is no greater single triumph of man in his march toward civilization than the discovery and utilization of smallpox vaccination. In man's baffling struggle to control his environment, Jenner taught us to utilize nature and its methods for the protection of the health and the promotion of the happiness of all the people. The simple discovery by Jenner of the natural means to control smallpox is one of the greatest of all achievements in the field of preventive medicine.

CHRONOLOGY OF SMALLPOX
Tenth Century
Rhazes described smallpox as a clinical entity.

Sixteenth Century

1518	Differentiated from Great Pox, or syphilis.
1520	Smallpox introduced into Mexico by Spaniards, killing nearly half the population (Rolleston, *History of The Acute Exanthemata*, 1937). (Spaniards arrived in 1507.)

Seventeenth Century

1616-19   Epidemic just preceding the arrival of the Plymouth Colony. (Cotton Mather says it killed 9 in 10.) Holmes thought it was smallpox. Williams suggests bubonic plague. They were "yellow all over," but the disease was not yellow fever, as it occurred in the winter. Indians were sure it was *not* smallpox.

1633   Massachusetts epidemic. Samuel Fuller died, also "whole plantations of Indians" (Thacher).

1663   Epidemic among Dutch in New York. English captured New York the following year.

1666   Epidemic transmitted from England to New England.

1677-78   Epidemic in New England. Date of Thacher's first medical publication: 1677.

1679   Sydenham distinguished features of measles and smallpox. He noted both were diseases of children.

1689-90   Epidemic in New England. Cotton Mather: "In about a twelvemonth, 1,000 of our neighbors have been carried to their long home"—in a town of 7,000.

Eighteenth Century

1702   Epidemic in New England.

1714   Timonius, a Greek, published an essay on smallpox inoculation in *Philosophical Transactions* (London). Read by Cotton Mather in 1716.

1721   Violent epidemic in Boston. 5,759 cases. Boylston, instigated by Mather, began inoculation.

1738   Dr. Mowbray, of Charleston, introduced inoculation—450 persons—with success. The disease had been brought to Charleston from Africa and was highly fatal.

1747   Governor Clinton of New York forbade the use of inoculation in New York City.

1752   Epidemic in Boston. Discussion in *Gentleman's Magazine,* June, 1753, of this epidemic and the effects of inoculation.

1759   Letter of Benjamin Franklin, written in London, concerning the value of smallpox inoculation in Boston in 1752.

1764   Epidemic year.

1776   Epidemic in Boston. Whole town inoculated in three days. 9,152 persons, 165 deaths. See table of this epidemic: Shattuck, *Census of Boston,* 1845, p. 144.

1776-78   Epidemic. American troops inoculated with success.

1792   Epidemic in Boston.

1798   Jenner developed cowpox vaccine.

1800   Benjamin Waterhouse introduced vaccination to America.

YELLOW FEVER

As already noted, three great epidemic diseases have menaced the American people. Smallpox dominated the seventeenth century, cholera was the great destroyer of the first half of the nineteenth century, and yellow fever was the "great avenger" during both the eighteenth and nineteenth centuries.

Our first record of an epidemic of yellow fever is the outbreak on the populous little island of Barbados in 1647. It struck with terrific force; over 5,000 died within a few months. Governor Winthrop of Massachusetts called the disease "Barbadoes distemper" and instituted the first ship quarantine regulations on this continent as a measure of protection against the disease. But the disease did not reach North America that year. In 1648 St. Kitts, another small West Indian island, was visited, and over one-third of the population of nearly 20,000 persons died of yellow fever within a short time. The North American continent was spared again, and for many years to come the disease remained in the islands of the West Indies but did not reach the mainland.

Yellow fever was brought to Jamaica from Panama in 1671; Pernambuco, Brazil, was ravaged by yellow fever from 1687 to 1694, and in 1690 the vessel "Oriflamme" brought the disease to Martinique. She had cleared originally from Siam, and thus the disease gained the name "Siam fever." It is certain, however, that the infection of the "Oriflamme" was not brought from Siam, but from a much more recent port of call.

Three years later the mainland had a narrow escape. A fleet under Sir Francis Wheeler was to go to "Martinico" to reduce the island. Having performed this service, it was ordered to go to Boston, take on additional land forces under Sir William Phipps, and proceed to conquer Quebec. The fleet arrived in Boston harbor on June 17. En route from the West Indies, Sir Francis Wheeler had buried at sea 1,300 of his 2,100 sailors and 1,800 of his complement of 2,400 soldiers.[9]

Hutchinson stated that the distemper which had been in the fleet spread to Boston and was even more malignant than ever the smallpox had been, or any other epidemical sickness that had been in the country before, and many families left the town and resided in the country until the infection ceased.

Despite Hutchinson's statement of actual yellow fever invasion of

[9] Hutchinson, Thomas: *History of Massachusetts Bay*, Vol. II, p. 72, 1767.

Boston, we have evidence that the epidemic never spread to the mainland.

Cotton Mather said: "There was an English fleet of our good friends, with a direful plague aboard *intending hither. . . . And that they did not come was the signal hand of heaven.*"[10] What probably occurred is given by Webster.[11] The vessels arrived in Boston harbor with the disease still on board, but the infection was not spread to individuals on shore.

The final arrival of the disease was postponed, but not for long.

Charleston had its first of many epidemics of yellow fever in 1699. In that small colony 150 persons died within a few days, the survivors saving themselves by fleeing to the country.[12]

That same year Penn returned to visit his seventeen-year-old colony of Philadelphia. It had a population of about 4,000 and was prospering. "Barbadoes distemper" arrived on a ship from Barbados. When Penn arrived he found the colony in great distress. Over one-third of the people had the disease, and 220 died within a few weeks. Penn instituted ship quarantine measures, but the disease disappeared as suddenly as it arrived and these measures were never enforced in an effective way.

By 1700 the colonies had developed to the point where yellow fever could find fertile soil in the main ports. During this century it struck again and again, always at the same time of year, always in the same way and at the same places. New York was the first victim in 1702. The disease was imported from St. Thomas in the Virgin Islands. We do not know how many had the disease, but at least 570 died from the infection. During this century Philadelphia suffered the brunt of the attacks in the North. There is a good deal of confusion as to the exact dates of the epidemic years, but the chronology is not important. Carey[13] says that Philadelphia had epidemics in 1732 and 1737. Others have mentioned epidemics in 1745, 1747, 1748, and 1762. New York had an epidemic in the summer of 1743 with 217 deaths. New Haven was invaded in 1742, Norfolk in 1747, and Charleston had an epidemic in 1748. Dr. John Lining of Charleston[14] wrote the first American article on the disease. He described

[10] Mather, C.: *Magnalia, Book VII*, p. 116, 1702 Edition.

[11] Webster, N.: *A Brief History of Epidemic and Pestilential Diseases*, Vol. 1, p. 208. Hudson & Goodwin, Hartford, 1799. (In subsequent references to Webster, title will read *On Pestilence*.)

[12] *Ibid.*, p. 212.

[13] Carey, Mathew: *A Short Account of the Malignant Fever*, Fourth Edition. Printed by the author, Philadelphia, 1794.

[14] Lining, J.: *Yellow Fever*, Charleston, 1748.

the disease in detail and pronounced it to be contagious and imported. Charleston, of all the colonies, was most frequently visited by yellow fever. In fact, the disease probably became endemic at times, carrying through the winter months in the mosquitoes and breaking out again in the early summer. In the northern ports each epidemic represented a new invasion, usually from the West Indies.

In order to understand the strange and baffling nature of these visitations, a simple review of the epidemiology of yellow fever is necessary. The disease is due to a filterable virus. The endemic host is a wild animal of the forest. The disease is transmitted from these forest animals to man through the bite of sylvan mosquitoes. The virus has an incubation period in the mosquito. Furthermore, a mosquito when once infected remains infected for the rest of its natural life. After a man has been bitten by an infected mosquito, there follows an incubation period of about ten days. The man who then becomes ill with the disease can infect, for a few days only, mosquitoes that bite him. The mosquito that transmits the disease from man to man in a village, town, or city is a domestic mosquito— *Aëdes aegypti*. It has a narrow flight range. Thus, an epidemic of yellow fever requires a very special situation.

There must be a large number of *Aëdes aegypti* mosquitoes and a large number also of persons in the community that have not had the disease. Thus, the disease occurred only in summer in the northern part of America and only in the ports where yellow fever was introduced from infected ships. The ships might have infected mosquitoes as well as infected persons aboard. Charleston and the West Indian ports were warm enough so that the mosquitoes did not hibernate, and thus the disease became endemic. The most confusing thing to our forefathers was that the disease obviously spread through the community, yet continuous contact of a sick person with a comrade who had never had the disease did not of necessity result in an infection. The disease was both contagious and not contagious. It never occurred to them that a simple intermediate step was necessary, namely, the transmission of the infection from person to person by a mosquito bite.

The decade in which the worst disasters occurred began with the tragic Philadelphia epidemic of 1793.[15] This epidemic was the greatest single disaster that ever occurred to an American city throughout our national history. Charleston also had an epidemic in 1793;

[15] For a description of this epidemic see Mathew Carey, *op. cit.*

Providence, Rhode Island, and Baltimore were invaded in 1794, and the disease returned to Philadelphia that year. New York had its epidemics in 1794, 1795, and again in 1798. In this latter year 2,086 persons died in New York of yellow fever. Boston had a small epidemic in 1798, and Philadelphia lost 3,506 persons during that same year. New Orleans was invaded for the first time in 1796.[16] But, as we have noted above, the worst disaster of all was the outbreak in Philadelphia in 1793.

Philadelphia had become quite prosperous after the war. It was the capital of a nation of 4,000,000 people and itself had a population of over 35,000. George Washington and his cabinet were there. Politics were rife; speculation was the order of the day. The housing situation was acute. The summer of 1793 was hot and dry. The city was full of French fugitives who had fled the terrors of the slave uprising in the West Indies. The first cases of "bilious epidemic fever" occurred in July and caused no great concern. The epidemic began to assume serious proportions by the middle of August, and by the end of the month the city was like a deserted city of the dead.

Everyone who could do so fled from the city. A Citizens' Committee,[17] formed to take charge of the emergency, rendered heroic service. Several of its members died from the disease, but the others carried on. There was a commodious mansion owned by William Hamilton on Bush Hill, which was suitable for an isolation hospital. The Citizens' Committee took possession and used it throughout the epidemic. Conditions were terrible there at first, but Stephen Girard, the wealthy merchant, took Peter Helm with him and went to live at the pesthouse. He brought order out of chaos. He showed great organizing talent and supreme fearlessness. Although over 500 persons died in the hospital, he gave the patients good care and saved many lives. The "Medical Committee" made certain sanitary rules that resemble, to some degree, our current regulations for diseases which we do not know how to control (poliomyelitis or influenza, for example):

1. Avoiding contact with a case.
2. Placarding all infected houses.
3. Cleanliness and "airiness" of the sickroom.

[16] Choppin, S.: "History of the Importation of Yellow Fever into the United States, from 1693 to 1878," *Reports and Papers of the American Public Health Association,* 4:190, 1878.

[17] See *Minutes of the Proceedings of the Committee Appointed by the Citizens of Philadelphia.* R. Aitken & Son, Philadelphia, 1794.

4. Hospital provision for the poor.
5. Keeping streets and wharves clean.
6. General hygienic measures, such as quick private burials; avoidance of fatigue of mind and body; avoidance of intemperance; accommodation of clothing to the weather.

Vinegar and camphor were used on handkerchiefs of those attending the sick—to combat the effluvia—and gunpowder was burned in the streets. An important edict was: "Stop tolling the bells."

The disease was dreadfully destructive to the poor; whole families were wiped out. It was dangerous to doctors; ten died, not including medical students. Drunkards and prostitutes had a very high death rate. The newly arrived French refugees were immune and were of great assistance in nursing the sick. The epidemic ended the week of October 23, and was officially closed by the commission on November 14. Of a population of 36,871, some 13,000 had fled the city. Practically all the nonimmunes of the remaining 23,775 had the disease. Six thousand were ill at the same time in early October (Rush). Deaths totaled 4,044. Mathew Carey, in discussing the cause of termination of the epidemic, finally concluded that it was an act of God. Temperature, he said, could not bring about an abatement of the disease, as there had been no cold and little rain. We find the answer to his question at this late date from his own temperature records on the frosty nights of October 17 and 18. We now understand clearly what happened. We know that the daytime temperature was not so important as the night temperature. It was on the night of October 18 that the frost either killed or drove the *Aëdes aegypti* mosquitoes into hibernation, thus ending the epidemic.

Benjamin Rush of Philadelphia was the leading clinician of his day, and was a heroic figure in the Philadelphia epidemic of 1793. He has left us a complete record of this outbreak in his *Inquiries.*[18]

CHRONOLOGY OF YELLOW FEVER

1607-1800

1647 Epidemic in Barbados and St. Kitts, West Indies: 6,000 died on each island. Governor Winthrop quarantined Boston against these islands.

---

[18] Rush, Benjamin: *Medical Inquiries and Observations,* Fourth Edition, Vol. III, p. 3, 1815.

1693 British fleet from Barbados, decimated by yellow fever, arrived in Boston. Disease did not spread to mainland.
1699 Philadelphia epidemic. Settlement only 17 years old—220 died.
1699 Charleston epidemic—150 died.
1702 New York epidemic—came from St. Thomas—500 deaths.
1732 Philadelphia invaded (Mathew Carey).
1737 Philadelphia invaded (Mathew Carey).
1742 New Haven invaded (Mathew Carey).
1743 New York epidemic—217 deaths.
1745 New York and Philadelphia.
1747 Norfolk and Philadelphia.
1748 Charleston invaded (John Lining).
1762 Philadelphia—severe epidemic.
1793 Philadelphia—the great epidemic—4,044 deaths.
1793 Charleston.
1794 New York, Providence, and Baltimore.
1796 New Orleans invaded for the first time (Samuel Choppin).
1797 Philadelphia—severe epidemic—also Providence.
1798 New York—2,086 deaths. Boston—for the first time, limited to a small section of the town—145 died. Philadelphia—3,506 deaths.

MEASLES

Our knowledge of the epidemiology of measles would lead us to expect that the colonies, once firmly established, would have suffered severely from epidemics of measles. The epidemiology of the disease is closely related to smallpox in that susceptibility is universal and the disease is highly contagious. Thus, in large populations with frequent contacts, the disease is strictly a disease of childhood. But, where communities are isolated, a relatively large part of the community may come to adulthood without exposure. When measles invades a community in which a large proportion of the young adults are susceptible, the results are devastating. An excellent example is the terrible epidemic of measles in the Faroe Islands described by Panum in 1846.[19]

We can be almost certain that some epidemics of measles did invade the colonies from time to time, but the records of these outbreaks are not well described. It is not at all impossible that some of the "smallpox" epidemics that caused such heavy loss of life were in reality measles.

Measles was clearly distinguished from scarlet fever by Ingrassino

[19] Panum, P. L.: *Measles in the Faroe Islands*, 1846, translated from the Danish by Mrs. A. S. Hatcher. Delta Omega Society, New York, 1940.

of Naples (1510-1580) in 1553, but confusion between the two diseases remained for at least two centuries.

Thacher, in 1677, in his *Brief Rule to guide the Common-People of New-England,* described how the people should order themselves in the "Small Pox, or Measels." Thus, it is clear that he considered the two diseases to be related, if not identical. Sydenham separated these two diseases, smallpox and measles, two years later (1679), but confusion remained in the minds of physicians and the public for another fifty years. Thomas Fuller in 1730 did more than any of his predecessors in distinguishing measles from smallpox. He emphasized the fact that both measles and smallpox are primarily diseases of childhood.

For the above reasons, we cannot be sure of the prevalence or importance of measles as an epidemic disease in the colonies. It is quite possible that the terrible epidemic that decimated the Indians just before the arrival of the Pilgrims at Plymouth may have been measles. The Indians were sure this epidemic was not smallpox. They should have known, for they had suffered repeatedly with smallpox, following the Spanish invasion.

One would anticipate that epidemics of measles during the seventeenth and early part of the eighteenth centuries would be relatively infrequent, with a high virulence when the invasion came. We have some evidence that this was the case. Lemuel Shattuck[20] stated that measles was very fatal in New England in 1713. He also wrote that, from 1759 to 1772, this disease caused many deaths in New England. In the year 1772 an epidemic of measles in Charleston, South Carolina, caused over 800 deaths, and in 1778 malignant measles invaded Philadelphia.

We may be sure that other extensive outbreaks of measles were of common occurrence during the eighteenth century, but the colonists had more important and distressing things to cope with than measles. As the country expanded and communications increased, the disease assumed less and less importance.

The Pestilence of the Indians in 1618

A terrible epidemic struck the North American Indians just before the landing of the Pilgrims at Plymouth. Their numbers were so reduced that they were unable to make even a slight resistance to this threat to their sovereignty.

[20] Shattuck, Lemuel: *Census of Boston,* 1845.

Cotton Mather[21] said:

The Indians of these Parts had newly, even about a Year or Two before, been visited by such a prodigious Pestilence: as carried away not a *Tenth*, but *Nine Parts of Ten* (yea 'tis said *Nineteen* of *Twenty*) among them: so that the Woods were almost cleared of these pernicious Creatures to make Room for a *better Growth*.

Noah Webster[22] made a careful study of this outbreak, gleaning material from all available sources. He summarized his information as follows:

Capt. Dermer, an English adventurer, who had arrived in America, in a fishing vessel, a year or two before, passed the winter of 1618-19 in Mon-higgan, an Indian town on the northern coast. On the 19th of May 1619 he sailed along the coast, on his way to Virginia, and landed at several places, where he had been the year before; and he found many Indian towns totally depopulated—in others a few natives remained alive, but "not free of sickness"; "their disease, the plague, for we might perceive the sores of some that had escaped, who described the spots of such as usually die." These are his words. He found some villages, which, in his former visit, were populous, all deserted—the Indians "all dead."

Purchas, vol. 4, 1778.

Richard Vines, and his companions, who had been sent by Ferdinando Gorges, to explore the country, wintered among the Indians, during the pestilence, and remained untouched, the disease attacking none of the English. Belknap's Life of Gorges, American Biography, vol. I, p. 355, but the year is not specified.

A sermon was preached by Elder Cushman at Plymouth, in 1620, just after the colony arrived, and sent to London to be published. In the Epistle Dedicatory which is dated December 21, 1621, the author has these words. "They [the Indians] were very much wasted of late, by a great mortality, that fell amongst them, *three years since,* which, with their own civil dissentions and bloody wars, hath so wasted them, as I think the twentieth person is scarce left alive."

Hazard's Collection, vol. I, p. 148.

This corresponds also with the accounts in Prince's Chronology from original manuscripts. This fixes the time in 1618, precisely agreeable to Capt. Dermer's account. This was the year of the principal mortality; but like other pestilential periods, this continued for a number of years; for some of the Plymouth settlers went to Massachusetts (now Boston), in 1622, to purchase corn of the natives; and "found among the Indians, a

[21] Mather, C.: *Magnalia,* Fourth Edition, Book I, Chap. 2, 1702.
[22] Webster, N.: *op. cit.,* pp. 176-78.

great sickness, not unlike the plague, if not the same." It raged in winter, and affected the Indians only.

See Purchas. 4, 1858. Prince's Chron. 124.

The time then is fixed. The disease commenced, or raged with its principal violence in 1618 and through the winter. So fatal was the pestilence in America, that the warriors from Narragansett to Penobscot, the distance to which the disease seems to have been limited, were reduced from 9000 to a few hundreds.* When our ancestors arrived in 1620, they found the bones of those who perished, in many places, unburied.

Magnalia, book I, p. 7.

* Hutchinson says 30,000 of the Massachusetts tribe alone were supposed to be reduced to 300.

The kind of disease is another important question. Dermer seems to think it a species of plague, and he saw some of the sores of those who had survived. Hutchinson, vol. I, p. 34-35, says some have supposed it to have been the smallpox, but the Indians, who were perfectly acquainted with this disease, after the English arrived, always gave a very different account of it, and described it as a pestilential putrid fever.

Fortunately General Gookin, in the passage above cited, has left us a fact, which leaves no doubt as to the nature of the malady. His words are—"What the disease was, which so generally and mortally swept them away, I cannot learn. Doubtless it was some pestilential disease. I have discoursed with some old Indians, that were then youths, who say, that the *bodies all over were exceeding yellow* (describing it by a yellow garment they showed me) both before they died and afterwards."

Oliver Wendell Holmes in his *Medical Essays*[23] discussed this "great and grievous plague" at some length. He pointed out that those who recovered from the purulent fever were left with unhealed places on their body. "The whole surface of the body both in the living and the dead was yellow, as though covered with a garment." He suggested that the most probable diagnosis was smallpox. "Confluent Variola is a hideous mark which may well have resembled the yellowness of a garment."

Since distances between villages were sometimes great and communications were slow, we must postulate an incubation period of at least six to seven days. Furthermore, the infection must have persisted in a carrier, human or other, through the summer months.

Holmes's suggestion of smallpox is a possibility. The Indians were well acquainted with smallpox, however, for they had suffered from

[23] Holmes, O. W.: *op. cit.,* p. 315.

successive epidemics since the appearance of the Spaniards. They were quite sure that this disease was not smallpox.

Williams[24] suggested that this epidemic was bubonic plague. If this were true, one would expect that the infection would persist in the country in a rodent host to devastate the colonists. This did not occur.

It was not yellow fever, as Noah Webster suggested, since it began in November. Malaria also is not a possibility for the same reason. Spirochetal jaundice (Weil's disease) does not present this epidemiological picture, and infectious hepatitis, though it may occur in serious epidemics in single communities, does not occur in widespread pandemics and does not produce sores on the surface of the body. Thus this disease is quite an unlikely diagnosis.

It is interesting, though perhaps fruitless, to speculate on the true cause of this outbreak.

The epidemiological characteristics are: A febrile disease that appeared in the early winter—November, 1618—and which struck the Indians with great violence. There was very little individual or community immunity to this infection among the natives. The few Europeans who were directly exposed to the infection were immune. Severe damage to the liver seems to have been a striking feature of the disease, and hemorrhage from the nose was one of the striking symptoms. The fever was high, and prostration was extreme. Apparently a rash accompanied the disease, but we do not have a good description of it. Unhealed lesions of the skin were noted in those who recovered from the fever. The fatality rate was over 90 per cent, and the incidence in each and every village was also almost 90 per cent. Highly contagious, it spread from one Indian village to another until all were invaded. The disease receded in the summer of 1619, only to return with unabated virulence in the winter of that year.

Meningococcus septicemia must be considered as a possibility, for its epidemiology has some of the attributes of this outbreak. Typhus fever may well explain the whole picture, but one would anticipate some susceptibility of the whites, and a prolongation of the infection into subsequent years, in endemic form. We have no evidence of endemic typhus in the colonies. We can be sure that it was not typhoid fever. Perhaps the best surmise is measles, which, in a nonimmune, primitive people, can produce the most devastating of all epidemics. One count against measles is the apparent disappear-

[24] Williams, H. U.: *Johns Hopkins Bull.,* **20**:340, 1909.

ance of the disease in the summer of 1619 with return of the epidemic in the late fall. On the other hand, the complete immunity of the whites is a strong argument in favor of measles.

We shall probably never know what destroyed the Indians in 1618. Whatever it was, this epidemic made possible the colonization of New England.

DYSENTERY AND OTHER INTESTINAL INFECTIONS

Bloody diarrhea is such a clear-cut entity that we can make at least an estimate of its prevalence during the Colonial period. Amoebic dysentery was not differentiated from bacillary dysentery. Other intestinal infections, such as typhoid fever, were sometimes confused with bacillary dysentery, at other times with typhus fever.

Dysentery in a pioneer community occurs in limited, sharp outbreaks with long periods of remission. Sporadic cases may occur at any time of the year, but the majority of infections occur in early summer in the southern part of the country, and in late summer in the colonies north of Chesapeake Bay.

The first settlement at Jamestown was devastated by dysentery in 1609, and the disease remained to plague this colony almost continuously. Dysentery was particularly prevalent during periods of war. The settlers had no clear idea of the importance of proper disposal of human wastes, nor of the necessity for protection of the drinking water from pollution. The stockade system of defense and the frequent danger of attack from Indians made it difficult to maintain good camp sanitation, particularly in a permanent camp. Flies were incredibly numerous, and the soldiers themselves "died like flies" during the summer months in the Jamestown camp.

There was one period of serious epidemicity of dysentery in 1749. It began apparently in Waterbury, Connecticut,[25] where 130 persons died. The disease did not appear to be very contagious, although it excited great alarm. Everyone avoided the sick if possible, but many who never came near the sick and who lived in remote places were seized and suddenly died. The summer had been very dry. The disease returned the following summer and was "epidemic and mortal in Hartford, New Haven, and in many places." It continued in epidemic proportions each summer until 1753 and then abated.

Dysentery occurred in very serious epidemic proportions at the outbreak of the Revolutionary War. That summer was hot and dry.

[25] Webster, N.: *op. cit.*, p. 241.

Dysentery was prevalent in all parts of the country and was "terribly fatal to the American troops at New York and Ticonderoga."[26] Of 13,000 troops at Mount Independence in October, one-half were unfit for duty because of dysentery.

The disease had appeared in epidemic proportion in 1773, two years before the onset of war. It was particularly malignant in New Haven, Connecticut, and Salem, Massachusetts. In Danbury, Connecticut, in 1775, over 100 persons died from the disease. During the years of peace, dysentery had been most prevalent and fatal among old persons and young children, but it spread to the encampments when war was declared on England, and continued to harass both British and American troops throughout the Revolutionary War.

The final dysentery epidemic of the eighteenth century occurred during the summer of 1793 and extended to various parts of the nation. It swept away many hundreds of inhabitants of Georgetown on the Potomac. Webster reports that in Coventry, Connecticut, in 1793, it "killed every person whom it seized." The disease raged in Duchess County, New York, in 1795. In Philadelphia, where it had not appeared for many preceding years, it began to attack children in the early summer of 1796. In August of that year dysentery increased to epidemic proportions in Wilmington, North Carolina. This outbreak was complicated, as were many others, by "bilious remittent fever"—e.g., malaria.

By this time some understanding of the relationship of polluted water to dysentery was developing. The dejecta of the patients was considered dangerous, but there was no real comprehension of the epidemiology of the disease, and no effective methods of control were applied. Even such simple precautions as isolation of the sick, burial of excreta, and boiling of drinking water were not utilized as preventive measures.

Diarrheal diseases of infancy took a very heavy toll every summer in all parts of the country. In Europe during the nineteenth century, this disease was called the "American disease of infants." As we shall see later, the industrialization of the country during the first half of the nineteenth century, with accompanying bad housing, together with heavy immigration, resulted in an appalling infant death rate, particularly from infantile diarrheas. During the Colonial period,

[26] *Ibid.*, p. 263.

however, these destructive diseases of infants, bad as they were, had not assumed true epidemic proportions.

Typhoid fever undoubtedly was highly prevalent during Colonial days, occurring every summer in each village and town. There were no striking outbreaks because there was no extensive common source of infection, such as a community-wide water system or a common milk supply. The epidemiology of typhoid fever in a frontier community was a series of small family or village outbreaks, and these attracted little attention because of their limited geographic distribution.[27] But the agent of infection was so constantly present that everyone in the community was exposed before he reached adult life, and thus an extensive degree of immunity was secured. For this reason the number of cases that occurred each year on the frontier was usually limited. Furthermore, malaria, which occurred during the same season as typhoid fever, confused the epidemiological picture to such a degree that we cannot evaluate the relative importance of these two diseases.

Asiatic cholera, which caused such devastation in the young nation during the first half of the nineteenth century, did not invade North America during the Colonial period.

INFLUENZA

Epidemic influenza did not play an important part in Colonial life during the seventeenth century, at least insofar as the records of the times indicate. The disease struck four times: in 1627 it appeared in Massachusetts and spread to the West Indies. This is the first record we have of epidemic influenza on the American continent. Winthrop[28] described a widespread outbreak in 1647, which did not cause many deaths. There was a general epidemic in June, 1655, and another in New England in the winter of 1697.

There were three epidemics of influenza in the first half of the eighteenth century—in 1732, 1737, and 1747—but apparently these caused no great concern. During the next fifty years there were seven epidemics of influenza, at least, according to the reports of Noah Webster. One is inclined to discount considerably the data on in-

[27] An excellent illustration was the epidemic of typhoid fever in New Salem, Illinois, which attacked young Abraham Lincoln, and was fatal to his sweetheart, Ann Rutledge. This village epidemic probably changed the course of American history, for if Lincoln had married Ann Rutledge he would never, in all probability, have become President of the United States.

[28] Winthrop, John: *History of New England,* Vol. 2, p. 310, 1647.

fluenza that were compiled by Webster, for he had a thesis which he was trying to prove and fitted his data to his theory. If Vesuvius erupted, or if a comet was seen in a certain year, then he searched assiduously for concurrent or subsequent epidemics; and it is almost always possible, of course, to report an influenza epidemic of some degree in some part of the world at some season of the year, if one searches far and wide for it.

The epidemic of influenza of 1789-1790, however, was probably quite troublesome. It was dispersed throughout the Western Hemisphere, and, though extensive, was mild in type. Rush[29] devoted a special chapter in his *Medical Observations* to this epidemic. Children under eight years and elderly people escaped the infection. The case fatality rate was low. Gallup[30] recorded this epidemic of 1789 as the first serious outbreak of influenza in Vermont. It came in the fall, accompanied by pneumonia. The disease returned the following spring and was more severe than it had been in the fall. Apparently the isolated settlements of Vermont suffered more from the pneumonia that accompanied the epidemic than did the larger centers, such as Boston and Philadelphia. In fact, this seems to have been a general rule in Vermont and the other rural pioneer northern states during the nineteenth century. Pneumonia was one of the most dreaded of all the diseases that attacked the isolated settlements.

James Thacher (1828) stated that influenza appeared nine or ten times in the colonies between 1733 and 1766. Whole communities were sick at the same time, but the death rate was low. Apparently the colonies never suffered from the devastating type of influenza that swept over the world in 1918.

CHRONOLOGY OF INFLUENZA AND PNEUMONIA
1600-1800

1627	Summer: Nieuw Amsterdam, Massachusetts, and Connecticut. First known in Western Hemisphere—spread to West Indies and South America. (Webster.)
1647	Description by Winthrop. Widespread, but not many deaths.
1655	June. New England states. General epidemic. (Webster.)
1697-98	Epidemic in New England described by Webster.
1732	October. First in New England states, then spread to West Indies. (Webster.)

[29] Rush, Benjamin: *op. cit.*, Vol. II, p. 266, 1815.
[30] Gallup, J. A.: *History of Epidemical Diseases in the State of Vermont*, 1815.

1737-38   Epidemic in North America (Webster).

1747   Epidemic all over North America.

1757   December to May. General diffusion in North America and West Indies. Very fatal to the aged. (Webster.)

1761-62   General diffusion in North America (Webster).

1767   General diffusion in North America (Webster).

1772   February. New England epidemic. (Webster.)

1780-81   March. North America. (Webster.)

1789-90   General diffusion, Western Hemisphere (Webster). Gallup reported this epidemic as extensive and mild. Rush also reported this outbreak.

1798-99   General diffusion throughout the United States of America (Webster).

SYPHILIS

Williams[31] has made a study of syphilis of the bones of Indians in North America and has presented convincing evidence that this disease afflicted the Indians before the arrival of the white man on this continent. In the United States these bones have come from New Mexico, Alabama, and Illinois. We have no convincing epidemiological evidence, however, that the colonists on the Atlantic seaboard contracted a virulent type of syphilis from the Indians during the early years of colonization of North America.

Beginning about 1598, a virulent epidemic of syphilis swept over all of Europe, causing a great deal of misery and suffering. The epidemiology of the disease was well comprehended, including an understanding of congenital syphilis. There has been a great deal of discussion concerning the possibility that the sailors of Columbus may have introduced this "new disease" into Europe from America. But there is ample evidence that syphilis was prevalent in Europe before the discovery of America and that it was not a new disease in 1600. However, it is quite possible that the adventurers who came to the New World returned with a virulent strain of *Spirochaeta pallida,* which, when introduced into a highly susceptible population, produced havoc.

During the seventeenth century the disease was introduced continuously by Europeans into all the various ports of the colonies in the New World.

Syphilis apparently was not a prevalent disease in the Puritan colonies, but as commerce developed and the seaports grew in im-

[31] Williams, H. U.: *Arch. Dermat. & Syph.,* 33:783, 1936.

portance, the disease became manifest. We have evidence of this fact through James Thacher,[32] who extracted from Governor Winthrop's *Journal* an account of a distressing epidemic of syphilis that occured in Boston in 1646:

The virtuous people of Boston were grieved by the discovery of a disease with which until then they were unacquainted, and which raised a scandal upon the town without just cause. The disease proved to be *lues venerea*. It originated in the wife of a seafaring man, who after childbirth was afflicted with an ulcerated breast. Many persons were employed to draw this woman's breast (by the common method of mouth suction), by which means about sixteen persons were affected by this new and odious disease. The nature of the complaint was at length discovered, but no physician could be found in the country who was acquainted with the method of cure. But it fortunately happened at that very season a young surgeon arrived from the West Indies who had been experienced in the disease, and he soon performed a cure. [With mercurials.]

We have many subsequent references to the ravages of gonorrhea and syphilis in the colonies, particularly in the seaports. Books on domestic medicine, which were found in every well-ordered home, discussed these diseases and their treatment in detail. James Ewell of Savannah in his famous *Planter's and Mariner's Medical Companion,* in 1807, gave an excellent discussion of the prevention, diagnosis, and treatment of gonorrhea and syphilis.

George Wallis in 1793 published *The Art of Preventing Disease and Restoring Health.* In his discussion of venereal disease, he stated that gonorrhea and syphilis were considered by some authorities to be different entities. "I shall treat them under the same head, perfectly persuaded that they are the same disease, occurring under different constitutional circumstances."

It is apparent that these venereal diseases were considered to be shameful, and that their contagious nature was well understood. The source of infection, Wallis stated, was in the most part from prostitutes. The general methods of treatment and the community attitude toward both syphilis and gonorrhea were no different in 1800 than in 1900. These diseases were considered as a just punishment for shameful sin, and their victims received little pity and scant consideration. Though the source of infection was understood, little effort was expended in preventing the disease, or in checking

[32] Thacher, James: *American Medical Biography.* Vol. 1, "History of Medical Science in the United States." Richardson & Lord, Boston, 1828.

its spread through the community. Treatment was empirical and symptomatic in gonorrhea; in syphilis, heavy reliance was placed on large, often toxic doses of the mercurials. This general attitude of the community and general policy of official health services in regarding venereal disease as a well-deserved punishment continued unchanged throughout the nineteenth century. It is hard to believe that an enlightened point of view concerning the prevention and treatment of venereal diseases has been achieved only during the past twenty-five years of our national history. As we shall see in subsequent discussions, the venereal diseases were considered, for generations, not as problems in public health but as punishment for wrongdoing—a matter of morals rather than hygiene.

SCARLET FEVER, DIPHTHERIA, AND OTHER TYPES OF THROAT INFECTIONS

Cynanche Trachealis, Angina Suffocativa, Scarlatina Anginosa, Angina Maligna, Throat Distemper, Angina Ulcerosa, "Plague of the Throat," etc.

During the Colonial period a great many descriptive names were used in attempting to classify the infections of the throat. We now know that practically all these diseases were due to infection with either the beta hemolytic streptococcus or the Klebs-Loeffler bacillus. The clinical descriptions of the various epidemics make it quite clear that some of them were severe outbreaks of diphtheria; others were, obviously, epidemics of scarlet fever. In the severe epidemic of 1735-1740, which began in New England, there is some reason to believe that both diphtheria and scarlet fever played a part in the heavy loss of life.

The prevailing opinion was that the "throat distemper" was not contagious, but was due to supernatural causes—a visitation of tribulation because of sin against God. (The minister of a local church in New Hampshire believed that the epidemic of 1735 started because the people had failed to pay his salary.)

The physicians of Boston insisted that bad air was the source of this particular epidemic and that no quarantine of the family of a victim was necessary. But the Boston City Council was much more realistic and responded to popular opinion with a rule which required isolation of the infected children.

No procedures were available which were effective either in pre-

vention or treatment of these infections, though vigorous therapy
of formidable proportion was applied.

The descriptive term, "scarlet fever," is supposed to have been
introduced by Sydenham (1624-1689) toward the end of the seventeenth century. He is also frequently credited with the differentiation
of scarlet fever from measles, though Ingrassino of Naples in 1553
made this distinction a century before Sydenham. The earliest use
of the term that I have discovered is that found in Pepy's *Diary*,
November 10, 1684: "My little girl Susan is fallen sick with the
measles, or at least of a scarlet Feavour." The disease must have been
prevalent during that century, and apparently was given a variety
of names. It was relatively mild, a disease of childhood, and little
feared. Thomas Fuller in the early part of the eighteenth century
considered it to be a benign fever, "nothing virulent in it, not
contagious, and chiefly a disease of children." Cotton Mather, in
Magnalia,[33] mentioned scarlet fever as a common and rather mild
disease.

As we have already noted, an extensive and severe epidemic began
in New England in 1735, which was called the "throat distemper of
New England." This epidemic began in Kingston Township, New
Hampshire, March 20, 1735, and raged throughout the summer.
Over 80 per cent of the deaths occurred in children under ten years
of age. It is reported that none of the first forty persons who developed this disease recovered. Several families in the rural districts
lost all their children. Twenty-seven persons in five families died
in one small community. The disease spread through New Hampshire to Portsmouth, and finally the epidemic reached Boston in
March, 1736. Here over 4,000 cases occurred in a population of
about 12,000. The case fatality rate in Boston was only 3 per cent,
whereas in the rural districts it had been 25 to 40 per cent. Douglass[34]
described the Boston outbreak, and considered the lower death rate
in the city to be due to the better treatment received there.

Ernest Caulfield[35] has advanced the very interesting theory that the
New England epidemic of 1735 was in reality two simultaneous epidemics—scarlet fever and diphtheria. He has presented convincing
evidence that the disease which began in Kingston, New Hampshire,
and which had a very high death rate, was diphtheria.

[33] Mather, C.: *Magnalia*, Book IV, p. 156, 1702 Edition.
[34] Douglass, W.: "The Practical History of a New Epidemical Eruptive Miliary Fever
with an Angina Ulcerosa Which Prevailed in New England in 1735-36," *New England
J. Med. & Surg.*, 14:1, 1825 (reprint).
[35] Caulfield, Ernest: *Yale J. Biol. & Med.*, 11:219, 1939.

There is no question but that the epidemic in Boston was scarlet fever. Douglass described the cases fully and unmistakably. He did not see the cases of sore throat that occurred in the country districts, according to Caulfield, but simply assumed that the two diseases were the same because the major symptom was sore throat.

It would seem to be a simple matter to distinguish scarlet fever from diphtheria, through absence or presence of a rash. But physicians did not consider a rash to be a significant diagnostic criterion. A rash was simply a symptom of a disease, and it might, or might not, appear. The rash might be "brought out" by appropriate treatment, or a patient might have a high fever with an "inward rash" and might die because it was never possible to bring out the rash. Thus, a severe case of diphtheria might be considered as a case of scarlet fever with an inward rash. The epidemiology of scarlet fever is quite similar to that of diphtheria. Both diseases occur at the same season of the year, are spread by direct contact, and frequently attack the youngest members of the family. Diphtheria, untreated with antitoxin, has a high case fatality rate. There is little reason to believe that it is less virulent today than before specific treatment became available in 1893, nor that it has changed its virulence at any time. In almost any outbreak 15 to 25 per cent of all untreated children die from this disease. Scarlet fever has, as a general rule, a much lower case fatality rate. There is good evidence, however, that scarlet fever has fluctuated in virulence from generation to generation and from place to place. In 1954 scarlet fever killed less than 1 per cent of its victims in the United States; yet in certain parts of the world the disease may still manifest itself with very high virulence, and with multiple cases in the same family. Thus, the high case fatality rate of the New England epidemic does not prove that the disease was not scarlet fever. It is most unusual, however, as Caulfield has pointed out, that in a given epidemic the disease should manifest a high virulence in one community and low virulence in another.

Studies of village records by Caulfield have shown that, during the epidemic of 1735 in the town of Kingston, New Hampshire, the ancestral home of Daniel Webster, over one-third of all the children died. The Webster family lost several children. The village of Kingston, with a population of about 1,000, lost 108 children during the first year of this epidemic, and 34 more died in this village during the second year of the outbreak.

In this same year an epidemic of sore throat occurred in New

Jersey and has been described by a minister, Jonathan Dickson[36] (1685-1747). His pamphlet is entitled, "The Observations on that terrible disease vulgarly called 'Throat Distemper.'" Dickson has given us a clear-cut description of a mild case of this disease. It is unquestionable that he is describing scarlet fever. He then goes on to describe the various manifestations of the disease, and has divided it into six types of infection. The severe form, type six, is certainly a case of laryngeal diphtheria. Thus, we cannot be sure whether this epidemic of 1735 in New Jersey consisted of one disease or two diseases. Probably both scarlet fever and diphtheria occurred simultaneously.

We can be sure of one thing—neither diphtheria nor scarlet fever was a *new disease,* since Cotton Mather had described an epidemic of "Cynanche Trachealis" in 1659, and scarlet fever was mentioned frequently by Mather and others as a mild disease of childhood. Apparently in 1735 these epidemic diseases found a fertile soil in a highly nonimmune population. The population was increasing gradually, with large families, which resulted in a high proportion of susceptible young children in the total population. This is always an inflammable situation.

A second great epidemic of throat distemper, which occurred in 1745 in New York and New Jersey, was described by Cadwallader Colden.[37] He considered the disease to be a continuation of the epidemic that had occurred in New England, as it probably was. Noah Webster noted that the disease began in New Hampshire in 1735, spread to Connecticut, New York, and then all over the country, lasting ten years. John Kearsley of Philadelphia, in an article in *Gentleman's Magazine,* London, in 1769, speaks of this "angina maligna" which prevailed in the colonies in 1746-1760. "Villages were almost depopulated. It seemed like a drawn sword of vengeance to stop the growth of the colonies."

Samuel Bard[38] described an epidemic of sore throat which occurred in 1769 in New York, which he considered identical with the disease described by Douglass at the time of the New England epidemic in 1735. From Bard's own description, one must conclude that the epidemic observed by him was diphtheria. Dr. J. A. Gallup, in his description of epidemics in Vermont, stated that malignant

---

[36] Dickson, Jonathan: Pamphlet on "Throat Distemper," 1736.

[37] Colden, Cadwallader: *Medical Observations and Inquiries,* Vol. I, p. 211, 1753.

[38] Bard, Samuel: "An Inquiry into the Nature, Cause and Cure of the Angina Suffocativa or Sore Throat Distemper," *Tr. Am. Philosophical Soc.,* Vol. I, 1771.

sore throat, or scarlet fever, prevailed in Vermont in 1773-1777 and again in 1787. By 1798, he stated, the scarlet fever had become endemic.

Benjamin Rush[39] described an epidemic of scarlet fever in Philadelphia in 1783. The disease began in September and lasted all winter. It was quite severe at first, then abated, but returned with increased vigor in March. The disease was limited almost entirely to children and was quite severe in some, very mild in others. The case fatality rate was low.

Rush also gave a description of "Cynanche Trachealis,"[40] which he did not consider to be contagious. His method of therapy was dreadful. "I once drew twelve ounces of blood at four bleedings in one day from a son of John Carroll, then in the fourth year of his age." He considered this to be relatively mild therapy, since his colleague, Dr. Bailie of New York, "used to bleed in this disease until fainting was induced." Rush also gave vomits every day, purges of jalap, and calomel in large doses, with "blisters to the throat, breast, and neck." Apparently this disease, in the great majority of cases, was diphtheria and particularly laryngeal diphtheria. Rush stated: "The vulgar name is 'Hives,' a corruption of heaves, because of the difficult breathing. 'Bowel heaves'[41] is the worst type of this disease because the abdominal muscles are required to aid the difficult respiration."

Lemuel Shattuck[42] stated that scarlet fever was severe in New England in 1735-1736, then it became quiescent for nearly a century and did not reappear in severe form until 1832. Its recrudescence in the nineteenth century will be described in a subsequent chapter.

The epidemiology of the group of throat infections that appeared at irregular intervals during the Colonial period indicates clearly that both streptococcosis and diphtheria were endemic in the larger centers of population. This is particularly true during the latter half of the seventeenth century. But transportation was laborious, and communication between settlements was quite infrequent. Most of the visiting was done by adults, chiefly the men. Thus, each scattered community with its high birth rate and stable stay-at-home families

[39] Rush, Benjamin: *op. cit.*, Vol. II, p. 243, 1815.

[40] *Ibid.*, p. 226.

[41] The author encountered the diagnosis of "bold hives" in the isolated southern communities of the United States in 1916. This term was undoubtedly derived from the "Bowel Heaves" of Rush. But "bold hives" in North Carolina was used to describe any severe eruptive fever.

[42] Shattuck, Lemuel: *Census of Boston*, 1845.

built up a high degree of community susceptibility to the communicable diseases of childhood. When an infectious agent invaded the community, a serious epidemic occurred in which a large proportion of the children developed the disease. As we have noted in the 1735 epidemic in New Hampshire, whole families of children lost their lives. However, the loss of life was limited in great part to children under ten years of age, which indicated a high degree of acquired immunity in the older age groups. For this reason we feel sure that those diseases which were called the infections of childood must have gone the rounds of the scattered communities at least every fifteen to twenty years.

From the data available it seems clear that the general epidemiological characteristics of both diphtheria and streptococcic infections of the throat were the same in Colonial times as at present. As we shall see later, however, there is good evidence that the streptococcic infections maintained a low virulence (3 to 5 per cent case fatality) until about 1835. Scarlet fever then became a very serious infection with a continuously high case fatality rate (20 per cent or higher) which persisted until about 1880. There then occurred the gradual and continuous decline in severity of this group of diseases, e.g., those due to the hemolytic streptococci, and this trend in the decline of virulence has continued even up to the present time. The decline of diphtheria will be discussed in more detail in a later chapter. (See pages 203-6.)

CHRONOLOGY OF "ANGINA MALIGNA," E.G., SCARLET FEVER AND/OR DIPHTHERIA

1679	The disease was differentiated from measles by Sydenham.
1684	Pepys' *Diary*, November 10, 1684: "My little girl Susan is fallen sick with the measles, or at least of a scarlet Feavour."
1699	Scarlet fever frequently mentioned as common and relatively mild disease (Cotton Mather, *Magnalia*, Book IV, p. 156, 1702 Edition).
1700	Thomas Fuller considered scarlet fever benign, "nothing virulent in it, not contagious, and chiefly a disease of children."
1735-36	New England epidemic (W. Douglass). Ernest Caulfield has studied this epidemic especially.
1735	Epidemic in New Jersey described by Jonathan Dickson.
1745	New York and New Jersey, second great epidemic, described by Cadwallader Colden, *Medical Observations and Inquiries*, Vol. I, p. 211, 1753.

1769	Article in *Gentleman's Magazine* by John Kearsley of Philadelphia. "Angina maligna"—"villages almost depopulated."
1769	Samuel Bard of New York: "An Inquiry into the Nature, Cause and Cure of Angina Suffocativa," *Tr. Am. Philosophical Soc.*, Vol. I, 1771.
1773-77	Malignant sore throat, or scarlet fever, in Vermont, described by J. A. Gallup, *History of Epidemical Diseases in the State of Vermont*, 1815.
1783	Epidemic of scarlet fever in Philadelphia, described by Benjamin Rush, *Medical Inquiries and Observations*, 1815.
1784	Malignant scarlet fever in Massachusetts and throughout New England in epidemic form.
1796	Scarlet fever in New England.
1798	Diphtheria and scarlet fever every winter—typhoid and dysentery every summer (J. A. Gallup, Vermont, 1815).
1821	Clear differentiation between scarlet fever and diphtheria (Bretonneau, Academy of Medicine of Paris).

MALARIA

There is abundant evidence that malaria did not exist in North America prior to the discoveries of Columbus.[43]

The disease was introduced by the Spaniards into the West Indies and flourished there. A Spanish colony was established near the present site of Jamestown, Virginia, in 1523, but an epidemic of fever, which was probably malaria, destroyed the colony, including its leader, Lucas de Pyllon.

The introduction of Negro slaves into the West Indies in 1563 certainly aggravated the malaria of those islands. Negro slaves were first delivered to the Jamestown colony from Africa in 1619. They brought the malaria parasite with them and undoubtedly intensified the infection, becoming the most important source of malarial infection on the American continent. The Jamestown settlement under John Smith, in 1608, suffered severely from illness, chiefly "flux and fever," which may be interpreted as bacillary dysentery and malaria or possibly typhoid fever. The site of Jamestown was poorly selected, for it was a marshy island with poor drainage. Malnutrition caused many deaths,[44] of course, and the Indians were a constant source of

---

[43] Carter, H. R.: *Yellow Fever: An Epidemiological and Historical Study of the Place of Origin*. Williams & Wilkins Co., Baltimore, 1931.

[44] During the Jamestown "starving time," in 1607, one husband is reported to have killed his wife, eaten half of the body, and salted down the remainder.

At the end of twelve years, Jamestown had a population of only 1,000. Five thousand settlers arrived during the next five years but, at the end of 1622, only 1,200 were left.

(*Footnote continued on page 56.*)

danger, but malaria was also one of the major foes. In fact, the whole area was so unhealthy that the colony was moved to Williamsburg in 1699.

Charlestown did not suffer severely from malaria until the introduction of the cultivation of rice in 1684. The disease then became so prevalent and so severe that rice cultivation became an occupation solely of the Negroes, who were relatively immune to the disease.

In fact, malaria played an important part in the establishment and development of slavery in the southern United States. In the heavily malarious zones, white labor could not compete with the partially immune Negroes, for the whites died of the disease, whereas those Negroes who developed malaria seldom died in consequence of their infection.

When the Pilgrims were debating whether they would settle in cold, bleak New England or in the tropical climate of the West Indies or South America, they decided on the colder climate because "such hott countries are subject to greevous diseases, and many noysome impediments, which more temperate climates are free from, and would not so well agree with our English bodys."

Webster[45] noted that within forty to fifty years after the settlement of New England, the infectious fevers of autumn had become endemic there. They were frequent in the villages and country areas, and were called *intermittent fever* and *remittent fever*. Later the appellation of bilious autumn fever was introduced. This latter term was usually reserved for epidemic yellow fever, but there is no question that yellow fever and malaria were frequently confused. Intermittent fever was almost always tertian malaria. Remittent fever was aestivo-autumnal malaria, as a rule, but might also be typhoid fever or even yellow fever.

Webster understood the relationship of malaria to the summer months. He also pointed out the high incidence of the disease in persons living near swamps and ponds, and noted the disappearance of these fevers with the first frost. The geographic distribution of the disease was well understood, and the relationship of the disease to swamps and ponds was so well known that the choice of a site for a settlement was determined, for the most part, by the terrain.

Soon 400 of these were killed by the Indians. (Adams, James T.: *Epic of America.* Little, Brown & Co., Boston, 1931.)

[45] Webster, N.: *op. cit.,* p. 179.

Blanton[46] has pointed out that malaria had a difficult time establishing itself endemically in the colonies during the seventeenth century. He has stated that malaria was *not common* in Virginia throughout the first century of Colonial life. Only by 1700 did the disease become endemic throughout the colonies. It reached a peak in New England about 1750 and then began to decline in prevalence.

Between 1700 and 1750 malaria occurred as far north as Maine, and was quite prevalent in the towns of Massachusetts, but in somewhat sporadic form, with only a short season, and no severe or extended epidemics. In 1763 the Indians on Nantucket Island were visited with "bilious plague" and their numbers were reduced from 385 to 136. "The epidemic was a very sharp one and terminated in early fall."[47] The disease occurred as far north as Lake Champlain, for J. A. Gallup[48] noted an epidemic there in 1798.

Rush[49] stated that the intermittent fevers prevailed in Philadelphia between 1760 and 1809. They occurred in the autumn and were encountered chiefly in the suburbs of the city. In 1765 the disease was epidemic in Southwark, a suburb of Philadelphia. "That year the disease was so general as to affect two-thirds of the inhabitants of the southern states." Rush was an ardent therapist. Though many people were afraid to take the Peruvian bark, he gave it freely in intermittent fever.

Peruvian bark had been introduced to the world early in the seventeenth century.[50] The first physician to use the "bark" in the colonies was the buccaneer, Lionel Hafer, who made frequent use of this drug in Virginia in 1682. Cinchona was not purified until 1811, and was not widely used in Colonial days except in the larger centers. There was no known method of prevention or control of malaria. The people clearly understood that the disease was related to low, swampy places, and Rush was certain that the "swamp fever" was due to miasmata arising from marshy places, particularly at night; but the people had no way of avoiding this menace except to close up all the windows and doors of sleeping quarters and to build

[46] Blanton, W.: *Medicine in Virginia in the Seventeenth Century.* Garrett & Massie, Inc., Richmond, Va., 1931.

[47] This may, of course, have been yellow fever.

[48] Gallup, J. A.: *op. cit.*

[49] Rush, Benjamin: *op. cit.,* Vol. IV, p. 230.

[50] Don Juan de Vega, a Spanish Physician in Peru, gave the wife of the Vice King of Peru, Countess Francisca de Ribera, an Indian remedy, quinquina, in treatment for a severe fever. The treatment produced a prompt and lasting cure. He introduced this drug into Spain on his return in 1641.

their houses on elevations as far as possible from swamps. Rush considered one and a half miles from the swamp as satisfactory. (This was a keen observation, for we know now that this is the approximate flight range of *Anopheles quadrimaculatus,* which has been the important transmitter of malaria in the United States.)

The Revolutionary War accentuated malaria. During the campaigns in Georgia and North Carolina, the British troops suffered severely from the infection, and at the Yorktown siege, where Cornwallis finally surrendered, the besieging New England troops were particularly affected by this disease.

Rush in his *Inquiries* spoke frequently of malaria in Philadelphia, but he confused the disease with both yellow fever and typhoid fever. He described one epidemic of malaria in his chapter on "Intermittent or Bilious Fever" which occurred in the fall of 1780. But from his description he was dealing quite obviously with an epidemic of *dengue*. The patients suffered from severe deep muscle pains, continuous fever for three days, and a rash. He stated that the people suffered so severely that they called the disease "break bone fever," and he noted the abundance of "moschetoes" that fall, which, as he frequently mentioned in his various writings, were always a certain sign of an unwholesome autumn.

We now have an exact knowledge of the bionomics of *Anopheles quadrimaculatus,* the transmitter of malaria in North America, and we have no reason to think that the habits and life history of this mosquito have changed through the centuries. Thus we can reconstruct the story of malaria in the colonies in detail. The malaria parasite was introduced continuously to America, largely through the slave traffic. After a long latent period of nearly 100 years, the disease became highly endemic throughout the southern states, for they had a long anopheles season and a heavy parasite prevalence, particularly in the Negro slaves. In the northern colonies, malaria occurred each fall in sharp epidemics, but those were of short duration. The parasite was carried through to the next summer in the blood of human carriers. We are sure of these epidemiological points because *Anopheles quadrimaculatus* does not appear in any considerable numbers in Massachusetts until late July and is gone by mid-September.[51]

By the middle of the eighteenth century malaria had begun to fade from New England. Below the Chesapeake it established itself firmly

[51] Author's studies with Massachusetts State Board of Health, 1933.

with a high endemic prevalence. Malaria did not really become "the American disease," however, until the opening up of the West after the Revolutionary War. This extraordinary invasion will be described in subsequent chapters. As an indication of what was to come, a French traveler reported in 1796, on a 700-mile trip from Cincinnati to Detroit in the early fall: "Not twenty families encountered on the whole trip were free from malaria."

CHRONOLOGY OF MALARIA

1593	Spanish colony near the site of Jamestown wiped out by malaria.
1619	Malaria brought by slaves to Jamestown colony (surmise).
1671	First outbreak of malaria in New England (O. W. Holmes).
1684	First epidemic of malaria in Charlestown.
1700-50	Malaria became highly endemic throughout the zone below the Chesapeake. New England widely invaded also by sharp, short ·summer epidemics.
1750	Malaria began to fade from New England.
1775-83	Great increase in malaria during Revolutionary War.
1800	With the opening up of the West, malaria became the *great American disease*.

RABIES

Rabies was fairly prevalent in Colonial days, particularly in the latter part of the eighteenth century. Webster noted that it was epidemic in all parts of the United States in 1785, and Gallup stated that rabies was frequent in Vermont in 1787. Its epidemiology was well understood, and the transmission of the disease from dogs to other animals was reported. The disease was greatly feared, for it was known to be highly fatal to man and animals. The long incubation period of the disease in man was emphasized.

Rush discussed rabies in some detail, and he admitted that it was a difficult disease to treat. Nevertheless, he was not daunted. He felt that strong diseases require strong remedies, so he tackled rabies with great vigor, using even stronger therapy, if possible, than he employed in yellow fever. He reported a few very satisfactory cures. One cannot but feel that Rush's patients merited the greatest pity when the famed physician really opened up his complete therapeutic armamentarium. Even the virus of rabies must have beaten a retreat at times before his assaults.

CEREBROSPINAL MENINGITIS

Cerebrospinal meningitis was not comprehended as a disease entity during the Colonial period. We are fairly sure, however, of its presence. Early in the nineteenth century it was most frequently confused with typhus fever, and was not distinguished as a separate entity until about 1830. Thus it is difficult to determine from the description of the victims of any epidemic the exact extent of the infection. We do know that this disease played havoc at various periods in the nineteenth century, and those episodes will be discussed in some detail in following chapters.

Noah Webster[52] described an epidemic in Fairfield, Connecticut, in 1697, which may well have been meningitis. He said: "This disease was doubtless that species of inflammatory fever, attacking the brain and ending in typhus, which has often proved a terrible scourge to particular parts of America." The first well-delineated epidemic of meningitis occurred in 1807, and this outbreak will be described in a subsequent chapter. (See Chapter 14.)

As we have already noted, it is not impossible that the great epidemic of the Indians in 1618 was due to meningococcus infection.

[52] Webster, N.: *op. cit.*, p. 210.

CHAPTER 4. *Public Health Administration*

So far as I know, no epidemic of measles, chickenpox, influenza, poliomyelitis, smallpox, and so forth has ever been adequately controlled by means of quarantine.

THOMAS M. RIVERS, *1948*

During the entire Colonial period or, to be more exact, from 1607 to 1797, the local American communities devised no permanent administrative machinery for prevention of disease, nor for promotion of the public health. The reason for this was quite simple. The authorities saw no particular advantage in the organization of an official health service for community protection. Except for temporary periods and particularly during serious epidemics, there was nothing for a health department to do.

The colonies got off to an excellent start in health legislation and health regulations with the public health law of the Virginia colony in 1610.

There shall no man or woman, Launderer or Launderesse, dare to wash vncleane Linne, driue bucks, or throw out the water or suds of fowle cloathes, in the open streete, within the Pallizadoes, or within forty foote of the same, nor rench, and make cleane, any kettle, pot, or pan, or such like vessell within twenty foote of the olde well, or new Pumpe: nor shall any one aforesaid, within lesse than a quarter of one mile from the Pallizadoes, dare to doe the necesseties of nature, since by these vnmanly, slothful, and loathsome immodesties, the whole Fort may bee choaked, and poisoned with ill aires, and so corrupt (as in all reason cannot but much infect the same) and this shall they take notice of, and auoide, vpon paine of whipping and further punishment, as shall be thought meete, by the censure of a martiall Court.

Euery man shall haue an especiall and due care, to keepe his house sweete and cleane, as also so much of the streete, as lieth before his door, and especially he shall so prouide and set his bedstead whereon he lieth, that it may stand three foote at least from the ground, as he will answere the contrarie at a martiall Court.

This regulation indicates a clear understanding of the importance of proper camp sanitation as a measure of community protection. A regulation of this sort could be enforced in a semimilitary community organization of the Jamestown type, but was not applicable to general colonization.

Some of the earliest acts relating to health protection concerned the regulation of medical practice. The Virginia Colony Act of 1639 and the Massachusetts Bay Colony Act of 1649 are illustrations of this principle. Quacks and charlatans abounded among the colonists, as in fact they are always found, in surfeit, among pioneer people. Thus it became necessary very early in our history to curb their dangerous activities by suitable laws.

COMMUNICABLE DISEASE CONTROL

Quarantine

A compilation of the public health acts of the colonies during the seventeenth century (see pages 80-83) shows clearly the prevailing concept during the period, e.g., that the major public health function of the community was the control of important contagious diseases. As we have already noted, these were smallpox and yellow fever.

The important measures that were employed were: (1) isolation of the patient, at home or in the pesthouse; (2) quarantine of the premises; and (3) a limited amount of disinfection. In seaports—and almost all of the larger settlements were seaports—maritime quarantine was an important local government function.

Since epidemics occurred only occasionally, no permanent health organization was required. When an epidemic occurred, a committee of citizens, usually with a physician as a member, was chosen to combat the epidemic. This committee was disbanded when the epidemic ceased. Usually these bodies were called "boards of health"— sometimes "health committees." In some instances the government paid a fee to the committee members, but they usually served voluntarily as a public duty. They were often given power to make expenditures and to employ personnel at community expense.

Noah Webster[1] is most famous for a dictionary, but he also wrote a large text on epidemiology and was very much interested in the

[1] Webster, N.: *On Pestilence,* 2 vols. Hudson & Goodwin, Hartford, 1799.

control of contagious diseases. He defined quarantine in one of the early editions of his dictionary as follows: "to compel to remain at a distance from shore for forty days, or for other limited period, on account of real or supposed infection, applied to ships or to persons or goods."

The forty days of detention were not dictated by caprice, but, as Hecker[2] noted, the fortieth day, according to most ancient ideas, was regarded as the last day of *ardent disease,* and the limit of separation of this type of acute disease from those diseases which are chronic.

The first "Laws of Quarantine" with a formal enforcement code were passed in Venice in 1448. However, there are records in existence that show that health officers (e.g., quarantine officers) were appointed as early as 1347.

A regularly organized lazaretto,[3] or pesthouse, was erected in 1423 by the Venetians. All persons arriving from places where the existence of plague was suspected were detained there. The Republic of Venice established the first board of health in 1485, and the northern cities of Italy, notably Milan, established quarantine in that year. It was customary to enforce very strict regulations during times of pestilence and, since the rules failed many times to bring about results, more and more rigorous restraints were imposed. These restraints, however, were so troublesome to commerce that as soon as the epidemic was over the regulations were ignored. Evasion and corruption in executing the regulations were so common as to render them almost useless.

House quarantine was common in England during the Great Plague of 1665. Infected houses were not only quarantined during the sickness period, but were shut up for one month after all the residents had died or recovered. A large red cross was painted on the door with the words: "Lord, have mercy on us."

Thus, the colonists of America, at the time of the very early settlements, were familiar to some degree with the principles of maritime quarantine, house isolation, and the *lazaretto* system.

Maritime Quarantine

The colonies consisted essentially of a series of seaports, with outlying dependencies scattered along the Atlantic coast. Practically the only intercommunication was by ship. There were long periods of

---

[2] Hecker, J. F. C.: *The Epidemics of the Middle Ages.* London, 1846.

[3] "Lazaretto" is derived from the name of the Biblical character Lazarus who was a leper. The monks of the early Christian era established special places of refuge for lepers. Later these lazarettos were used for isolation in other types of pestilence.

isolation from Europe, from the West Indies, and from each other. Isolation of a whole community then, as today, gave relative freedom from communicable disease; but it also built up large numbers of susceptible people, so that when any one of the contagious diseases was imported, it wrought havoc, both because of the intensity and the extent of the invasion.

It was obvious to the colonists that when an infected vessel touched at a port, the contagious disease that was on board would almost invariably be transmitted to the people on shore and would spread throughout the settlement, with disastrous results. Thus, the only recourse was maritime quarantine. Since the whole life of the community was absolutely dependent on shipping and open trade, it was necessary to facilitate the voyage of the ship and to disturb its passengers as little as possible.[4] Naturally, the merchants of the community were very much opposed to quarantine restrictions and their attitude interfered with effective contagious disease control measures. At first the infected ships were quarantined in the harbors, but later pesthouses for infected mariners were erected at isolated places near the ports.

Governor Winthrop of the Massachusetts Bay colony, in 1647, quarantined ships from Barbados and other West Indian islands against "the plague or grievous infectious disease that had raged extensively in those islands" (yellow fever). Two years later, in 1649, the "Court doth think meete that the order concerning the stopping of West India ships at the castle shall hereby be repealed, since it pleased God to stay the sickness there."

In 1689 we find an order of the City Council of New York relating to the quarantine of vessels; and in 1698 one notes an order to the effect that the pilot of any vessel touching at Charleston, South Carolina, be requested to ascertain from the captain of the vessel concerning any contagious disease aboard. If such was discovered, the vessel was quarantined in the roadstead. "All vessels are forbidden to pass to the east of Sullivan's Island by one mile without permission of the Governor, under penalty of being fired at by the gunner."

The foundation for maritime quarantine was established by the Massachusetts Quarantine Act of July, 1701. This stringent quar-

---

[4] Adams in his *Epic of America* has pointed out that the rich and leading men of the community believed that if the law interfered with business and profits it need not be obeyed. Thus they disobeyed quarantine laws despite the heavy penalties for infraction. (Adams, James T.: *Epic of America*. Little, Brown & Co., Boston, 1931.)

antine act was entitled "An Act for the Better Prevention of the Spread of Infectious Diseases." It contained the important provision which compelled parties bringing infectious diseases within the colony to pay all costs and damages. Any seaman or passenger who brought a contagious disease ashore was subject to forfeit in the sum of 20 pounds, and provisions were made for the confinement of individuals who were infected with pestilential sickness until they were well. The Act of 1701 also required that the selectmen of the various towns provide for the care of persons suffering from contagious diseases. The diseases recorded in this category were, apparently, smallpox, plague, and yellow fever.

William Penn, returning from England to Philadelphia in 1699, found the colony which he had established only seventeen years before, in terrible distress because of its initial invasion by yellow fever. He realized that the disease had been brought in from Barbados, and immediately passed "An Act to prevent Sickly Vessels from coming into this Government."[5] This primitive law required that vessels coming from "unhealthy" or "sickly" ports should not be permitted to land persons or goods until the vessel had obtained a license for landing from the governor of the colony.

[The law established] in the year of our Lord one thousand seven hundred (1700), by William Penn, Esq., Absolute Proprietary and Governor-in-Chief of the provinces of Pennsylvania, is entitled "An Act to prevent Sickly Vessels from coming into this Government," and reads as follows:

Whereas, It hath been found, by sad experience, that the coming and arriving of unhealthy vessels at the ports and towns of this province and territories, and the landing of their passengers and goods, before they have lain some time to be purified, have proved very detrimental to the health of the inhabitants of this province: *Be it therefore enacted, by the authority aforesaid,* That, from and after the publication hereof, no unhealthy or sickly vessels, coming from any unhealthy or sickly place whatsoever, shall come nearer than one mile to any of the towns or ports of this province or territories without bills of health; nor shall presume to bring to shore such vessels, nor to land such passengers or their goods at any of the said ports or places, until such time as they shall obtain a license for their landing at Philadelphia, from the Governor and Council, or from any two justices of the peace of any port or county of this province or territories, under the penalty of ONE HUNDRED POUNDS for every such unhealthy vessel so landing, as aforesaid, to the use of the Pro-

[5] *Proceedings and Debates of Third National Quarantine and Sanitary Convention.* Edward Jones & Co., Printers to Board of Education, New York, 1859, p. 279.

prietary and Governor; and that suitable provision be ordered by the Governor and Council for their reception, if they be permitted to land or come on shore.

This law apparently was a dead letter, and was not enforced until twenty-eight years later, when a vessel arrived in the river from Bristol, England, having cases of "malignant fever" on board. This vessel was quarantined at a convenient distance, and nine days later the cargo was put ashore after the ship had been smoked with tobacco and washed with vinegar, the goods exposed to the air on deck, while the vessel remained in the stream of the river until sufficiently cleansed.

His Majesty's Colony of Rhode Island, in 1711, passed an act to prevent the spread of infectious diseases. Smallpox was specifically mentioned in the act, as well as "any other contagious disease which shall come from any place or port where any contagious distemper is brief or prevalent." The vessels were to be quarantined until it was shown that there was no contagious disease aboard. Provision was made for fining offenders, and if the act was violated persons might be arrested and required to work out their fines. The act also provided that "if mariners, passengers, or slaves, notwithstanding the precautions, shall after being landed be taken sick with smallpox or any other infectious distemper, these persons may be removed by the Government to such convenient place as appears to be necessary to prevent the spread of the disease." In this act the principle was established that the shipowners were responsible for all expenses incurred for inspection of each ship by the authorized agent of the colony.

Charleston appointed Dr. Gilbert Guttery as health officer of the Province of Carolina in 1712. He was the first provincial health officer of the colonies. His duties were essentially those of a quarantine officer. He was "to inquire into the state of health of all persons as arrived on shipboard." He was to go on board all vessels as soon as they crossed the bar and inquire concerning illness and death on the passage, search the ship, and order all men on deck for that purpose. He could send persons to the pesthouse at Sullivan's Island, have the vessel fumigated, and detain her for twenty days. The diseases then specified were "plague, smallpox, spotted fever, Siam distemper, and Guinea fever." The penalty for violation of these regulations was 100 pounds.

The next step in the development of maritime quarantine was the establishment on shore of quarantine stations for care of the infected passengers and crew. Quarantine in the roadstead did protect the colony, but was cruel and inhuman, particularly in the southern ports during the hot summer season.

Isolation[6] of Persons Ill with Contagious Disease

Persons with contagious disease have been isolated from their fellows down through the ages, often by most barbarous methods. The first legal act providing for isolation, of which we have any record, is that of Viscount Bernabo of Reggio, Italy, who decreed on June 17, 1374, that "every plague patient be taken out of the city into the fields, there to die or recover." Their attendants, who were specifically appointed, were forbidden to associate with anyone for a period of ten days after their last exposure. This first legal act for the isolation of communicable disease shows clearly that the incubation period of contagious disease was comprehended even at that early date.

In the American colonies the isolation, in designated buildings, of persons who were sick with contagious disease was initiated primarily for those who arrived in a port from a foreign land. These "quarantine stations" were located on some remote sandspit or small island, where contact with the mainland could be controlled.

People who were resident in the community and who developed contagious disease were treated—and isolated—in their homes. But some of these poor people were homeless. Sometimes a whole family became ill, with no member left to nurse the sick. Thus there grew up the system of "pesthouses."

The pesthouse was not a hospital in any sense. Usually it was a temporary structure located outside the community in a remote, often inaccessible place with few facilities for adequate care of the sick. Medical and nursing care was often carried out on a voluntary basis. These voluntary nurses usually were immunes who had already had the disease (the colonists realized that one attack of smallpox or yellow fever gave a lifelong protection). Clothing and food were donated by individuals or by the community. Sometimes the whole structure of the pesthouse, including furniture and bed

[6] The term "isolation" refers to restrictions upon the individual who is actually ill with the infection. Quarantine is imposed on those who have been exposed to the infection and presumably are in the incubation stage of the disease. The colonists did not make this distinction.

clothing as well, was burned to the ground after the epidemic was over.

The first Colonial orders of governor and council concerning isolation of residents who became ill with communicable disease were those of Boston and Salem in 1678. Not only were the persons isolated who were sick with smallpox, but their families were prohibited from selling any goods whatsoever.

The basic contagious disease control act of Massachusetts in 1701 required each town to make provision for smallpox isolation. The town selectmen were officially authorized to provide food, shelter, and medical care for those who were isolated with smallpox. In 1731 Massachusetts authorized "a red cloth to be hung in places infected with smallpox," while in Charleston in 1738 it was ordered that a white rag be tied to the house or gate of a home that was infected with smallpox, and that all such infected homes in the county be advertised on the public road and at the church.

During epidemics of yellow fever and smallpox, whole settlements would be evacuated. Since it was understood that persons who had had these diseases would not suffer from another attack, these immune people remained to care for the sick; but the only sure protection for the nonimmunes was flight. Frequently one community would set up "shotgun" patrols against an infected community to prevent immigration by the refugees. For example, during the epidemic of yellow fever in Philadelphia in 1793, New York closed all roads from Philadelphia to New York and stationed guards to prevent any citizen of Philadelphia from bringing the disease to New York.

The people understood the general epidemiological principle of an incubation period in infectious diseases. Many persons who were perfectly well would flee from a source of pestilence to an uninfected area. Soon some of these people would become ill, and in turn they would infect their associates in the new community. The obvious solution of this situation was to restrain forcibly all those who attempted to flee from an infected community into an uninfected area.

The people might be in doubt about the contagious nature of many diseases, but they were never convinced that smallpox was not a contagious disease, despite the teachings and theories of the doctors. Thus, even at the height of the popularity of the environmental origin theory of contagion, cases of smallpox were always isolated.

Disinfection

The colonists of the seventeenth century had some conception of the role of intermediate factors in the transmission of the two most important contagious diseases—smallpox and yellow fever. Although they believed that direct contact and transmission from person to person was the most important mode of contagion, nevertheless they also felt that there was ample evidence that clothing, bedding, and, in fact, the whole environs of the sick person became contaminated with the disease. Thus it was quite logical to institute some form of disinfection for the purification of the environs of the sick.

Mariners who fought in the West Indies had a tradition that the best way to escape yellow fever was to launch an immediate attack on shore. They believed that exploding gunpowder dispelled the disease. Thus it became common practice to explode gunpowder between decks as a suitable method of ship disinfection.

During epidemics of yellow fever, fires were kept burning constantly in the streets. Mathew Carey,[7] who reported the epidemic of yellow fever in Philadelphia in 1793, did not believe in the effectiveness of this practice, but he did have great faith in the value of frequent explosions of gunpowder in the region of houses in which yellow fever patients were confined.

The most common method of disinfection was the burning of all clothing, bedding, and indeed, in some instances, the bed and furniture and even the dwelling that had been visited with pestilence.

Tar was burned extensively in disinfection of ships, and tar was burned also in infected dwellings, but the commonest fumigation procedure was the burning of sulfur. The colonists had plenty of precedent for sulfur dioxide as a disinfectant, for it had been used for this purpose for over 2,000 years.

Rhode Island passed an act in 1721 which required disinfection of goods that were removed from infected ships. The rule was quite sensible, namely, "exposure of the materials for six days to the rays of the sun."

At the end of the eighteenth century, "smokehouses" were built at ferries and other strategic places where the clothing and goods of travelers from presumably infected places would be disinfected with the smoke of tar or sufur.

[7] Carey, Mathew: *A Short Account of the Malignant Epidemic in Philadelphia,* Fourth Edition. Printed by the author, Philadelphia, 1794.

Pesthouses

Jones,[8] in his "History of Quarantine," stated that Connecticut had a pesthouse for mariners, and quarantine officers as well, as early as 1710. Dr. Guttery of Charlestown built a pesthouse in 1712, and here he established a quarantine period of twenty days. The penalty for leaving the pesthouse without permission was a fine of 50 pounds.

The Massachusetts Bay colony established a hospital for sick mariners on Spectacle Island in Boston Harbor. The exact date is unknown, but it was between 1715 and 1717.[9] In Massachusetts, in 1736 Rainsford Island was set aside for a lazaretto, and "a good and convenient house was provided at the charge of the Province for the reception of such persons as shall be visited with any contagious sickness."

The Philadelphia Colonial Assembly in 1743 provided for a lazaretto for sick passengers on Fisher's Island.[10] Between 1700 and 1774, Philadelphia made several minor changes in its original quarantine act (see page 65). In this latter year new features were added to the act. By this time the city had a health officer (the term was synonymous with "ship quarantine officer") who was responsible for the examination of all vessels coming from pestilential ports. A fine of 100 pounds was exacted for concealing a sick passenger. Any person escaping from Fisher's Island (now called Province Island) was arrested and fined 50 pounds. If unable to pay he was to receive "any number of lashes not exceeding twenty, on his bare back well laid on."

In 1744 Charleston appropriated 1,000 pounds for the pesthouse on Sullivan's Island. "No ships from Africa shall pass the city without leaving the Negroes ten days in the pesthouse. Vessels violating the quarantine laws may be fired upon."[11]

New York was much slower than the other colonies in the protection of her citizens against the importation of disease by vessels from foreign ports. There were several acts relating to the importation of smallpox or malignant fever from the West Indies in 1702, 1714, and 1742, but the first real quarantine act was that of the Colonial

[8] Jones, Joseph: *Medical and Surgical Memoirs*, Vol. III, Part II, pp. 3-30. L. Graham & Son, New Orleans, 1890.

[9] Shattuck, Lemuel: *Report of the Sanitary Commission of Massachusetts, 1849*. Dutton & Wentworth, Boston, 1850.

[10] Jewell, Wilson: "Quarantine—Historical Sketches," presidential address, County Medical Society. Philadelphia, 1857.

[11] Jones, Joseph: *op. cit.*

legislature in 1755, to prevent "infectious distempers from being brought into this colony and to hinder the spread thereof." This act provided for the inspection of vessels by some surgeon, and Dr. John Bard was appointed quarantine officer. He continued in this office until 1773. Through his personal activity a pesthouse was established on Bedloe's Island for smallpox, yellow fever, and other contagious diseases. The money for the pesthouse was raised by a lottery provided for by an Act of 1756, "to *build* a *pesthouse* and *erect* a *medical college*." This was the medical school of King's College, later to become the medical school of Columbia College.

Quarantine after the Revolution

During the Revolutionary War practically all quarantine and isolation procedures were completely abandoned, but immediately at the close of the war the various states again assumed responsibility for the protection of their citizens by ship quarantine. In New York, for example, in 1784 the state legislature passed a strict quarantine law similar to the Colonial law of 1758, but much more rigorous. In 1791, following the renewal of commerce with the West Indies and the breaking out of yellow fever in New York, the act was extended "to all vessels."

In May, 1796, an attempt was made by Representative Smith of Maryland to regulate the quarantine of the whole United States by federal law. The bill was strenuously opposed by the representative from Pennsylvania, who stated that the principle of the bill was to take the power from the individual states to regulate "what respected the health of their citizens, and to place it in the President of the United States." One objection was that the measure would be very inconvenient, because most states lay very distant from the seat of government; thus, disease might be introduced and cause great havoc among the citizens before the federal government could take action. Pennsylvania considered that the governor of each state was better qualified to regulate quarantine, because he was on the scene.

Pennsylvania was supported by Mr. Lyman, of Massachusetts, who thought that the individual states should possess the sole control over the regulation of quarantine. The bill was vigorously debated and finally defeated, since the national legislature was not willing to place the right of quarantine in the hands of the general government, nor to give the President authority to direct the particular periods of time that vessels arriving from foreign ports and other places might be quarantined. It was held that quarantine is based on the inalienable *right* of self-preservation, and thus it became the duty of each state to protect its citizens from foreign pestilence.

Congress did, however, authorize the President to direct revenue officers and the commanding officers of forts and revenue cutters to aid in the execution of quarantine, and also to aid in the execution of the health laws of the states in "such matters as to him may appear necessary." This conflict of authority between the federal government and the various states in relation to maritime quarantine was continued for nearly 100 years, and the final relinquishment of the rights of the states to quarantine the vessels which entered their ports was achieved only after a great deal of acrimonious dispute and rivalry.

GENERAL SANITATION

Community Cleanliness

The early settlements gave little heed to community hygiene and sanitation. Land was to be had for the clearing. Houses were widely separated, and the dangers of transmission of disease from one family to another through unsanitary living conditions were minimum.

The growth of the towns was very slow. Boston's population by 1700 was about 6,500 persons, and fifty years later it had reached only 17,000. When the great epidemic of yellow fever struck Philadelphia in 1793, it had a population of less than 35,000 and yet it was the second largest metropolis of the land.[12]

From their cultural contacts with the cities of Europe, the colonists realized the necessity for community cleanliness. For example, the local justices of Boston in 1692 assigned proper places in the community for stillhouses, slaughterhouses, tanneries, and places for rendering tallow, but this order was a community planning measure to insure good community housekeeping; it did not have any particular sanitary significance. Charleston, Carolina, in 1698 enacted a nuisance ordinance which ordered the filling of offensive privies, and which related also to the cleanliness of pigpens and slaughter-

[12] Adams has given us the following population estimates for the colonies:
In 1640 there were about 65,000 English settlers in America—two-thirds in the West Indies and one-third or about 20,000 on the mainland. All the colonies on the Atlantic coast were settled by the English except the Dutch colony of New York and the Swedish colony in Delaware. By 1700 there were 260,000 persons on the Atlantic seaboard, 90 per cent of whom were farmers. The populations of the towns were approximately: Boston 7,000, New York 4,000, Philadelphia 4,000, and Charleston 1,500. (Adams, James T.: *op. cit.*)

houses; but these were esthetic rather than disease-prevention regulations. In 1702 the City Council of New York passed an ordinance which required the cleansing of the streets, following an epidemic of yellow fever. This is the first direct evidence we have that the prevalence of this disease was considered to coincide with filthy conditions. A New York City ordinance which required citizens to keep the streets clean was passed in 1760, and Philadelphia's civic activities in 1762, which were concerned with paving the streets, building of sewers, and cleaning the alleys and highways, were inaugurated as matters of improvement and tidiness.

It apparently never occurred to the people that water and milk were important vehicles of disease transmission. As a matter of fact, they were not of major, community-wide importance as disease vehicles at that period. Each family had its own well, its own cow, its own garden, and its own meat supply. It also disposed of its own wastes. Thus food and drink were not important factors in the production of infection. Even when sewers were built in Boston, it was forbidden to connect cesspools or privies to them. The sewers were built to drain the land and to carry off surplus surface water from the streets. They were not built for sanitary purposes.

The concept of miasmata as a cause of disease, that is to say, the dangers from bad odors, and the theory of the importance of decaying vegetable and animal matter in the causation of illness and even epidemics, apparently did not gain headway until the latter part of the eighteenth century. Noah Webster was one of the great proponents of this theory,[13] and Benjamin Rush, convinced by Webster's arguments, was a champion of this dogma. Rush refused to believe that yellow fever is contagious. He listed the important sources of yellow fever and related diseases as:

1. Exhalation from marshes.
2. Rotten cabbage.
3. Putrid potatoes, onions, and Indian meal.
4. Rotten coffee (cause of the yellow fever epidemic of 1793).
5. Cotton, hemp, flax, and straw, wet and rotten.
6. Bilge water and stagnating rain water.
7. Duck ponds and hogsties.

[13] "The acquiescence of all descriptions of men, learned and unlearned, in the opinion that epidemic diseases are to be ascribed solely to infection or specific contagion, has proved extremely injurious to philosophy and to medicine." (Webster, N.: *On Pestilence*, Vol. 1, p. 264.)

8. Unburied human bodies.
9. Old books and old paper money.
10. Salt beef and pork.
11. Raw hides.
12. Entrails of fish.
13. Fetor from privies.

These are only a few of the sources. Many others are cited. He specifically noted the relationship of drought to yellow fever. This is a key observation, for drought and long storage of rain water offered most favorable opportunity for propagation of yellow fever mosquitoes.[14]

When the Board of Health was first established in New York in 1796 the enabling act was comprehensive, for it covered both theories of infection, namely, (1) quarantine of contagious disease, and (2) the control of miasmata in the prevention of epidemics. But the Massachusetts Public Health Act of 1797 assigned to the health officers as their sole duty "to remove filth, if in their judgment it endangers lives and health of inhabitants." The rules of the Boston Board of Health of 1799 refer to nothing except nuisances and offensive trades. Bad-smelling establishments such as tanneries were considered to be most dangerous. Pigpens were a very serious danger, and cesspools were worse than privies—because they had a worse odor.

Nuisances

Nuisances were of chief concern to municipalities during the early Colonial days because of their bad odor and not because they were considered dangerous to health. As we have mentioned earlier, we do not encounter the concept that "nuisances," e.g., *bad odors*— decaying animal and vegetable matter, effluvia from ponds, drains, and bad air of all sorts—were actual causes of disease until the end of the century.

Gradually, the concept developed that all epidemics were due to a combination of unfavorable evironmental factors. At the beginning of the nineteenth century, the consensus of scientific opinion was that fevers and most other illnesses as well were directly due to miasmata which were air-borne and usually were bad smelling.

---

[14] Rush, Benjamin: Report of the yellow fever epidemic of 1794 in Philadelphia, as recorded in his *Medical Inquiries and Observations,* Fourth Edition, Vol. III, p. 195, 1815.

Thus, from about 1800 through the next seventy-five years, more and more attention was given to environmental factors as important elements in the production of disease. In fact, the pendulum swung far away from the individual patient as a source of infection, and a maximum of emphasis was placed on the environment as the actual cause of illness.

For this reason the sanitation of the environment became the major activity in the prevention of disease throughout the greater part of the nineteenth century. Public health regulations and practically all public health procedures from 1800 through 1875 were concerned primarily with the abatement of nuisances, particularly with destruction of causes of bad odors. These traditions which relate to the importance of bad odors as important factors in the production of illness became so firmly fixed in the minds of the people that they still prevail, 150 years later, in many parts of the United States.

Community Water Supplies

During the Colonial period the major sources of water for the family and the community were surface waters from springs, streams, lakes, and ponds. As the towns increased in size, shallow wells which were scattered at convenient intervals became an essential part of the village water system. In 1799 a bill was passed in New York giving the Manhattan Company the privilege of supplying the city "with pure and wholesome water." Both Alexander Hamilton and Aaron Burr, later mortal enemies, were influential in forming this company. Dug wells provided the supply and bored logs were used to transport the water. Lead pipes carried the water from the street into the houses. John Stevens was the engineer for this unique project. "From actual experiment," he states, "there is no doubt that one of the wells already opened will yield five thousand families a daily supply of at least fifty gallons each."

BOARDS OF HEALTH

Chapin[15] has stated that Petersburg, Virginia, was the first community to organize a local board of health. Since the courthouse of Petersburg was burned and all the records were lost, we have been unable to trace Chapin's authority for this priority claim of the city of Petersburg.

[15] Chapin, Charles: "History of State and Municipal Control of Disease," *A Half Century of Public Health*. American Public Health Association, New York, 1921, p. 133.

CHAP.
LV.

Petitioner, &c.
may apply to
the court, &c.

III. And be it enacted, That in all petitions now depending, or hereafter commenced, for freedom, either the petitioner or defendant may apply to the court for the benefit of a trial by jury, and that the court shall thereupon charge, as the law directs, the attending jury to determine each and all of the allegations contained in the said petition, which may be controverted, any law, usage or custom, to the contrary notwithstanding.

There shall be
no appeal, &c.

IV. And be it enacted, That there shall be no appeal from the judgment of the county court upon such petitions, except as to matters of law, where the facts shall have been tried by a jury; and the master, mistress or owner, of such petitioner, or the petitioner, at the election of either, shall have the right of appeal as to matters of law only, in all cases so tried, to the general court of their respective shore, any thing in this law contained to the contrary notwithstanding.

Master, &c.
may chal-
lenge, &c.

V. And be it enacted, That either the master, mistress or owner, of such petitioner, or the petitioner, shall have the right and privilege of challenging peremptorily to the number of twelve jurors impannelled to try the facts in issue, and for want of a sufficient number of jurors remaining upon the original pannel, a *tales*, at the prayer of either party, shall be awarded by the court, to try the said issue or issues.

C H A P.   LVI.

Passed De-
cember 28.

An ACT to appoint a health officer for the port of Baltimore-town, in Baltimore county.

Preamble.

WHEREAS, to prevent the ingress of the plague, or other malignant contagious diseases, is an object of great importance to the welfare and commerce of the citizens of the state; till, therefore, proper arrangements and establishments shall be made by congress in the premises,

Governor to
appoint, &c.

II. Be it enacted, *by the General Assembly of Maryland*, That the governor, with the advice of the council, shall and he is hereby authorised to appoint one or more persons, being able and skilful physicians, whose duty it shall be to visit and examine all foreign vessels, and other vessels coming from suspected places, and where it shall appear necessary, to oblige the same to perform quarantine, not less than ten days nor exceeding twenty; and in all such cases the visiting physician shall give a certificate to the captain or master of the vessel, signed with his name, expressing the number of days the said vessel is to ride quarantine; and at or before the end of each quarantine, the physician is hereby enjoined to make a second visit to the said vessel, and should it appear to him that a farther quarantine is necessary, he is hereby authorised to enjoin the same for any number of days not exceeding ten.

Masters of ves-
sels having
passengers dis-
ordered, not
to land, &c.

III. Be it enacted, That if the master, or other person having charge of any vessel bound to the port of Baltimore, having on board altogether, when the said vessel departed from port, above thirty passengers on board, disordered with any contagious disease, or coming from any sickly port or place, without a clean bill of health, shall bring his vessel, or suffer or permit the same to be brought, nearer to the port of Baltimore than Hawkins's Point, or shall land, or bring on shore, or cause or suffer to be landed or brought on shore, any of such infected persons, or any part or parcel of their goods or effects, or any other goods, until he has obtained a licence or permit so to do from the physician, or his assistant aforesaid, such master, or other person having charge of such vessel, shall forfeit and pay, for every such offence, the sum of one thousand dollars.

Penalty on
masters, &c.
for conceal-
ing, &c.

IV. Be it enacted, That if any master, or other person having charge of any vessel, at the time of inquiry by the aforesaid physician or his assistant, shall have on board any person infected as aforesaid, and shall knowingly conceal the same, or shall not make a just and true discovery to the physician, or his deputy, of the sickly and disordered state and condition of all and every person on board, from the time the said vessel departed from the port or place from whence she last sailed,

---

Fig. 4. "An ACT to appoint a health officer for the port of Baltimore-town, in Baltimore county." (From "Baltimore's Health Service 150 Years Old," *Baltimore Health News*, 20:200, [Dec.] 1943.)

Baltimore has claimed that it was the first community to organize a local board of health in 1793 and has submitted documents to prove this point. Philadelphia organized a temporary board of health during the yellow fever epidemic in 1793 and again in 1798. In 1796 New York City formed a local board of health consisting of three commissioners, together with the health officer. The health officer was both quarantine officer and physician to the pesthouse.

It should be emphasized that these various claims to priority of establishment of local boards of health are not significant, since these boards were appointed only for a temporary period because of the menace of an epidemic and were disbanded when the epidemic ceased.

It is true that the health officer (e.g., the quarantine officer) was a part-time government official with tenure and this gave some continuity to public health activities. He either had a salary or served the community on a fee-for-service basis.

In 1797 the Massachusetts state legislature passed a state-wide act providing for the establishment of local boards of health, on a permanent basis, in each township. This act is the foundation stone of local health service in the nation. It was a permissive, not a mandatory act.

The Boston Board of Health was established in 1799, with Paul Revere as its chairman. The important duties of this board of health were to control unfavorable environmental factors that might produce disease. It was empowered to abate nuisances and to promote community cleanliness. These primitive functions, together with the initial structure of local boards of health in Massachusetts, remained practically unchanged for more than 150 years.

Thus the ideas of Webster and Rush, according to Chapin,[16] "became crystallized in the wording of the Massachusetts Health Act of 1797."

These ideas of state responsibility in health promotion were not widely accepted. As we shall learn in subsequent chapters, most of the states did not authorize the establishment of local health services on a permanent basis for many years. For the most part, local boards of health throughout the country during the entire first half of the nineteenth century were established on a casual, informal, impermanent basis.

[16] Chapin, Charles: *op. cit.,* p. 139.

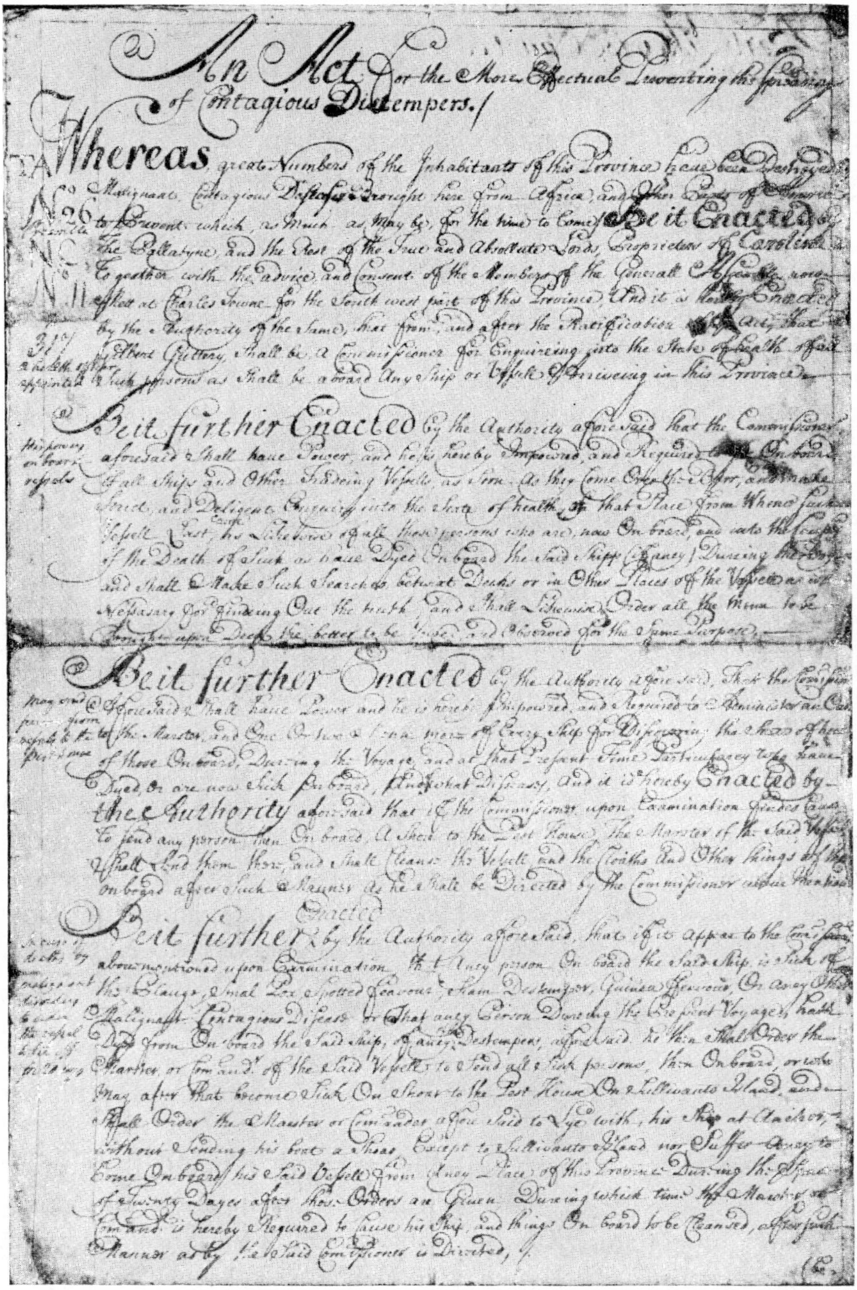

An Act for the More Effectual Preventing the Spreading of Contagious Distempers.

Whereas great Numbers of the Inhabitants of this Province have been Destroyed by Malignant Contagious Diseases brought here from Africa and Other Parts of America to Prevent which as Much as May be for the time to Come Be it Enacted by The Pallatyne and the Rest of the True and Absolute Lords Proprietors of Carolina Together with the advice and Consent of the Members of the Generall Assembly now Met at Charles Towne for the South west part of this Province And it is Hereby Enacted by the Authority of the same that from and after the Ratification of this Act that Gilbert Guttery shall be a Commissioner for Enquireing into the State of health of said Such persons as Shall be aboard Any Ship or Vessell Arriveing in this Province

Be it further Enacted by the Authority aforesaid that the Commissioner aforesaid Shall have Power and he is hereby Impowred and Required to go On board of all Ships and Other Tradeing Vessells as Soon As they Come Over the Barr and make Strict and Deligent Enquiry into the State of health of that Place from Whence such Vessell Last came his Likewise of all those persons who are now On board and into the Cause of the Death of Such as have Dyed On board the Said Shipp (if Any) During the Voyage and Shall Make Such Search as between Decks or in Other Places of the Vessell as may be Necessary for finding Out the truth and Shall Likewise Order all the Men to be brought upon Deck the better to be Viewed and Observed for the Same Purpose

Be it further Enacted by the Authority aforesaid That the Commissioner aforesaid Shall have Power and he is hereby Impowred and Required to Administer an Oath to the Master and One Or two or more of Every Ship for Discovering the State of health of those On board During the Voyage and at that Present Time Particularly who have Dyed Or are now Sick On board and of what Diseases And it is hereby Enacted by the Authority aforesaid that if the Commissioner upon Examination finds Cause to Send any person then On board A Shore to the Pest House The Master of the Said Vessell Shall Send them there and Shall Cleanse the Vessell and the Cloaths And Other things of those On board after Such Manner As he Shall be Directed by the Commissioner aforesaid

Be it further Enacted by the Authority aforesaid that if it appear to the Commissioner abovementioned upon Examination that Any person On board the Said Ship is Sick of the Plauge Small Pox Spotted Feavour Siam Destemper Guinea Feavour Or any Other Malignant Contagious Disease or that any Person During the Present Voyage hath Dyed from On board the Said Ship of any Destemper aforesaid he then Shall Order the Master or Commandr of the Said Vessell to Send all Sick persons then On board or who May after that become Sick On Shore to the Pest House On Sullivants Island and Shall Order the Master or Commander aforesaid to Lye with his Ship at Anchor without Sending his boat a Shore Except to Sullivants Island nor Suffer Any to Come On board his Said Vessell from Any Place of this Province During the Space of Twenty Dayes after those Orders are Given During which time the Master or Commander is hereby Required to Cause his Ship and things On board to be Cleansed after Such Manner as by the Said Commissioner is Directed

Fig. 5. Appointment of Dr. Gilbert Guttery as health officer of the Province of Carolina (1712). (From Mustard, Harry S.: *Government in Public Health*. The Commonwealth Fund, New York, 1945. Reproduced by permission of the Fund and the Harvard University Press.)

Health Officers

Reference is made frequently, during the eighteenth century, to the selection of a *health officer* for a community. These health officers were physicians (usually) who were appointed to enforce the maritime quarantine laws. Thus the terms "health officer" and "quarantine officer of the port" were interchangeable.

The first "health officer" of a local community in the colonies was Dr. Gilbert Guttery, who was appointed in 1712 as health officer of the Province of Carolina. He was, in actual fact, quarantine officer of the port of Charleston.

John Bard was the first health officer of New York. He was selected in 1755 and he enforced the maritime quarantine against smallpox and yellow fever in New York harbor. During the period of 1750 to 1800, practically every seaport selected a maritime quarantine officer to enforce the community regulations concerning contagious disease. At the time of the Philadelphia yellow fever epidemic in 1793, Dr. Hutchinson was so unfortunate as to be quarantine officer of the city (he died of yellow fever during the epidemic). Dr. Rush abused Dr. Hutchinson unmercifully for permitting the epidemic to generate at Ball's Wharf in a cargo of rotting coffee.

Thus, as we noted above, the term "health officer," as used during the Colonial period and for a long time thereafter, referred to the physician who was appointed by the community to enforce maritime quarantine. He had practically no other functions.

In summary, public health administration during the Colonial period was not an important function of government. The community authorities selected temporary health committees in time of serious epidemic. These men acted as consultants, rather than administrators, and served only during the emergency. The enforcement of sanitary regulations, and the maintenance of community cleanliness as well, were not functions of the health officer but were the responsibility of the police authorities of the towns. In time of disaster, voluntary citizen associations did valiant service in caring for the sick poor, and as the cities grew in size, medical, hospital, and nursing care of the poor were provided for, in some degree, by the local government. But for the most part, these services were provided by charitable citizens and were not an official governmental function.

It is quite understandable, therefore, that protection of the public health as a function of government is not even mentioned in the

Constitution of the United States. Benjamin Franklin, wise and farsighted as he was, never thought of it.

ENACTMENT OF PUBLIC HEALTH LAWS

This chronology of enactment of public health laws is not all-comprehensive, but does, in itself, give an interesting index of the development of community concepts in relation to health protection.

The approximate dates of the establishment of the various colonies are as follows:

1607 Virginia colony at Jamestown.
1620 Pilgrims landed at Plymouth on Massachusetts Bay.
1623 Colonization of Nieuw Amsterdam (New York).
1630 Massachusetts Bay colony at Boston.
1634 Maryland colony established.
1636 Providence settled by Roger Williams.
1662 Connecticut colony founded.
1664 Nieuw Amsterdam, which had been settled by the Dutch, was taken by the English.
1670 Carolina colony at Charlestown.
1681 Pennsylvania colony at Philadelphia.

Legislative Action that is Related to Public Health
1600–1650

1610 Virginia: first public health law of the colonies. (See page 61.)
1631 Virginia: an act to provide for registration of vital statistics.
1639 Virginia: an act to regulate the practice of medicine, and to curb irregular practitioners.
1639 Massachusetts: first vital statistics law.
1647 Massachusetts: an act preventing the pollution of Boston Harbor.
1647 Massachusetts: Governor Winthrop quarantined certain ships from Barbados against plague or Guiana infection, "a disease that had raged exceedingly in the West Indies."
1649 Massachusetts: an act to regulate the irregular practitioners of medicine.

1650–1700

1672 Massachusetts: Boston and Salem passed ordinances relating to nuisances and regulating offensive trades.
1678 Massachusetts: Salem and Boston isolated those who were sick with smallpox and prohibited the selling of goods by infected families. Disinfection was also provided for in these acts.
1689 New York: an act relating to the harbor quarantine of vessels.

1692 Boston: regulations relating to the suitable location of places for leather and tallow making, which were considered offensive trades.

1695 New York: an act permitting physicians to travel on the Sabbath and to conduct their medical visits on Sunday.

1698 Charleston: a regulation requiring the pilot to ascertain from the ship's captain of any vessel, concerning contagious disease aboard; if found, the vessel was to be quarantined at the roadstead.

1699 Massachusetts: Boston enacted a stringent quarantine regulation "to prevent the spread of contagion." This act was soon disallowed by the Privy Council.

1700–1725

1700 Philadelphia: strict quarantine of vessels by Governor William Penn.

1701 Massachusetts: an act to provide for those who were ill with contagion. It required the town to isolate persons with smallpox. It also prevented persons on board ship, who had smallpox, yellow fever, or plague, from coming ashore.

1702 Massachusetts: an act relating to drains and sewers, amended in 1709, 1744, 1763, 1796, and 1797.

1702 New York: a ship quarantine act, amended in 1714, 1716, and 1725, and many times thereafter.

1710 Massachusetts: a regulation prohibiting the use of lead in worms and in heads of distillery equipment, because of the danger of lead poisoning from rum (letters of Benjamin Franklin).

1711 Connecticut: an act which provided for the care of those who were sick with contagious diseases.

1712 Charleston: ship quarantine against plague, smallpox, spotted fever, Siam distemper, Guiana fever, and other malignant fevers. Dr. Gilbert Guttery was appointed health officer of the Province.

1712 Pennsylvania: a regulation providing for a penalty for obstruction of streets with filth and rubbish.

1716 New York: an act to regulate the practice of midwifery.

1717 Massachusetts: an act providing for the erection of a pesthouse on Spectacle Island. Transferred to Rainsford Island in 1757.

1721 Rhode Island: a regulation requiring compulsory disinfection of infected ship's cargo (sun's light recommended).

1725–1750

1726 Massachusetts: an act to prevent distillation of rum through lead pipes, for prevention of lead poisoning.

1731 Massachusetts: a regulation prohibiting the concealment of a case of smallpox. A red cloth must be hung on places infected with the disease.

1738　Charleston: a regulation that in a house quarantined with small-pox a white rag was to be tied to the house gate.

1742　Massachusetts: an act concerning smallpox quarantine.

1743　Pennsylvania: an act establishing a pesthouse at Fisher's Island for ship passengers who were ill with smallpox or yellow fever.

1744　Charleston: 1,000 pounds appropriated for the Sullivan's Island pesthouse.

1750–1799

1755　New York: a quarantine act intended as a protection against small-pox and yellow fever. John Bard selected as health officer.

1756　New York: an act providing for a lottery, the proceeds to be used to build a pesthouse and to erect a medical college. Medical school of King's College, later medical school of Columbia College.

1758　New York: Bedloe's Island established as a location for a pesthouse for mariners ill with contagion.

1760　New York: a city ordinance requiring citizens to keep the streets clean.

1763　New York: an act to regulate and to curb the practice of inocula-tion against smallpox.

1774　Charleston, Carolina: an enforcing regulation which required ves-sels bearing "contagious distemper" aboard, to perform proper quarantine.

1776　Massachusetts: a bill to license smallpox inoculation.

1780　Petersburg, Virginia: formation of the first local board of health (according to Chapin in *A Half Century of Public Health*).

1785　Massachusetts: an act relating to the control of unwholesome and adulterated food.

1793　Baltimore: an act to form a local board of health.

1793　Philadelphia: formation of a temporary local board of health to take charge of the great epidemic of yellow fever.

1796　New York City: formation of a local board of health (during yellow fever epidemic). Three commissioners of health, together with the health officer who was also physician to the pesthouse.

1797　Massachusetts: permissive legislature authorizing towns to appoint local boards of health and to formulate health regulations.

1799　Boston: organization of the Boston Board of Health with Paul Revere as its chairman.

1798　*Federal:* President John Adams signed a bill which provided for medical care of American seamen (July 16, 1798).

1799　*Federal:* a bill which authorized the federal authorities to aid states in enforcing quarantine regulations. The first session of Congress in 1790 appointed a committee of five to prepare a bill which would establish federal quarantine officers in the principal ports of the nation, but no act was passed at that time.

CHAPTER 5. *Medical Care*

Our education has made our calling exclusively a curative, and not a conservative one, and the business of our responsible lives has confined us to it. Our thoughts are devoted to, our interests are concerned in, and our employments are connected solely with, sickness, debility, or injury,—with diminution of life in some of its forms. But with health, with fullness of unalloyed, unimpaired life, we, professionally, have nothing to do.

EDWARD JARVIS, *1850*

MEDICINE IN THE COLONIES

Medicine as a profession had little recognition during the early Colonial period. Physicians had scanty formal training and charlatans abounded. The new settlements did not attract well-trained European doctors, for there was little opportunity for remunerative employment. For example, in 1647, Giles Firman in writing to Governor Winthrop stated, "I am strongly sett upon to study divinities, my studyes else must be lost for physick is but a meene help."

As late as 1685, a Connecticut colonist writing to his brother in England advised him as follows: "If you desire to come hither yourself, you may come as a Planter or a Merchant, but as a Doctor of Medicine I cannot advise you, for I hear of no diseases here to cure but some Agues, and cutted legs and fingers, and there is no want of empirics for them already!"

This statement was, for the most part, quite true. The isolation of the colonists provided a protection from many of the diseases of European civilization. The pioneer became hardy, resourceful, vigorous, and inured to privation. He absorbed the stoicism and indifference to pain and suffering which were such striking characteristics of the native Indian, and he took care of the injuries and sickness of his family without outside help.

The Virginia colony at Jamestown employed a surgeon to care for the wounds and ills of the colony. The first of these was Dr. Thomas

Wooten, who was appointed surgeon general of the colony in 1607.[1] He was followed by a succession of contract surgeons who came to America for adventure, but had no intention of settling permanently in the colony.

Savage,[2] in his *Genealogical Dictionary* of the seventeenth century in America, has included 134 medical practitioners, of whom twelve practiced surgery. One of these doctors was a woman—Ann Moore. Most of these physicians had received scanty medical training, and there was little legislative protection or encouragement of ethical practice. Quacks and charlatans were prevalent as early as 1631, for in that year Nicholas Knapp of Boston was sentenced to be fined or whipped for "taking upon him to cure the scurvey by a water of noe value which he solde atte a very deare rate." Many of the ministers also practiced medicine. Thomas Thacher, who came to Boston as minister to Old South Church in 1635, was also an eminent physician, and had the confidence of his people for his skill as a doctor as well as a divine. He issued the first medical publication in America—a broadside which was published in 1677 and was posted on the door of Old South Church. A copy of this publication is reproduced on page 23.

The combination of the profession of medicine and ministry was a most natural one. Both required a knowledge of Latin; and neither profession alone provided sufficient income to support a family. Furthermore, what could be more advantageous, when a minister visited the sick to give religious comfort, than to take with him the simple remedies that were available to relieve the patient's physical suffering? Cotton Mather in *Magnalia* says of Charles Chauncy's sons: "All of these did, while they had opportunity, Preach the Gospel, and most, if not all of them, like their excellent Father before them, had an eminent skill in physic added to their other accomplishments."

Practically all these early physicians received their training in Europe and then migrated to America. William Douglass, for example, arrived in Boston from Scotland in 1718. He was the only university graduate practicing in Boston at the time. He had the following opinion of his confreres: "In general, the physical practice

---

[1] Thacher says that Dr. Walter Russel was the first physician to the Jamestown colony, and that he accompanied John Smith on his voyages of discovery. Dr. Anthony Bagnal is also mentioned by John Smith.

[2] See Holmes, O. W.: "The Medical Profession in Massachusetts," Lowell Lecture, January 29, 1869.

in our colonies is so perniciously bad, that excepting in surgery and some acute cases, it is better to let nature take her course than to trust to the honesty and sagacity of the practitioner; our American practitioners are so rash and officious that the saying of the Apocrypha may, with propriety, be applied to them: 'He that sinneth before his Maker, let him fall into the hands of the physician.' Frequently there is more danger from the physician than from the distemper."

Dr. Alexander Hamilton of Annapolis, Maryland, who met Dr. Douglass on a journey he made to New England in 1744, says: "Douglass, the physician of Boston, is a man of good learning, but mischievously given to criticism, and the most compleat snarler ever I knew. He is loath to allow learning, merit, or a character to any-body." While in Albany Dr. Hamilton met the surgeon of the fort "who, by his own conversation, seemed to have as *little of the quack* in him as any half-hewn doctor ever I had met with. The doctors in Albany were mostly Dutch, all empirics, having no knowledge or learning but what they have acquired by bare experience. They study chiefly the virtues of herbs, and the woods there furnish their shops with all the pharmacy they use. A great many of them take the care of a family for the value of a Dutch dollar a year, which makes the practice of a physick a mean thing, and unworthy of the appli-cation of a gentleman. The doctors here are all barbers."

Dr. William Bell (1709-1791) was the first white person born in Charleston, Carolina, and is frequently said to be the first white American to win a medical degree. He studied under Boerhaave, and defended his thesis in 1734. He soon went into politics and was, for many years, lieutenant governor of the Province of Carolina.

During the eighteenth century, the young Americans began to go to Europe for their medical education. This was particularly true of the Carolina colony, for in 1786, according to Dr. David Ramsey (1748-1815), ten native Carolinians had graduated in medicine at the University of Edinburgh. Dr. Ramsey, who came from Philadel-phia, had been trained in the more conventional way as an apprentice under a praeceptor. He was a pupil of Benjamin Rush, who thought very·highly of his ability. Ramsey wrote *The History of the Revolu-tion* and *The Life of George Washington*. He was killed in his office by a maniac in Charleston in 1815.

Dr. Benjamin Rush has described medical practice in Philadelphia in 1760 as follows:

The system of Dr. Boerhaave then governed the practice of every physician in Philadelphia. Of course diseases were ascribed to morbid acrimonies, and other matters in the blood, and the practice of those years was influenced by a belief in them. Medicines were prescribed to thin, and to incrassate the blood, and diet drinks were administered in large quantities, in order to alter its qualities. Great reliance was placed upon the powers of nature, and critical days were expected with solicitude, in order to observe the discharge of the morbid cause of fevers from the system. This matter was looked for chiefly in the urine, and glasses to retain it were a necessary part of the furniture of every sickroom. To ensure the discharge of the *supposed morbid matter of fevers through the pores, patients were confined to their beds, and fresh, and even cool air, often excluded by closed doors and curtains.* The medicines to promote sweats were generally of a feeble nature. The spiritus Mindereri, and the spirit of sweet nitre were in daily use for that purpose. In dangerous cases, saffron and Virginia snake-root were added to them.[3]

James Thacher, in his *American Medical Biography,* of 1828, listed the following physicians as the most outstanding in Colonial America:

JOHN BARD (*1716-1799*) New York. First quarantine officer of New York Port. (Founder of medical school of King's College, later medical school of Columbia College.)

SAMUEL BARD (*1742-1821*) Son of John Bard—one of the founders of the New York Hospital.

JOSIAH BARTLETT (*1729-1795*) New Hampshire. Signed the Declaration of Independence. Governor of state.

BENJAMIN S. BARTON (*1766-1815*) Philadelphia. Botanist.

RICHARD BAYLEY (*1745-1801*) New York. Health officer of the Port.

THOMAS BOND (*1712-1784*) Philadelphia. One of the founders of the first medical college in the colonies.

ZABDIEL BOYLSTON (*1680-1766*) Boston. Introduced smallpox inoculation.

CADWALLADER COLDEN (*1688-1776*) Lieutenant governor of New York.

This list is quite selective, for it does not include all the founders of the Philadelphia Medical College, and none of the Virginia or Carolina doctors are in the group. William Douglass and Benjamin Waterhouse of Boston and Benjamin Rush of Philadelphia should certainly have been included. Practically all of the physicians on this list were trained in Europe.

[3] Miller, Genevieve: "Medical Education in Colonial America," *Ciba Symposia,* 8:516, (January) 1947. Reproduced by permission.

Government assumed little control over the quality of medical practice. A medical practice act was promulgated in Massachusetts in 1649. "Chirurgeons, midwives, and physicians to use no force or violence in their respective callings without the consent of adepts in the same art."

The Massachusetts colony assumed responsibility for medical care of the sick poor by 1671. Thacher[4] has stated that Dr. Daniel Stone of Boston contracted to give medical care to the town poor for 20 shillings annually, and remission of his taxes. Toner[5] has noted that: "Few acquired fortunes solely from medical practice during the Colonial period. The few wealthy physicians acquired their fortunes through inheritance or by investments and fortunate speculations. New countries are overrun by adventurers. New fields invite the most adventurous and often the least qualified persons. For the first century, medicine received little consideration from legislature and as a profession was left without recognition, protection, or encouragement. Professional education requires leisure, means and reasonable prospect of remunerative employment."

We have no accurate knowledge of the prevailing diseases that gave greatest concern to the very early colonists. We do know that among the important contagious diseases that caused greatest havoc were smallpox and measles (see chapter on communicable diseases). These were primarily diseases of childhood, occurring in the various settlements at irregular intervals and causing great suffering and loss of life. Scurvy killed a number of the Pilgrims at Plymouth, and from time to time this disease caused serious trouble in the various settlements. Governor Winthrop knew that fresh lemons would prevent as well as cure this disease, for he notes this fact in his journal. Malaria was one of the important illnesses experienced by the settlers, but did not become highly prevalent until the eighteenth century. The colonists were well aware that it occurred in the vicinity of ponds, particularly when a miller put in a new milldam.

Consumption is mentioned in the early records and influenza, accompanied by pneumonia, apparently struck the isolated colonies from time to time with severity. Accidents were of common occurrence, but the physician was not called except for very grave injuries. Only in major obstetrical crises was a physician called, for obstetrics was handled by midwives.

[4] Thacher, James: *American Medical Biography*. Richardson & Lord, Boston, 1828.
[5] Toner, J. M.: *Annals of Medical Progress*. Government Printing Office, Washington, D. C., 1874.

HOSPITALS IN THE COLONIES

Establishment of institutions for the care of the chronically ill had been an accepted practice in Europe from medieval times. But these were really *hospices,* which were organized usually under church supervision, and which gave food and lodging to lepers, to persons with mental disease, to the destitute, and to orphan waifs. There was no urgent need for this type of organization in a pioneer community.

In America people who were acutely ill were cared for in their homes. The very definition of a hospital was a *place where a destitute person went to die.*

There is a record of a small hospital erected in Nieuw Amsterdam, now New York, by the Dutch in 1658. It was intended for sick sailors, but was also used for sick Negro slaves. The building was sold in 1689 by the British for 200 pounds.

Pesthouses were erected in the colonies for the control of smallpox and other plagues, but these were, in no true sense, hospitals. (See discussion of smallpox, Chapter 3.) Following the introduction of smallpox immunization by Zabdiel Boylston in 1731, *inoculation stations* were established in many towns for the specific purpose of smallpox immunization. The subjects had, of course, to be isolated during the entire period of immunization and throughout their subsequent illness. For example, Dr. Uriah Rogers advertised in the *Hartford Courant* in 1767, on November 13, that he had prepared a special hospital for this purpose, which would be open until the following March.

At least two small private proprietory hospitals were opened during the eighteenth century in Virginia,[6] by prominent surgeons, for care of their private patients. The first hospital for the care of the sick poor[7] was built in Charleston in 1738. St. Philip's Parish had asked the legislature for funds to build a hospital, a workhouse, and a house of correction in 1734. An act was passed for this purpose, granting 2,000 pounds for the current year, and 1,000 pounds annually thereafter. The patients cared for were chiefly the chronically ill and destitute. This hospital was discontinued in 1789.

The first provincial institution for the care of the insane was built at Williamsburg by the Province of Virginia in 1773.

[6] Blanton, Wyndham: *Medicine in Virginia in the Eighteenth Century.* Garrett & Massie, Inc., Richmond, Va., 1931.

[7] Ransom, John E.: "The Beginnings of Hospitals in the United States," *Bulletin of the History of Medicine,* 13:531, (May) 1943.

Thomas Bond of Philadelphia initiated the oldest general hospital in North America in 1751 "for the reception and care of poor sick persons, whether inhabitants of the province or strangers." Dr. Bond was greatly aided by Benjamin Franklin, who became sponsor for the whole project. Franklin introduced the system of "matching funds" for philanthropic purposes, a system that 150 years later was to be utilized extensively by universities and hospitals, as well as voluntary health and welfare agencies.

According to Franklin's own account:

I inquired into the nature and probable utility of his scheme [Dr. Bond's] and receiving from him a very satisfactory explanation, I not only subscribed to it myself, but engaged heartily in the design of procuring subscriptions from others. Previously, however, to the solicitation, I endeavored to prepare the minds of the people by writing on the subject in the newspapers, which was my usual custom in such cases, but which he had omitted.

The subscriptions afterwards were more free and generous; but beginning to flag, I saw they would be insufficient without some assistance from the Assembly, and therefore proposed to petition for it, which was done. The country members did not at first relish the project; they objected that it could only be serviceable in the city, and therefore the citizens themselves should be at the expense of it; and they doubted whether the citizens themselves approved it. My allegation on the contrary, that it met with such approbation as to leave no doubt of our being able to raise two thousand pounds by voluntary donations, they considered as a most extravagant supposition, and utterly impossible.

On this I formed my plan; and, asking leave to bring a bill for incorporating the contributors according to the prayer of their petition and granting them a blank sum of money, which leave was obtained chiefly on the consideration that the House could throw the bill out if they did not like it, I drew it so as to make the important clause a conditional one, viz.: And be it enacted, by the authority aforesaid, that when the said contributors shall have met and chosen their managers and treasurer, and shall have raised by their contributions a capital stock of ——— value (the yearly interest of which is to be applied to the accommodating of the sick poor in the said hospital, free of charge for diet, attendance, advice and medicine), and shall make the same appear to the satisfaction of the speaker of the Assembly for the time being, that then it shall and may be lawful for the said speaker, and he is hereby required, to sign an order on the provincial treasurer for the payment of two thousand pounds, in two yearly payments, to the treasurer of the said hospital, to be applied to the founding, building, and finishing of the same.

This condition carried the bill through; for the members, who had opposed the grant, now conceived they might have the credit of being charitable without the expense, agreed to its passage, and then, in soliciting the subscriptions among the people, we urged the conditional promise of the law as an additional motive to give, since every man's donation would be doubled; thus the clause worked both ways. The subscriptions accordingly soon exceeded the requisite sum, and we claimed and received the public gift, which enabled us to carry the design into execution. A convenient and handsome building was soon erected; the institution has by constant experience been found useful, and flourishes to this day; and I do not remember any of my political maneuvers, the success of which gave me at the time more pleasure, or wherein, after thinking of it, I more easily excused myself for having made use of cunning.[8]

New York Hospital

The graduating exercises for the first recipients of a degree by medical students of King's College were held in New York in 1769, in Trinity Church. Dr. Samuel Bard, only twenty-seven years of age, and professor of the practice of medicine at the college, was the principal speaker at those exercises. He made a ringing appeal for the establishment of a hospital in New York for the care of the sick poor, for there were over 300,000 people in the province, with no hospital to serve them. He insisted that the hospital was also needed for instruction of students. He pointed out the fact that "a hospital affords the best and only means of properly instructing pupils in the practice of medicine."

The governor of the province was in the audience. He took immediate action, and pledged his aid and a substantial sum of money. King George III granted a charter in 1771, and the hospital was completed in 1775. Promptly it burned to the ground. It was rebuilt in 1776, was occupied briefly by Revolutionary soldiers, and after the Americans were driven out of New York, was used by the British as a barracks. It was not reopened as a hospital until 1791.

This brief history represents our total initial efforts at hospitalization during the Colonial period excepting, of course, the emergency pesthouses that have been described elsewhere.

COLONIAL DISPENSARIES

Governor John Winthrop (1606-1676) was America's first pharmacist. He took a great interest in chemistry, and this led to his

[8] Pepper, William: *The Medical Side of Benjamin Franklin.* William J. Campbell, Philadelphia, 1911.

interest in medicine. He compounded many of his own medicines, and studied the medicinal qualities of the herbs that were used by the Indians. During his later years, he devoted a good deal of time to pharmacy, and dispensed remedies to the colonists, usually gratuitously.

Medicines were dispensed to patients by physicians during Colonial days, but, in addition, apothecaries were established for dispensing of drugs. When Benjamin Franklin opened a general store in Philadelphia in 1730, his advertisements show that he sold herbs and "secret prescriptions" over the counter. Dr. Douglass of Boston wrote in 1731 that there were fourteen apothecary shops in the city (with a population of about 13,000 persons).

The first dispensary of medicine for the poor was established in Philadelphia in 1786. Samuel Bard,[9] who was to contribute so much to community service for the sick, established a dispensary in New York in 1790. In Boston the physicians were accustomed to dispense medicines freely from their offices to the indigent, but in 1796 they agreed that it would be more efficient to establish a central free dispensary and consultation service for the poor, each physician in town to take his turn as dispensary physician. Thus the Boston Dispensary was organized and has continued down through the years, and is still one of the important medical-care facilities of New England. Medical students got much of their practical training in these dispensaries, for Thacher[10] stated that by 1828 "some 2,000 young men had received instruction in the Philadelphia Dispensary for Medical Relief." From this simple plan of dispensaries for the poor there developed the extensive system of out-patient services for the indigent in all parts of America. Later these were incorporated into the services of general hospitals and the combination of an in-patient and out-patient hospital service became a universal procedure throughout the nation. Gradually, each hospital developed its own dispensary and free out-patient system. The out-patient service, for a great many years, was essentially a charitable function of the hospital, and remained so, long after the in-patient facilities of the hospital were utilized by all income groups.

After 150 years the out-patient service of many hospitals is still basically a dispensary of medicine for the indigent. Often, however, the medical services provided for these out-patients by the hospital

---

[9] See Langstaff, J. Brett: *John Bard of Hyde Park*. E. P. Dutton & Co., Inc., New York, 1942.

[10] Thacher, James: *op. cit.*

are not at all comparable to the quality of service given to the in-patients.

NURSING AND MIDWIFERY IN COLONIAL TIMES

One of the best indices of the nature and quality of nursing during the Colonial period is a priceless statement of the proper qualifications of a communicable disease nurse, as set forth by Dr. Thomas Fuller in 1730 in *Exanthematologica*. These requirements may well be given in their entirety.

Impossible to meet with a nurse every way so qualified for the Business as to have no Faults or Failings, yet the more she cometh up to the following Particulars, the more she is to be liked. It is desirable that she be:

1. Of Middle Age, fit and able to go through the necessary Fatigue of her Undertaking.
2. Healthy, and especially free from Vapors and Cough.
3. A good Watcher that can hold sitting up the whole Course of Sickness.
4. Quick of Hearing, and always ready at first call.
5. Quiet and still so as to talk low and but little, and tread softly.
6. Of Good Sight to Observe the Pocks, their color, manner and Growth, and all alterations that may happen.
7. Handy to do everything the best way, without Blundering and Noise.
8. Nimble and quick, at going, coming and doing everything.
9. Cleanly, to make all she dresseth acceptable.
10. Well tempered to humor and please the Sick as much as she can.
11. Cheerful, pleasant, to make the best of everything without being at any time cross, Melancholy or Timorous.
12. Constantly careful and diligent by Night and Day.
13. Sober and Temperate, not given to Gluttony, Drinking or Smoaking.
14. Observant to follow the Physicians orders fuly and not to be so conceited by her own Skill so as to give her own Medicines privately.
15. To have no Children or others to come much after her.

As basic qualifications, these might serve admirably in selection of a bedside nurse today, even though over 200 years have elapsed since these rules were formulated. Obviously, this type of nurse had no training except that of experience. Nursing was not a profession, but simply an accommodation to a neighbor or friend. Many years were to pass before nursing was to assume any importance or dignity as a separate profession with specific techniques and essential procedures in the care of the sick.

The first course of lectures for the practical instruction of nurses in America was inaugurated by Dr. Valentine Seaman at the New York Hospital in 1799, but over sixty years were to pass before a formal course of training was provided for them by the hospital. It is a sad but true commentary that most of the nursing for community hospitals was furnished by prisoners, vagrants, and the most degraded and dissolute men and women of the community.

Midwifery, as we have noted elsewhere, was almost entirely in the hands of women during the seventeenth and eighteenth centuries. These women were professionals, but were self-taught, or learned their trade from elder midwives. Many of them were ignorant of even the simple principles of childbirth, and some of them were meddlesome, careless, and cruel. Puerperal infection was common in their patients. In the more remote communities, the wives of the colonists followed the Indian plan of self-delivery. In this they were encouraged by their husbands, as is evidenced by a quotation from a Dutch minister from Nieuw Amsterdam, who in 1644 wrote *A Short Account of the Mohawk Indians,* in which he noted that the Indian women go about immediately after delivery, "and be it ever so cold, they washed themselves and the young child in the river or snow. . . . they walk, they stand, they work, as if they had not lain in, and we cannot see that they suffer any injury by it; and we sometimes try to persuade our wives to lie-in so, and that the way of lying-in in Holland is mere fiddle-faddle."[11]

The first publication that one encounters which deals with midwifery was distributed in America in 1663. It was a reprint of a London pamphlet which was entitled *A Present to be given to Teeming Women by their Husbands or Friends,* "containing Scripture-Directions for Women with Child, how to prepare for the hour of Travail." The pregnant woman was admonished to care for her health by avoiding excesses, and was urged to "prayer, repentance, reading of the Scripture, meditation, resignation, and preparation for death."[12]

Since medical practitioners as well as midwives were unlicensed in the colonies, there was no sharp line of distinction between them and charlatans.

[11] Heaton, Claude E.: "Obstetrics in Colonial America," *Ciba Symposia,* 1:389, (March) 1940. Reproduced by permission.
[12] See above reference.

Anne Hutchinson of Boston was a midwife as well as a spiritual leader. She was expelled from the Massachusetts Bay colony because of her religious fanaticism. She helped to found Rhode Island and later was killed in an Indian massacre in Pelham, New York. In 1638 Jane Hathaway was also banished for "notorious familiarity with the devil" and ordered to stop meddling "in oyles, plaisters, surgery or physick."

Bridget Fuller, wife of Samuel Fuller of the Plymouth colony, was an expert midwife who also helped her husband in letting blood. In her widowed old age she was invited to the town of Rehoboth "to come and dwell among us to attend to the office of midwife, and to answer the town's necessity." Ann Moore was primarily a midwife but also practiced medicine. The same is true of Margaret Barnard, who practiced medicine quite successfully in Nantucket. As far as we know, the first community that licensed midwives was the city of New Orleans in 1722.

MATERNAL AND CHILD CARE IN COLONIAL TIMES

Instruction of physicians in midwifery began in Britain as early as 1726. But in the colonies a physician was not called in childbirth, except in cases of serious emergency. Some of the young American physicians studied obstetrics in Europe under William Smellie and John Hunter. John Moultrie of Charleston, South Carolina, was a real pioneer in this field in the colonies. He came to Charleston in 1733, and was the dean of the medical profession there for forty years. He was designated as America's first male midwife. His death in 1773 was regarded in that community as a great public calamity.

Teaching in obstetrics was initiated by Dr. Shippen of Philadelphia in 1765. In that year he established a "convenient lodging for the accommodation of a few poor women who otherwise might suffer from want of the common necessities on those occasions, to be under the care of a sober, honest matron, well acquainted with lying-in women, and employed by the Doctor for that purpose." This lodging was a separate building and not a section of the general hospital. At the New York Almshouse, out of which Bellevue Hospital developed, an official midwife was employed from the very beginning—in 1736.

A lying-in ward was established at the New York Almshouse in 1799. Here, Dr. Valentine Seaman gave lectures on midwifery, exclusively to women. Dr. David Hosack established the New York Lying-In Hospital in 1799.

Midwives with some pretense of training were available in the larger towns throughout the colonies but, for the most part, they were self-trained and "grossly ignorant."

Child Health Promotion

Very little can be said concerning the promotion of child health during the Colonial period. We know that the birth rate was high, probably more than thirty-five per 1,000 population, with a correspondingly high infant mortality, averaging year by year well over 250 deaths per 1,000 live births. The chief causes of infant death were the diarrheal diseases of infancy. Tetanus due to infection of the umbilical cord was prevalent, and acute respiratory infections caused many deaths. Most of the babies were nursed for at least one year, and the transition from mother's milk to the rough pioneer food was the period of difficulty and danger. At the present time the neonatal death rate, e.g., infant deaths during the first thirty days of life, is far higher than the death rate during the entire subsequent eleven months of infant life. In 1750 the ratio was exactly reversed, since a high proportion of infant deaths occurred after the neonatal period, and the second year of life was almost as hazardous as the first.

In our discussion of contagious diseases we have noted the importance of the infectious diseases of childhood as a cause of death. Smallpox was fundamentally a disease of childhood and was the most dreaded of all the childhood infections. No child could escape this terrible affliction. The death of a child was considered the will of God. "The Lord giveth and the Lord taketh away." In a pioneer community where life was hard and resources limited, marriages occurred at an early age. Girls customarily married before sixteen years of age and pregnancies followed in quick succession. The average woman gave birth to eight children, but even though eight to twelve children might be born to one mother, seldom did more than four or five of these children survive to adulthood.[13] At the beginning of the nineteenth century, the average span of life in America has been estimated at about thirty-two years. This can mean but one thing—a very high mortality of infants and young children.

[13] Napoleon once said when bemoaning the fact that Josephine, his wife, had given him no heirs: "Every woman should have six children, for three will perish before they reach adulthood, two are required to replace their parents, and one remains to serve the state."

The pioneers of the West had a saying that "pioneering is heaven for men and dogs but hell on women and oxen." To this might have been added, "And worst of all, on young children."

MENTAL HYGIENE IN COLONIAL TIMES

There is good reason to believe that mental aberration was as common in Colonial days as at the present time. Certainly the epidemic of witch-burning at Salem, Massachusetts, gives ample evidence that hysteria might and did become a mass phenomenon. Frequent references are found which relate to the prevalence of mental disorder and mental deficiency. However, no special provision was made by the community for the care of those who were ill with mental disease. The violent patients were confined in the jails, otherwise they were cared for by relatives and friends. The Philadelphia Almshouse began to provide custody for the mentally ill in 1729.

The Philadelphia Hospital, which was founded in 1751, was the first permanent general hospital in America. It was a voluntary, philanthropic enterprise. From the very onset it admitted the mentally ill to its wards. The first state-supported mental disease hospital was established at Williamsburg, Virginia, in 1773 by the provincial government. In New York City, the New York Hospital[14] treated the mentally ill on the general medical service as early as 1792 but the "medical asylum" of the hospital was not established until 1808. These institutions were, of course, totally inadequate to carry all, or even a small part, of the burden of care of mental disease, but development of special hospitals to care for mental illness was slow. In fact, most of the states did not assume any responsibility for the care of the insane until well into the middle of the nineteenth century.

Psychiatry as a special field of medical science was completely uncultivated, although the general practitioner of medicine utilized a very practical form of pioneer mental hygiene with excellent results. Benjamin Rush gave much thought to mental disease and his book on this subject became a classic. But, by and large, the individual with a twisted personality had to untwist it himself. He got little help from his family, his physician, or his community. As Holmes said:

[14] Russell, William: *The New York Hospital.* Columbia University Press, New York, 1945.

What has come down to us from that first century of medical practice in America is comparatively simple and reasonable. The conditions of the rude, stern life in which the colonists found themselves in the wilderness took all the nonsense out of them. Good food and enough of it, pure air and water, cleanliness, good home nursing, an anesthetic, an opiate, a stimulant, quinine, a purge or two, and a few common drugs proved to be the marrow of good treatment. The rest went the way of white kid gloves and a malacca cane.[15]

[15] Holmes, O. W.: *op. cit.*

CHAPTER 6. *Medical Education*

The training of students adequately to meet the new philosophy of medical responsibility can only be brought about through a shift in the interests and the point of view of those in charge of medical education.

FINAL REPORT OF THE COMMISSION
ON MEDICAL EDUCATION, *1950*

We have included in this text a brief discussion of physicians, medical schools, and medical education during the Colonial period in order to illustrate the primitive state of medical care in the colonies. When we realize how little knowledge existed concerning disease and its prevention, we can more readily understand why public health made so little progress during this whole period. It is quite true that public health and medical education as well made real progress in Europe during this epoch, but the colonists were so fully concerned with the sheer necessity of maintaining life, and the establishment of safe settlements in the wilderness, that they had little time for consideration of the refinements of civilization.

PRAECEPTOR SYSTEM OF THE EDUCATION OF PHYSICIANS

Most of the young men in the northern colonies were trained as apprentices. The most famous teacher was Dr. John Kearsley, who came to Philadelphia in 1711. His office was called "the first medical college of America." His pupils included both William Shippen and John Bard, and these two, in turn, aided in the founding of the first medical college in the country—Shippen in Philadelphia in 1765, and John Bard with his son Samuel in New York in 1768. John Redman was another famous praeceptor, who was responsible for the training of John Morgan, Benjamin Rush, and Caspar Wistar.

Apprenticeship training was exacting and arduous, as is well shown by the following indentures which were drawn in the colonies early in the eighteenth century for apprentices in medicine:

Indenture Drawn up in Marlboro, Massachusetts, in 1734. Hollister Baker, a minor, aged about sixteen. . . . Of his own free will and accord and with the consent of . . . his guardian, doeth put and bind himself to be an apprentice unto Benj'n Gott, . . . physician, after the manner of an apprentice to dwell and serve from the day of the date hereof, for and during the full and just term of five years and four months next ensuing, and fully to compleat and ended. During all of which said term the said apprentice his said master and mistress honestly and faithfully shall serve; their secrets keep close; their lawful and reasonable commands everywhere gladly do and perform. Damage to his said master and mistress he shall not willfully do; his master's goods he shall not waste, embezel, purloin or lend unto others, nor suffer the same to be wasted or purloined: but to his power shall forthwith discover and make known the same to his said master and mistress.

Taverns nor alehouses he shall not frequent, or cards or dice, or any other unlawful games he shall not play. Fornication he shall not commit, nor matrimony contract with any person during said term. From his master's service he shall not at any time unlawfully absent himself, but in all things as good, honest and faithful servant and apprentice shall bear and behave himself towards his said master during the full term of five years and four months, commencing as aforesaid.

And the said Benj'n Gott for himself doeth covenant, promise, grant and agree unto and with his said apprentice in manner and form following, that is to say, that he will teach the said apprentice, or cause him to be taught by the best ways and means that he may or can trade, art or mystery of a physician according to his own best skill and judgment (if the said apprentice be capable to learn), and will find and provide for and unto said apprentice good and sufficient meat, drink, washing and lodging during said term, both in sickness and in health; his mother all said term finding said apprentice all his clothing, of all sorts, fitting for an apprentice during said term; and at the end of said term to dismiss said apprentice with good skill in arithmetick, Latin, and also in the Greek through to the Greek grammar.[1]

Dr. Rush described medical education in Philadelphia in 1760 most graphically:

In the month of February 1761, I began the study of medicine, and continued constantly in my master's family and shop 'till July 1766. During this period I was absent from his business but eleven days and never spent

---

[1] Miller, Genevieve: "Medical Education in Colonial America," *Ciba Symposia,* 8:508-9, (January) 1947. Reproduced by permission.

more than three evenings out of his house. My master at this time was in the most extensive business of any physician in the city, and as he had at no time more than two apprentices, he kept them constantly employed. In addition to preparing and compounding medicines, visiting the sick and performing many little offices of a nurse to them, I took the exclusive charge of his books and accounts. It may not be amiss to mention here that before I began the study of medicine, I had an uncommon aversion to such sights as are connected with its practice. But a little time and habit soon wore away all that degree of sensibility which is painful, and enabled me to see and even assist with composure in performing the most severe operations in surgery. The confinement and restraint which were now imposed upon me gave me no alternative but business and study, both of which became in a short time agreeable to me. I read in the intervals of business and at late and early hours all the books in medicine that were put into my hands by my master, or that I could borrow from other students of medicine in the city. I studied Dr. Boerhaave's lectures upon Physiology and Pathology with the closest attention, and abridged a considerable part of Van Swieten's commentaries upon his practical aphorisms. I kept a commonplace book in which I recorded everything that I thought curious or valuable in my reading and in my master's practice. To him I am indebted for the estimation in which I have always held the works of Dr. Sydenham. He put them into my hands soon after I went into his shop, and frequently alluded to his opinions and practice, particularly in the treatment of Epidemics. However laborious and self-denied my situation was during my apprenticeship, I owe much to it. It produced in me habits of industry and business which have never left me. It rendered diseases in all their forms and symptoms familiar to me, and gave me a facility in knowing them which is to be acquired in no other way. During my residence in Dr. Redman's shop, he was one of the physicians of the Pennsylvania Hospital by which means I was admitted to see the practice of five other physicians besides his own in the hospital.[2]

No medical colleges existed in North America until 1765. A few of the more prominent physicians gave occasional courses of lectures, but there were no hospitals, and teaching by physicians was formal and didactic.

ESTABLISHMENT OF MEDICAL COLLEGES IN AMERICA

Two young men born in Philadelphia, who had been trained at the University of Edinburgh, established the first medical school in the colonies. John Morgan, born in 1735, received his medical degree

[2] Miller, Genevieve: "Medical Education in Colonial America," 8:515-16, (January) 1947. Reproduced by permission.

from Edinburgh in 1763. His associate, Dr. William Shippen, Jr., first studied with his father, then went to Europe and graduated from Edinburgh in 1761. On his return to America, he began a series of private lectures in anatomy. These two men opened the Medical College of Philadelphia in 1765.

Morgan lectured on theory and practice of physic and materia medica, and Shippen gave sixty lectures on anatomy. Thomas Bond began his clinical lectures at the Pennsylvania Hospital in 1766, but was never appointed a professor in the medical college. Each student was required to give one year's attendance at Pennsylvania Hospital in addition to following the courses of lectures. If they did not have a bachelor's degree they were required to show proficiency in Latin and mathematics, together with natural and experimental philosophy.

Each student also had to serve an apprenticeship with a reputable practitioner and to have a general knowledge of pharmacy. A candidate for a medical degree had to be at least twenty years old. The doctorate in medicine was given not less than three years after the bachelor's degree, and each candidate was required to defend a thesis publicly in the college and to pass a public examination. These requirements were as high as those of most of the medical colleges in the United States in 1950. The schools produced a small group of well-trained physicians, but their professors were not realistic in that they did not meet the needs of a pioneer Colonial society, and the high requirements of the few Colonial schools were not widely accepted as essential qualifications for the average medical practitioner.

Morgan and Shippen were jealous of each other and quarreled. Both were able and ambitious, but they did not unite in their original purpose to make a strong medical faculty. During the Revolutionary War, leadership of the Medical Department of the Continental Army was first given to Dr. Morgan, then taken from Dr. Morgan and given to Dr. Shippen. This caused a great deal of bitter contention and recrimination.

Dr. Adam Kuhn in 1768 was appointed third member of the Philadelphia faculty. He taught materia medica and botany, and was a splendid addition to the staff. Benjamin Rush was appointed professor of chemistry in 1769. The place had been held open for him while he completed his education in Edinburgh, and in other parts of Europe. He was to become the most famous of all practitioners of medicine throughout the colonies. On June 21, 1768, the first class in medicine in North America was graduated. Ten students qualified for their degrees.

Samuel Bard initiated the steps that resulted in the organization of the medical school of King's College in New York in 1768 (see page 98). But the Revolutionary War put an abrupt end to all these splendid plans for medical education in the colonies.

At the end of the Revolutionary War there were about 3,000,000 people in the nation. There had been two medical schools, but both were closed. Toner estimates that there were about 3,500 practitioners of medicine in all the thirteen states, one to every 800 population in the towns, and one to every 1,200 in the rural areas. But less than 400 of these physicians had received a medical degree. Quacks abounded, and many of the physicians were little more than charlatans. Only fifty-one medical diplomas had been issued by the American medical colleges. All others with a degree were trained in Europe, but most physicians had no formal training at all.

Harvard opened a medical school in 1782, and Dartmouth in 1798, but by 1800, Harvard had given only 9 medical diplomas, Dartmouth 5, Columbia 29, and the University of Pennsylvania 131.

MEDICAL PUBLICATIONS DURING THE COLONIAL PERIOD

Since the best of the Colonial physicians were educated in Europe, they depended upon the mother country for medical literature. Almost all texts were in Latin. The texts of Sydenham and Boerhaave were the essentials of every physician's library, around which his meagre bookshelf was built.

Thacher's "Broadside" (see page 23) stands almost alone as an American medical publication in the seventeenth century. Descriptions of drugs that were utilized by the Indians are found in many Colonial reports, even including those of the explorer, John Smith. In 1726 Zabdiel Boylston published an historical account of inoculated smallpox in New England, following his controversy with the physicians in Boston on this matter. His major opponent, William Douglass, was the author of essays on "Smallpox" in 1722, and he also wrote a treatise on eruptive miliary fever in 1736. (This is his description of the epidemic of scarlet fever in Boston of that same year.) Nathaniel Williams in 1742 wrote on "The Method of Practice in Smallpox," and a clergyman, Thomas Howard, wrote on

"Pharmacy." According to Josiah Bartlett,[3] those were *all* the medical writings in Massachusetts in more than a century and a half.

Dr. John Walton of Boston published an "Essay on Fevers" in 1743, and Dr. John Lining of Charleston gave us our first accurate clinical and epidemiological picture of yellow fever in 1748.[4]

In 1769 Dr. John Kearsley, Philadelphia's leading physician, published, in *Gentleman's Magazine* in London, an article relating to the angina maligna which prevailed in the northern colonies from 1746 to 1760.

The first publication of medical society transactions was the essay of Dr. Everett Hubbard of the County Medical Society of New Haven, Connecticut, on "A Case of a Deformed Foetus."

The first medical journal in America was the *New York Medical*

MEDICAL PUBLICATIONS DURING THE COLONIAL PERIOD[5]

YEAR	SUBJECT	AUTHOR	PLACE
1677	A brief guide on smallpox and measles	Thomas Thacher	Boston
1722	Essays on smallpox	William Douglass	Boston
1726	Inoculated smallpox in New England	Zabdiel Boylston	Boston
1730	Essays on smallpox	William Douglass	Boston
1736	Miliary eruptive fever (scarlet fever)	William Douglass	Boston
1740	Pleurisy	Dr. Tennent	Virginia
1740	Illiac passion	Dr. Cadwallader	Philadelphia
1742	Smallpox	Nathaniel Williams	Boston
1742	Yellow fever	John Mitchell	Virginia
1743	Malignant fever	Cadwallader Colden	New York
1748	Yellow fever	John Lining	Charleston
1749	Malignant pleurisy	John Bard	New York
1750	Smallpox inoculation	Benjamin Gale	Connecticut
1753	Epidemical sore throat (scarlet fever)	Cadwallader Colden	New York
1754	Tetanus	Lionel Chalmers	Charleston
1760	Smallpox inoculation	Dr. Thompson	Philadelphia
1764	Malignant sore throat	Dr. Ogden	Long Island
1767	Essays on fevers	Lionel Chalmers	Charleston
1769	Angina maligna	John Kearsley	Philadelphia

[3] Bartlett, Josiah: *Progress in Medical Science*, 1810.

[4] Toner, J. M.: *Annals of Medical Progress.* Government Printing Office, Washington, D. C., 1874.

[5] Cited by Thacher, James: *American Modern Practice.* Cottons & Barnard, Boston, 1826, pp. 10-13.

Repository, which was inaugurated in 1797. Editors were Doctors Sam Mitchell, Edward Miller, and Elihu H. Smith.

These few medical publications are cited, not because they are an all-inclusive list, but to illustrate the paucity of medical literature of the period, and the necessity for the physician to use his own judgment and initiative in the care of his patients, without recourse to consultation with his colleagues or reference to current medical literature.

Without exception, these medical papers, which were published throughout a whole century of Colonial life, were devoted to discussions of acute contagious disease that occurred in epidemic form. What better evidence can we have that the most important diseases of this period were acute infections? Very little effective knowledge existed either in treatment or in prevention of these diseases. Preventive medicine was as yet unborn.

CHAPTER 7. *Medicine, Curative and Preventive, among the Indians*

Man is largely indebted to his social surroundings for the degree of his physical perfection.

E. H. JANES, *1876*

Benjamin Rush, in his essay on the "Natural History of Medicine Among the Indians," noted: "Their remedies are, like their eloquence, full of strength; if they are few in numbers, they are accommodated as their languages are to their ideas to the whole of their diseases."[1] A statement of this sort, coming from a man who gave vigorous, even drastic, treatment, is ample evidence that Indian therapy was potent indeed. There was, of course, a great variation in the details of treatment among the various tribes, but the general pattern was quite similar throughout the nations.

Preventive medicine was not a clearly developed concept among the Indians. Certain tribes had excellent sanitary practices; for example, when they camped along a river, their water supply was always secured upstream from the camp, and individual discharges and camp wastes as well were always disposed of below the camp. They understood the value of fresh fruits and vegetables in the prevention of scurvy, and took some pains to secure a diet rich in vitamins A and B.

The cranberry, which has a high vitamin C content, was well known as an antiscorbutic, and cod livers were a sovereign remedy for malnutrition. But for the most part, preventive medicine was a system of necromancy. Fetishes were frequently utilized in disease prevention. The commonest were amulets or necklaces containing a mixture of abhorrent substances that were supposed to ward off

[1] Rush, Benjamin: "Natural History of Medicine Among the Indians," *Medical Inquiries and Observations,* Fourth Edition, Vol. I, p. 68, 1815.

disease and prevent invasion of the body by evil spirits. Certain tribes believed that the four brother gods (Manitou) lived at the four corners of the universe. They had a brother who was an evil spirit, and thus corresponded to Satan. Manitou taught both the use of remedies and the prevention of disease. The latter was achieved chiefly by the casting out of evil spirits.

Thus the medicine men who served Manitou were a special cult, and received long and careful education. They had two major functions—to prevent disease, largely by incantations, and to cure illness. In some cases, the power of suggestion was a potent factor in curing illness, as well as a measure for warding off disease.

The profession of a medicine man was most hazardous, for if the patient died, a member of his family frequently took his revenge by killing the doctor.

The Indian medicine men were very skillful in *treatment* of illness, and were particularly adept in surgery. As time passed, white pioneers learned to have a high respect for the Indian doctors or medicine men. In fact, the tradition grew among white fur traders and trappers that the Indian medicine man was frequently to be preferred to his illiterate, badly trained white colleague, and this tradition has persisted in some degree in certain parts of America, right down to the present day.

The Indians used a very large number of roots and herbs in treatment of disease. Some of them were most effective, and some are still in use. John Josselyn, who wrote "New England's Rarities Discovered" in 1672, mentioned the use by Indians of turpentine in seriously infected wounds, the treatment of the weak with oil of cod livers and "sounds," and the use of a hot poultice of leaves in an infection of a woman's leg. Ipecacuanha as an emetic was well known by the Indians, and they had many other drugs to produce vomiting. It was the Indian custom to go for long periods without food. At the end of the chase they ate enormously, with resultant bellyache that required both vomits and purges. These purges were severe, but they had mild laxatives as well. Senna is one of these that became a household remedy throughout the nation, and is still used each spring in many country households as "Indian spring tonic." Sassafras became a famous remedy, which was adopted from the Indians, and soon developed into one of the Colonies' major exports to Europe. Among other of its qualities, sassafras was supposed to be of special value in the treatment of syphilis. The fat from bears, wildcats, rattlesnakes, and other animals was highly prized. These greases were used to treat rheumatism, bruises, burns, and general aches and pains. The Indians also knew the value of oil of chenopodium in the treatment of roundworms, as well as pumpkin seed in removal of tapeworms. Astringents were used very successfully, and wild lettuce was a favorite remedy for diarrhea. Diuretics were often quite drastic, and blisters as counterirritants were often worse than the disease. We now know that most of the roots, herbs, and concoctions that were employed in the treatment of disease had little therapeutic value. However, the various systems of steam baths and hot packs which the medicine man used undoubtedly were of real aid and comfort to the sick.

The Indians knew the value of hot springs in the treatment of arthritis, and considered mineral springs to be a special gift of the gods. (Manitou Springs, Colorado, is an example.)

But in surgery they had developed their highest skill. They used sutures in the treatment of wounds, employing animal tendon for thread. They understood the part that the heart and arteries played in the circulation of the blood, and applied the tourniquet effectively. They were very skillful in applying splints to fractures of the legs and arms. They knew the value of immobility in fractures, and also understood the necessity of applying traction. They did not amputate a limb in case of a severe injury or infection, but tried their best to save at least a functioning member. If an amputation had occurred, as in battle, for example, they knew the importance of skin flaps to protect the stump of the wound. Suction was employed for boils and local infections. They also used cupping and counterirritants for relief of pain. Poultices were used also to relieve pain, and abscesses were incised. Foreign bodies were removed from all wounds, and the principle of wound healing from the base was well understood. Thus it is readily understandable that the early pioneers who lived among the Indians developed a high respect for the surgical skill of the tribal medicine man, and often consulted him when suffering from fractures, injuries, and other wounds. But the Indians had no remedies for the prevention or treatment of smallpox, syphilis, or tuberculosis—the white man's diseases that invaded and devastated their tribes and destroyed whole nations.

SECTION II. *The Pioneer Period*

1790 TO 1861

CHAPTER 8. *Introduction to the Pioneer Period*

*Public health was entirely without the purview of the fathers
of the Republic and lay unrevealed in the womb of the future.*

CRESSY L. WILBUR, *1911*

In our discussion of the development of public health and medical
care during the Colonial period of America, we followed the course
of events in a more or less chronological order. The colonies grew
slowly and the evolvement of their social organization occurred in
a fairly logical and orderly sequence.

Each Colonial problem was solved as it developed. Each community hazard was met as it appeared. The health of the people was
protected during periods of emergency insofar as existing knowledge
permitted.

It is very true that little progress was made in the field of public
health in nearly 200 years of Colonial growth, but medical care and
health protection kept abreast of other social advances and maintained an orderly and progressive course.

The period from 1790 to the Civil War will be presented as a
series of episodes. Each of these episodes will represent a specific
event in the advance of the health protection of the nation. They
will not be described in chronological order since this gives no
coherence or logic to our discussion.

We can best describe this period of the growth of the nation as the
period of adolescence. In the period of adolescence of a child or of
a nation there is no coherence and no logical chronology. It is an
episodic period—a series of startling and apparently unrelated
events. One part of the body may develop with great rapidity at the
sacrifice of other parts—the physical development often surging far
ahead of a sluggish and incoherent mental apathy. What is true of a
growing boy is true of a growing nation.

The major characteristics of the *pioneer period* were:

1. Rapid growth of the population due to the high birth rate, and heavy immigration.
2. The industrialization of the eastern seaboard, with sudden increase in municipal population, which resulted in over-crowding, bad housing, inadequate sanitary facilities, polluted municipal water supplies, contaminated food, myriads of flies, and general prevalence of filth.
3. An explosive expansion of the West with continuous movement of population. In fifty short years the nation extended from the Appalachian Mountains to the Pacific, and from the Canadian border to the Gulf of Mexico.

We were a virile, dynamic, exuberant, careless, restless pioneer people, with little regard for security or for human safety, willing to do or die—and many died. Life was cheap. Recklessness was a virtue. Every young man was anxious for adventure, willing to take his chances of survival, and to risk the hazards. The risks were great, but the rewards of individual initiative were enormous. The watchword was: "Each man for himself; the devil take the hind-most"—and the devil in the form of cholera, typhoid fever, and yellow fever often took many of the strongest and the best as well.

Canals, railroads, and highways together with innovations such as the telegraph, the steamboat, and the cotton gin were put to speedy use by the eager, pulsing, progressive spirit of the people. Europeans charged Americans with execrable taste, unbounded vulgarity, unlimited bigotry, and colossal ignorance. We were called a materialistic, gross, undisciplined people, devoid of all the elements of greatness. Sydney Smith, writing in the *Edinburgh Review* in 1820, complained bitterly about our cultural shortcomings.

During the thirty or forty years of their Independence, the Americans have done absolutely nothing for science, nor for the arts, for literature or even for statesman-like studies of Politics or Political Economy.

What does the world owe to American Physicians and Surgeons? What new substances have their chemists discovered? Or what old ones have they analyzed?

Urbanization of the nation without proper understanding of the problems and hazards of crowded community life was one of the most important factors in the high death rate. The newly urbanized people utilized the same type of sanitary facilities and followed the same habits and customs that had been common in the sparsely settled rural communities from which they had come. The results were disastrous.

Stephen Smith[1] in 1865 clearly understood the relation of sickness to poverty, overcrowding, and bad social conditions. He says, "And when we remember that the great excess of mortality and of sickness in our city occurs among the poorer classes, and that such excessive unhealthiness and mortality is a public source of physical and social want, demoralization and pauperism, the subject of needed sanitary reforms in this crowded metropolis assumes such vast magnitude as to demand the most serious consideration of those who have regard for the welfare of their fellow beings, and the interests of their community."

Bolduan, in his essay on "The Public Health of New York City," has said:

New York appears to have been a reasonably clean and tidy town during the first quarter of the nineteenth century. The general death rate was about twenty-five per thousand, and the infant mortality ranged between 120 and 140 per thousand live births.

The second quarter of the century brought profound changes. Population growth became accelerated. Factories multiplied, immigration from Europe increased rapidly, standards of living were lowered, the housing situation became acute and conditions became more and more unsanitary.[2]

Let us for a moment view a cross section of the population of the United States in the year 1850 as revealed by the United States Census reports of that year. The total population was just over 23,000,000. Fifteen per cent were Negroes, of whom 11 per cent were free and 89 per cent slaves. The occupations of this population are shown in Table 2. Nearly half of the free male population over fifteen years of age were employed in agriculture. If we add the Negro field workers, it is estimated that there were about 3,500,000, out of a total of 6,500,000 employed persons, working on farms. Industry occupied only 30 per cent of the total labor, and professions classified as "requiring an education" occupied only 4 per cent of

[1] Smith, Stephen, and associates: *Report of the Sanitary Condition of the City of New York.* D. Appleton & Co., New York, 1865.

[2] Bolduan, C. F.: "The Public Health of New York City," *Bull. New York Acad. Med.*, 19:437, (June) 1943.

Table 2

Employment of Free Male Population over 15 Years of Age*
1850 Census

OCCUPATION	AMOUNT	RATE (PER CENT)
Agriculture†	2,400,583	45.1
Industry—e.g., commerce, trade manufacturing, mechanical arts	1,596,265	29.9
Common labor—not agriculture	993,620	18.7
Seamen and navigation	116,341	2.2
Law, medicine, and divinity	94,515	1.8
Other occupations requiring an education	95,814	1.8
Government service	24,966	0.5
TOTAL	5,322,104	100.0

* SOURCE: Smillie, W. G.: "The Period of Great Epidemics in the United States," *The History of American Epidemiology*. Ed. by F. H. Top. Copyright 1952 by the C. V. Mosby Co., St. Louis.

† NOTE: We have made an approximate estimate of an additional 1,000,000 Negroes over 15 years of age, engaged in agriculture—giving a total of about 3,500,000 agriculture *workers* in a total of 6,500,000.

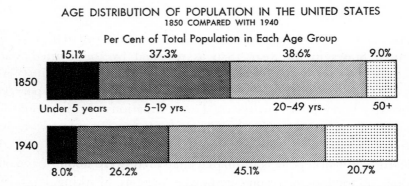

Fig. 6. Comparison of the age distribution of population in the United States of 1850 with 1940, as based on reports of the Bureau of the Census. The shift to the left in this graph represents a major social change. (From Smillie, W. G.: "The Period of Great Epidemics in the United States," *History of American Epidemiology*. Ed. by F. H. Top. Copyright 1952 by the C. V. Mosby Co., St. Louis.)

the working population. The very small proportion of persons in government service is striking.

We have compared the age distribution of the population in the 1850 census with a similar age distribution in 1940 (see Figure 6). This graph is, perhaps, the key to the high rate of epidemic disease.

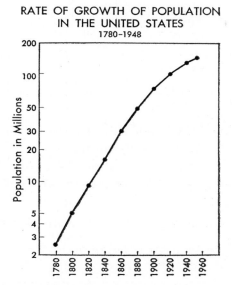

Fig. 7. The *rate of growth* of population in the United States (as indicated on a semilog scale drawn from data of the Bureau of the Census) was most rapid during the early part of the nineteenth century. (From Smillie, W. G.: "The Period of Great Epidemics in the United States," *The History of American Epidemiology*. Ed. by F. H. Top. Copyright 1952 by the C. V. Mosby Co., St. Louis.)

Over 50 per cent of the population was under twenty years of age, less than 10 per cent was over fifty years. Epidemics, of course, strike hardest at the children and young adults.

We have no accurate data concerning migration, but the distribution of foreign-born in our largest cities gives us some insight into the social problems of the day (see Table 3). The great proportion of immigrants were of German and Irish origin. The immigrants

Table 3

Nativity of Population: Four Largest Cities*†
1850 Census

CITY	TOTAL	FOREIGN-BORN	PER CENT FOREIGN-BORN		
			TOTAL	IRISH	GERMAN
New York	513,485	235,783	45	20	11
Philadelphia	408,045	121,699	30	17	5
Baltimore	165,983	35,492	21	7	11
Boston	135,625	46,677	34	26	1.3

* NOTE: No accurate summaries for nation as a whole.
† SOURCE: Smillie, W. G.: "The Period of Great Epidemics in the United States," *The History of American Epidemiology*. Ed. by F. H. Top. Copyright 1952 by the C. V. Mosby Co., St. Louis.

made up from one-third to one-half of the total population of New York, Philadelphia, Boston, and Baltimore.

The *rate* of the growth of the nation is shown in Figure 7. It will be noted that the greatest rate of growth occurred during the first

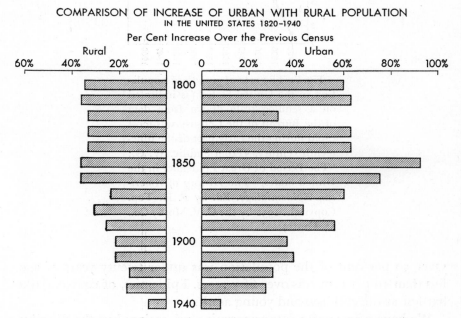

Fig. 8. The rate of increase of urban as compared with rural population is an index of the industrialization of the nation. Our cities grew so rapidly that sanitary facilities could not keep pace. (From Smillie, W. G.: "The Period of Great Epidemics in the United States," *The History of American Epidemiology*. Ed. by F. H. Top. Copyright 1952 by the C. V. Mosby Co., St. Louis.)

part of the nineteenth century. Figure 8 compares the *rate* of increase of rural and urban population of the United States from 1800 to 1940. Urbanization began about 1820, and increased rapidly during the first half of the century. Overnight we became a nation of city dwellers.

A comparison of proportion of deaths by age groups is given in Figure 9. We have compared Wigglesworth's famous table of 1789 with 1850, and 1850 with 1945. It will be seen that conditions were worse in 1850 than during the Colonial period, with a particularly high fatality of children of school age.

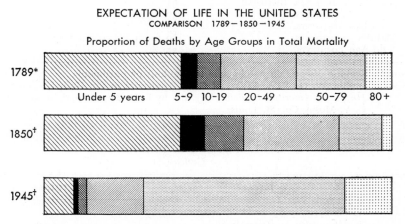

EXPECTATION OF LIFE IN THE UNITED STATES
COMPARISON 1789—1850—1945

Proportion of Deaths by Age Groups in Total Mortality

* Data from Wigglesworth's table.
† Data from United States Bureau of Census; however, some interpolations have been made because of difference in selected age groups.

Fig. 9. The health situation in America was not improved but worsened during the first half of the nineteenth century. By 1945 the death rate in the age groups under 20 years had been reduced strikingly. (From Smillie, W. G.: "The Period of Great Epidemics in the United States," *The History of American Epidemiology.* Ed. by F. H. Top. Copyright 1952 by the C. V. Mosby Co., St. Louis.)

There were over 300,000 deaths in 1850, and over 40 per cent of these deaths were due to "zymotic" diseases. These diseases took their heaviest toll in the younger age group for, in children from five to nine years of age, 56 per cent of the deaths were from pestilential diseases. (See Table 4.) We have no true measure of infant mortality since there were no accurate records of birth, but we have some idea of the appalling death rate in infants from the ratio of

Table 4

Deaths from Zymotic Diseases*†
1850 Census

Total deaths	323,023
Deaths from zymotic diseases	131,813
Per cent of deaths from zymotic diseases	40

Deaths from Zymotic Diseases by Age Groups
1850 Census

AGE GROUP	PER CENT OF TOTAL DEATHS FOR EACH AGE GROUP
Children under 1 year	32
" 1- 4 yrs. inclusive	54
" 5- 9 yrs. "	56
Youths 10-19 yrs. "	45
Adults 20-49 yrs. "	39 (men 44—women 33)
Old Age 50-79 yrs. "	25

* NOTE: Zymotic diseases do not include tuberculosis or pneumonia.
† SOURCE: Smillie, W. G.: "The Period of Great Epidemics in the United States," *The History of American Epidemiology*. Ed. by F. H. Top. Copyright 1952 by the C. V. Mosby Co., St. Louis.

Table 5

Deaths from Zymotic Diseases*
1850 Census

DISEASE	TOTALS
1. Cholera	31,506
2. Dysentery and diarrhea	26,922
3. Fever—remittent, intermittent, intestinal	19,220
4. Typhoid fever	13,099
5. Croup (diphtheria)	10,706
6. Scarlet fever	9,584
7. Cholera infantum and Cholera morbus	5,528
8. Whooping cough	5,280
9. Measles	2,983
10. Erysipelas	2,786
11. Smallpox	2,352

IMPORTANT INFECTIOUS DISEASES NOT INCLUDED AS ZYMOTIC

Consumption (pulmonary tuberculosis)	33,516
Pneumonia (lobar)	· 12,130
Cephalitis—in children under 5 (chiefly cerebrospinal meningitis)	6,422
Convulsions and *teething*, chiefly in children under 2	6,072

* SOURCE: Smillie, W. G.: "The Period of Great Epidemics in the United States," *The History of American Epidemiology*. Ed. by F. H. Top. Copyright 1952 by the C. V. Mosby Co., St. Louis.

infant deaths to total deaths. This ratio was 17 per cent in 1850, as compared with 7 per cent of total deaths in 1945.

The deaths from zymotic diseases in 1850, by cause, are shown in Table 5. Cholera led the list that particular year, for it was a cholera year, but the deaths from other intestinal infections held a high rank. Table 6 gives a tabulation of all causes of death of infants; intestinal infections lead all the rest.

Table 6

Intestinal Infections of Infancy*†
Deaths in Children under 1 Year

DISEASE	TOTALS
Cholera infantum	1,111
Cholera morbus	908
Diarrhea	1,467
Dysentery	3,311
Cholera	1,417
Enteritis	645
Teething	836
Typhoid fever	391
TOTAL	10,686
Total deaths in children under 1 yr.	54,265
Total deaths from zymotic diseases in children under 1 yr.	20,064

* NOTE: Convulsions—2,844 deaths due in great part to intestinal infections have been omitted.
† SOURCE: Smillie, W. G.: "The Period of Great Epidemics in the United States," *The History of American Epidemiology.* Ed. by F. H. Top. Copyright 1952 by the C. V. Mosby Co., St. Louis.

In a social organization of this order it is inevitable that the people will be devastated from time to time by overwhelming epidemics of infectious disease. No alternative can be anticipated. This is exactly what occurred. Furthermore, we shall show that the epidemics were themselves the *activating force which led to the development of comprehensive, effective health services.*

CHAPTER 9. *The Period of Great Epidemics*

A Pestilence speaks to nations in order that greater calamities
than the untimely death of the population may be avoided.

ELISHA HARRIS, *1878*

During the first part of the nineteenth century America experienced a series of great epidemics. They were initiated by the dreadful attack of yellow fever in the national capital of Philadelphia in 1793, and continued unabated for over half a century. These epidemics began to decline in extent, frequency, and virulence about 1870 and within a generation they had vanished completely.

Why did the nation suffer from these devastating plagues? What were the factors that were responsible for these disasters? Why did the epidemics disappear?

During the Colonial period there had been many epidemics, but they did not have the magnitude of the disasters of the following century. It seems probable that the colonists did not suffer from repeated, overwhelming epidemics because of their geography and their social structure. The population consisted of small groups, living on scattered farms and in villages. The communities were quite stable. Transportation was slow and difficult. A person was born and lived his entire life in the same house, often never leaving his village. There were no large cities and there was relatively little contact with the outside world.

As we have just noted, the period of great epidemics really began in 1793, in the capital city of Philadelphia, then the largest city in America. Yellow fever proved to be the cause of the outbreak which resulted in the death of nearly one-eighth of the population. This epidemic has been described in detail by Philadelphia's leading physician, Benjamin Rush,[1] who attributed it to a pile of rotting coffee on Ball's wharf.

[1] Rush, Benjamin: "The Phenomena of Fever," *Medical Inquiries and Observations,* Fourth Edition, Vol. III, p. 43, 1815.

We can best understand the epidemiological concepts of this whole period from a study of Rush's essay on "The Phenomena of Fever."[2] Epidemic diseases were called "zymotic" diseases from the Greek word *zymos* meaning "fermentation." These zymotic diseases were believed to be due to a fermentation of the tissues, and were always produced by an external stimulus. This stimulus was often cosmic in origin and was almost always transmitted through the air. The miasma might be produced by man himself, by the products of his household, by any type of decaying vegetable or animal matter, or by cosmic phenomena. Zymotic diseases were always accompanied by fever.

The basic theory of Rush was that "there is but one fever. However different the predisposing, remote, or exciting causes of fever may be, whether from cosmic forces, marsh or human miasmata, there can be but one fever. Furthermore, there is but one exciting cause of fever, and that is *stimulus*. This proposition cuts the sinews of the division of diseases from their remote causes. Thus it establishes the sameness of pleurisy, whether it be excited by heat following cold, or by the contagion of measles or smallpox, or the miasmata of yellow fever."

Noah Webster,[3] who had a great influence on Rush's theories relating to epidemic diseases, published in 1799, as we have seen, his *Brief History of Epidemic and Pestilential Diseases*. In this unique treatise of two volumes, he attempted to show a relationship between cosmic forces, such as volcanic eruptions, showers of meteors, and other environmental factors in the production of serious epidemics and pestilential diseases. According to Webster, epidemics were due to an accumulation of special unfavorable factors which combined to affect large numbers of people at the same time, and thus produce overwhelming disaster. This extraordinary theory kept its firm hold on the minds of medical men for more than half a century.

A general summary of the opinions of the physicians who met at the Sanitary Conference of Paris in 1851 is illuminating. The conclusions of the conference as presented by Clot-Bey[4] were:

1. Epidemics are always the result of cosmic conditions.
2. Isolated, e.g., individual, ill persons attacked by contagious

[2] *Ibid.*, pp. 3-36.
[3] Webster, N.: *On Pestilence*, 2 vols. Hudson & Goodwin, Hartford, 1799.
[4] Clot-Bey, Le Dr.: *Sur la Peste*. Paris, 1854.

diseases, virulent or miasmatic, are absolutely unable to produce epidemics.

3. Even epidemic diseases of essential contagious character are never spread through transmission, e.g., from person to person.

4. The essential—the specific—in epidemics is produced by a certain "state of affairs," unknown meteorological conditions, invisible and unfathomable.

The conference defined *virulent* diseases as variola, vaccinia, syphilis, and perhaps scarlet fever. *Miasmatic* diseases were typhoid fever, dysentery, cholera, intermittent fevers, and malaria. Plague, it was stated, does not fall in any group and thus cannot be contagious.

Epidemiological concepts of this type did not require the isolation of the sick person, and quarantine was not enforced against individuals who arrived in a port upon a "sickly vessel," but against their effects and against the ship's cargo.

This theory is clearly expressed by the Quarantine Act of London of 1825,[5] and in the records of the famous Quarantine Convention of 1857,[6] which was called by Wilson Jewell of Philadelphia.

This first convention was followed by similar conventions in 1858, 1859, and 1860. Their deliberations dealt almost exclusively with maritime quarantine and with environmental sanitation.

It is clear that the average person of the street was not as firmly convinced as were the physicians that individuals with smallpox, cholera, and yellow fever were not dangerous to others. Thus the regulations of the lay boards of health of the period did concern themselves with isolation of the sick during epidemic periods, as well as with removal of dead animals and with the location of cemeteries.[7]

Medical science, however, held strictly to the dogma that zymotic diseases are not transmitted from person to person, and that epidemics are due to natural phenomena which are, for the most part, uncontrollable.

One is led to the conclusion that epidemics must, perforce, have

[5] *Act for Making Provision for the Effective Performance of Quarantine.* London, 1825.

[6] *Proceedings of the Quarantine Convention.* Philadelphia, 1857.

[7] J. H. Rauch of Chicago, in 1866, in a privately printed pamphlet, pointed out the great dangers of burial of those dead with contagious disease within the city limits. Burial should be far from populous places and at a depth beneath the surface sufficient to prevent contamination of the air.

prevailed in a community which held such a tragically fallacious philosophy. Certainly these beliefs did not aid in the prevention or control of infectious diseases. However, we are willing to advance the theory that these fallacies were not entirely responsible for the prevalence of the great epidemics. With some temerity, we suggest that these epidemiological fallacies were not even very important factors in the production of epidemics. The great epidemics during the nineteenth centry were an integral, almost essential, part of the development of the economy and the social structure of the nation in such a degree as to make high death rates, with periodic disastrous epidemics, almost inevitable. Furthermore, we shall show that the great epidemics disappeared and the over-all death rate declined because of changes in social conditions. They declined before the causes of infectious diseases were known, before the epidemiological factors producing epidemics were understood, and before effective official health services were established.

What were the real causes of the great epidemics? What were the factors that produced during that period a continuously higher annual death rate in the American cities than the death rate of any other civilized nation of the globe?

The great *epidemic peaks* of the crude death rate curve were caused by recurring invasions of Asiatic cholera, by smallpox, and in the seaports by yellow fever. Worst of all was cholera. The epidemic of cholera from 1845 to 1855 swept over the nation at the time of the California gold rush, with its great movement of population and pioneer expansion to the far West. Thousands and thousands of young, vigorous, hardy men, who started to California to make their fortune, left their bones on the plains along the western trails, struck down by cholera. Time after time, cholera invaded the ports of New York, Philadelphia, Baltimore, and New Orleans; then, swinging from the focal point in ever-widening circles, invaded smaller cities and rural communities.

The epidemic disease that was dreaded even more than cholera was yellow fever. New Orleans fared worst of all the port cities, but none of these were spared from invasion, even the ones as far north as Halifax. The disease, after invading New Orleans, would sweep up the Mississippi River to the interior towns, spreading terror as it came, but it almost never invaded the towns and rural areas that were removed from the main waterways. The situation became so serious that New Orleans, with its great wealth of natural resources,

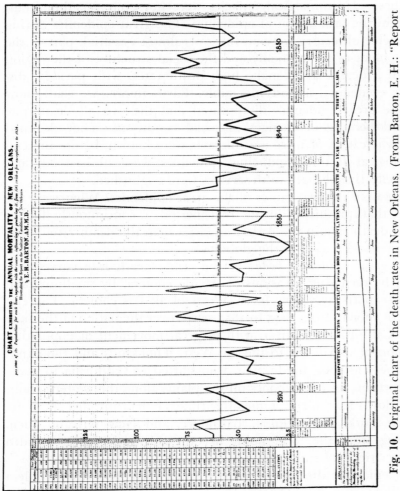

Fig. 10. Original chart of the death rates in New Orleans. (From Barton, E. H.: "Report upon the Sanitary Condition of New Orleans," *Report of the Sanitary Commission of New Orleans on the Epidemic Yellow Fever of 1853*. Published by authority of the City Council of New Orleans, 1854.)

had a much higher death rate than birth rate for nearly a century, and maintained her population only by the immigration of those hardy adventurers who were willing to take the great risk of their lives for the unparalleled financial opportunities that were offered by this fabulous city.

Smallpox recurred in epidemic waves and took a heavy toll of lives. Vaccination had been introduced in 1800, but was not widely accepted, and thus the disease always found ample susceptible material in the rapidly shifting, rapidly growing, unstable, pioneer community. We often forget the chief reason for the prevalence of smallpox in America during the nineteenth century. It is true that cowpox vaccine was introduced in our nation by Benjamin Waterhouse in 1800, and one would assume that this protective method would have met with almost instant and unqualified acceptance. But *calf lymph* did not become available until 1870. The method of vaccination was from arm to arm, with all its attendant difficulties and dangers. Many outbreaks of syphilis occurred, which were due directly to transmission by vaccination.[8] Frequent transmission of erysipelas and other virulent human infections resulted from arm-to-arm vaccination, and thus this method of prevention became justifiably unpopular.

Negri of Naples produced a good quality of calf lymph in 1834. The technique was introduced into France by Lanoix in 1864, and to Prussia and Brussels in 1865. In 1870 H. A. Martin of Boston distributed, on dried quill points, the first calf lymph in America for vaccination against smallpox. The method was not too successful, as the dried vaccine soon lost its potency.

Although the pestilential diseases of cholera, smallpox, and yellow fever were held in horror by the people, the real enemies which were producing the enormously high death rate caused little concern. These monstrous undertones of death were of everyday occurrence; for these diseases invaded every family, and their very familiarity brought about casual and inevitable acceptance.

The principal causes of death during the period of the great epidemics were not cholera, smallpox, and yellow fever, but were pulmonary tuberculosis, diarrheal diseases of infancy, bacillary dysentery, typhoid fever, lobar pneumonia, and the infectious diseases of childhood, particularly scarlet fever and diphtheria.

[8] In the Rialta, Italy, syphilis epidemic in 1861, forty-six children and twenty nurses were infected with syphilis from an initial arm-to-arm vaccination.

Shattuck, in his report for the Sanitary Commission of Massachusetts appointed in 1849,[9] noted that the most common infectious disease of all was malaria. It invaded every city, every town, every hamlet, and almost every home throughout the vast continent. Boyd[10] has emphasized the fact that, to our forefathers, malaria was the most familiar of all the fevers. This disease rose to its greatest height during the middle of the nineteenth century. It became somewhat stabilized in the 1850's, only to break out with increased violence during the Civil War, extending through the period of postwar recovery well into the twentieth century.

"The extent to which zymotic diseases prevail is the great index of public health," said Shattuck in 1849; "when the proportion is comparatively small, the condition of public health is favorable; when large, it is unfavorable."

But *"Diseases* of the *Respiration Organs* furnish one of the largest classes of causes of death. . . . *Consumption,* that great destroyer of human health and human life, takes the first rank as an agent of death. It destroys *one-seventh* to *one-fourth* of all that die. . . . The occasional visit of the cholera, or some other epidemic disease, creates alarm and precautionary means are adopted for prevention. But where is the alarm and precaution against a more inexorable disease over which curative skill has little or no power?"[11]

An index of the supreme importance of tuberculosis as a cause of death in pioneer times is secured from the death records of some of the larger cities, where the rates of 350 to 400 per 100,000 population were the rule during the fifth decade of the nineteenth century.

A report of the New York Sanitary Association in 1857[12] stated that New York City had the highest death rate (36.8 per 1,000 population) of any of the large cities in the world. The reasons for this were manifold. The city had increased very rapidly in population and harbored over 600,000 people. In the previous twelve years, a horde of immigrants had poured into the Port of New York. Many of these poor people were destitute, starving Irish fleeing from their potato famine. They arrived without resources, in a terrible state of

[9] Shattuck, Lemuel: *Report of the Sanitary Commission of Massachusetts, 1849.* Dutton & Wentworth, Boston, 1850.

[10] Boyd, Mark: "A Historical Sketch of the Prevalence of Malaria in North America," *Am. J. Trop. Med.,* 21:223, 1941.

[11] Shattuck, Lemuel: *op. cit.,* pp. 92-98.

[12] *Report of the New York City Sanitary Association.* Academy of Medicine, New York, 1859.

malnutrition, and were crowded into basement tenements under desperately filthy and foul conditions, where they died in appalling numbers. Deaths from diarrheal diseases of infancy had increased 250 per cent. Smallpox, typhus fever, cholera, even erysipelas and cerebrospinal meningitis swept through these wretched hovels, slaying the helpless victims by the thousands.

The city of New York, as late as 1858, had no sanitary protection whatever. It is true that the health inspector's office had been established early in the century, and until 1844, there had been medical men in charge of those municipal functions that related to ship quarantine. These civic responsibilities then fell into the hands of politicians. In 1858 the board of health consisted of the mayor, the aldermen, and the councilmen. There was no health officer. Six commissioners of health—all physicians—were appointed by the mayor, but their duties pertained to *quarantine* only, and they had no powers to regulate the sanitary condition of the city. This important function was delegated to twenty-three health wardens, whose duty it was to supervise the sanitary conditions of the various wards. There was not a physician in the group. Indeed, these wardens were an ignorant, vicious collection of ward heelers who had no knowledge of, or interest in, the health protection of the people.

Everett Dick, professor of history at Union College, Nebraska, in *The Sod House Frontier*[13] has noted that in the 1850's on the western plains, cholera, typhoid fever, the ague, pneumonia, and smallpox were the prevailing diseases. Diphtheria took a heavy toll of children. Hardly a family escaped diphtheria and, in some instances, whole families were wiped out. Water was obtained from springs, sloughs, water holes, and buffalo wallows. This supply was frequently contaminated. Water was scarce and hard to get. It was often necessary to dig 200 feet to obtain an adequate household supply. In the early days there was no equipment for drilling and no pumps.

"A contributing factor to illness," says Dick, "was lowered vitality from improper clothing, exposure and unbalanced rations. The common diet was salt pork, corn bread, and dried foods. Settlers searched the fields for 'greens' and used weeds of all sorts to supply their vitamins.

"Malaria was the disease of the young, and caused more deaths than any other illness. Pneumonia was a common cause of death

[13] Dick, Everett: *The Sod House Frontier, 1854-1890.* Appleton-Century, New York, 1937.

among the older people, but certainly the most prevalent disease was malaria. Typhoid epidemics were very common. Every community had typhoid fever every fall."

In retrospect it becomes quite clear that the prevalence of the great epidemics and, in fact, the very high over-all death rate were not primarily due to deficient epidemiological theories of physicians nor to lack of understanding of causal factors in illness.

Rather the epidemics were due, in great part, to the social and economic factors that dominated the lives of all the people. Why did these epidemics disappear, and the crude death rate begin its steady decline before health services were organized and before the advent of bacteriology with its knowledge of the cause of infection and its incrimination of the individual patient as the important source of transmission of infectious diseases?

Our data show that the great proportion of deaths was due to unfavorable environmental factors, to polluted water supplies, indescribable systems of feces disposal, overcrowding, with resultant disreputable housing conditions, bad milk, bad food, flies by the millions, poor nutrition, long hours of overwork, and gross ignorance and carelessness.

The sanitary reform began about 1845. It was greatly aided by the sanitary conventions of 1857-1860. Though this reform was checked by the Civil War, it again gathered momentum at the end of the war, and by 1870 had gained great impetus. The effects of these changes became apparent almost at once.

Our forefathers were misled by their theories that disease was transmitted by miasmata, and therefore that community cleanliness was the only sure road to good health. The sanitary survey of New York City by Stephen Smith[14] and his associates was concerned almost wholly with bad housing conditions, with no understanding of the immediate causes of illness and death. But they concluded rightly that the "fever nests" of typhus which they encountered were due to the indescribably overcrowded, damp, dark basement housing of the recently arrived Irish immigrants, and that the enormous infant death rate of the summer months was a component part of poverty, ignorance, slums, and filth.

An awakening insight concerning those matters resulted in an

[14] Smith, Stephen, and associates: *Report of the Sanitary Condition of the City of New York.* D. Appleton & Co., New York, 1865.

aroused public consciousness. The newspapers, the church, business-men, and the local sanitary services that were rapidly being formed, educated the people in the simple laws of community sanitation. Ener-getic efforts were undertaken to clean up the cities and to promote wholesome surroundings. "A clean city is a healthful city," was the slogan, and although it was only a part truth and based on faulty premises, nevertheless the results were most gratifying. Indeed, within a short period of time, the reduction of illness and death was really astounding.

Even malaria began to become circumscribed, not as a result of quinine, nor because of a knowledge that mosquitoes transmitted the disease. The decline of malaria was a social and economic phenomenon. It was due to a transition from pioneer conditions to improved cultivation of the land, better rural housing, more cattle, more drainage of the bottom land, rapid transportation, replace-ment of the village mill and its millpond by centralized milling, and all the other components of an advancing civilization.

The period of the great pestilences was on the wane, the period of exact bacteriological and epidemiological knowledge was about to dawn. Important as this new epoch was to be in saving life and preventing suffering, nevertheless, the most important factor of the whole century in reduction of illness and death was an awaken-ing of a social consciousness in the nation. A development of com-passion for the suffering of the poor, an aroused sense of public decency, a finer feeling for the value of human life, all of these re-sulted in the development of a sanitary consciousness, and this, in turn, culminated in the adoption and the establishment of the simple principles of family and community cleanliness. In truth, it was common-sense, down-to-earth community housekeeping which led the way out of the wilderness of disease and disaster. The period of great epidemics was over.

This whole concept of epidemic prevention may be summarized in a few words:

As we look back through the years in our attempt to analyze the factors that brought about the disappearance of the great epidemics, certain clear-cut patterns emerge. We are driven to the conclusion that community invasion by epidemic disease is, in itself, an irre-sistible force in the initiation of improved health services and in the promotion of general social betterment. Thus, the great epidemics of the nineteenth century in America were of paramount importance because of the impetus they gave to the initiation and consummation of sound and comprehensive health services for the nation.

An epidemic is an unexpected and dramatic deviation from the normal. We have all observed the striking social phenomenon that any abrupt upheaval, any rapid and sharp deviation from the accustomed state of affairs, will arouse the people to an astounding degree. This may result sometimes in an overwhelming panic. The existing "normal" conditions may represent a very bad situation, for "normal" does not mean "optimum." In fact, it may not mean satisfactory conditions at all. A normal situation is simply one to which the individual or the community is accustomed and to which he or it is adjusted. The unhappy situation in which the American people found themselves from 1800 to 1865 had become acceptable to them. It was recognized, of course, that the unsanitary living conditions, the gross overcrowding in cities, the poverty and ignorance of great masses of people, contributed to the high general morbidity, the appalling mortality in childhood, and the over-all high death rate. But these matters were regarded with equanimity as burdens to be borne, for they were omnipresent, of everyday occurrence, and certainly of no direct concern to government—local, state, or national.

But the epidemics, though comparatively infrequent and relatively unimportant as causes of illness and death, were regarded as terrifying disasters for the reason that they appeared so insidiously, so suddenly, and struck with such dramatic force. As a result of these epidemics, immediate and vigorous action was taken to improve the whole sanitary situation.

Thus we learn that it is the sudden and rapid deviation from the normal in our social or economic system which first causes consternation of the people, and then serves as the catalyst in bringing about extensive social reforms.

CHAPTER 10. *Asiatic Cholera*

My people are destroyed for lack of knowledge.

HOSEA, IV:6

Asiatic cholera did not enter America until 1832. Despite great vulnerability, the American colonies were never invaded by the two greatest scourges of mankind—bubonic plague and cholera. How fortunate for the young country, struggling to establish a foothold, that the East India Company did not open up the great Asiatic continent to commerce until the end of the eighteenth century! For central Asia is the home of cholera and probably has been its dwelling place for a great many centuries. From there it has spread in a series of pandemics to other parts of the world.

It is a fantastic disease from every point of view. It lurks, hidden and slumbering within a small area, for a long period of time; then quietly and for no known reason makes its inroads, still within a narrow zone and by a series of forays. Suddenly it lashes out, invading larger and larger areas, until it assumes the qualities of a great raging fire, which becomes impossible to control until it burns itself out. Like a forest fire, it starts with a small spark in dry leaves, gradually grows and leaps into flame, perhaps destroying one valley completely. It may pass over a single farmhouse or small settlement without touching it, only to burn more fiercely than ever in the adjoining forest. Terror spreads before, with everything fleeing the onslaught, only to be surrounded and licked up by the flames. The incubation period of the disease is short. Death strikes quickly and is inevitable; whole families are perfectly well and at peace in their home in the morning, all unaware of danger. A stranger passes by to ask for a drink of water and falls dying at their feet. Next day the whole family sickens—the following day all are dead.

The disease is most devastating among the poor, the miserable, and the unfortunate; but no one, rich or poor, is immune. It has been called the disease of criminals, prostitutes, wretches, and sinners. In part this is true, for examples may be given of whole streets of prostitutes being completely destroyed by cholera, insane asylums standing empty with flapping doors, all the miserable patients dead or dying, deserted by their attendants. Jails and prisons are a holocaust, the slums a festering mass of dying and dead. The drunkard dies in the gutter, the homeless vagabond is found at the roadside as though asleep.

But not all deaths occur in the homes of the poor and lowly. Through the kitchen of the wealthy the servant enters and with her enters the specter of death. The rich and well-favored, though they may flee the city to escape destruction, will be followed and slain. The enemy strikes so silently, so ruthlessly, and with so little warning. How Death must have laughed when the port authorities of New York, in order to calm the people, denied that cholera was within the city gates! True, one or another new arrival, a wretched, ignorant immigrant who had just embarked, had died from a most mysterious "putrid diarrhea" and had been surreptitiously buried. The very men who viewed the body, who lied about the known cause of death, and who had ordered the secret disposal of the corpse, would themselves, within a day's time, be stricken and perish. Within a week hundreds of families in the city would be in mourning and the countryside in terror and abject panic.

It is a disease of youth and particularly of strong and vigorous young men. The analysis of over 7,000 cases that were reported from eighteen states in the epidemic of 1873 gave a case fatality ratio of 51 per cent. Every other victim attacked by the disease died. And this was considered a mild epidemic. Negroes were more susceptible than whites, with a 61 per cent death rate. Male patients preponderated over females three to two. Forty-six per cent of the cases were between twenty and forty years of age, although they made up less than 25 per cent of the total population. Very few infants developed the infection and people over sixty years of age were relatively safe. But no one was secure from danger. Most vulnerable of all were those who volunteered to care for the sick and to bury the dead.

The disease is so horrible. A young man who is perfectly strong and healthy in the morning begins to feel dizzy and weak. By noon he is dreadfully ill with intractable vomiting, continuous diarrhea, a cold and clammy skin, sunken eyes, and skin drawn tight over the cheekbones. He has parched lips, a dull lusterless expression, and the

weakness of an infant. Soon he becomes covered with his own ex-
crement—helpless, hopeless, and stuporous. Death strikes quickly
and mercifully—not within a few days, but within a few hours.
This is cholera.

For reasons that no one understands, the terrible pestilence sweeps
over the land and then is gone completely. Unlike almost every
other disease that we know, it strikes with incredible power, then
retreats to its ancestral home in far-away Hindustan, and remains
silent, smoldering, perhaps for years, perhaps for a century.

America has had four and only four invasions. The first began in
1832, and the infection remained three years, though it gradually
diminished after the first year. The second and greatest pestilence
began in 1849 and died down within two years, but was reactivated
in 1854, and then completely disappeared about 1857. A small but
very serious and short epidemic occurred in 1866, directly after the
Civil War. The last disaster occurred in 1873 and lasted two years.
The disease has never returned—down to the present day.

Though records were poorly kept and many attempts were made
to hide the source and mode of the infections, the disease is so devastating, so ruthless and overwhelming, that today we know the exact
port where each invasion occurred. We even know the very ship of
destruction, and the very day that the epidemic began. The actual
names of the persons who were its first victims and who brought the
pestilence ashore are recorded. Furthermore, the mode of transmission, the manner of spread, the rapidity of invasion, all could be
traced like the crimson glare of the forest fire—traced even today
by the blackened ruins of the devastation that remained.

Cholera has undoubtedly been, from the beginning of the history
of mankind, one of the major plagues. From early historical records
there is convincing evidence that great epidemics of a peculiar disease, characterized by terrible vomiting, severe diarrhea, rapid wast-
ing, complete stupor and death, all occurring within a few hours,
have swept over the world at irregular intervals. There is undoubted
evidence that cholera has prevailed in its homeland in central Asia
from time immemorial. Lack of communication with Europe, poor
transportation, desert barriers and impassable waterways, readily
explain the maintenance of the disease within bounds, even during
the active awakening of commerce in the sixteenth century. The
very nature of the disease explains its failure to spread. The incubation period is so short and the course of the disease so swift. Large

numbers of susceptible and recently exposed hosts are required to keep the flame burning. Wars or other great movements of people are required in order that the disease may propagate and spread. A great pilgrimage to Mecca was required to enable the disease to burst its bounds and invade Europe in 1830. A great immigration to America was under way, with relatively rapid means of transportation, carrying hundreds of wretched potential victims, who were crowded in the steerage under bad sanitary conditions, and who had been met by cholera at the port of embarkation. This chain of circumstances was essential in order to produce a cholera invasion of America.

THE EPIDEMIC OF 1832

Following the British occupation of India, the disease had spread abroad first in 1816. An outbreak occurred in the delta of the Ganges in 1826. It crossed the desert by caravans to the Caspian Sea. Cholera reached Russia and the Near East about 1830. In 1831 a great number of Mohammedans met at Mecca. In a pilgrimage of over 50,000 persons, nearly one-half perished with cholera en route. Approaching both from the east and south, the epidemic arrived in central Europe that same year. It appeared in England in the summer of 1831 and reached Scotland, Ireland, and Wales by January of 1832. The Irish at this time were just beginning their migration to America, the land of promise, a migration that was to increase with a crescendo which was to reach its full force twenty years later, and which was to modify the whole social structure of the new country. The young, adventuresome, carefree immigrants encountered cholera at the heavily infected ports of embarkation. The disease accompanied them on their voyage, when many died en route. It was first established in the New World in Quebec in the spring of 1832, spreading rapidly to Montreal—thence down the canals to Albany and west to the Mississippi Valley. By July all the canal cities, Utica, Syracuse, Rochester, Buffalo, and the smaller towns as well, were having a heavy death toll. By July 4 the disease was well established in New York City.

There is substantial evidence, however, that cholera arrived in New York before it came to Quebec, brought there by one or more immigrant-laden ships from Ireland. The board of health is said to have suppressed the news, and all records that could have any bearing on the matter were destroyed or "mislaid." However, the epi-

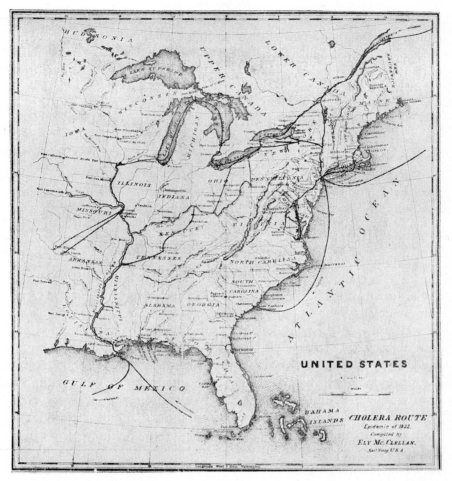

Fig. 11. Map from Woodworth's report on cholera. The 1832 epidemic entered at the ports of New York, Quebec, and New Orleans and spread along the main lines of travel. (From McClellan, Ely: "A History of the Travels of Asiatic Cholera in North America," *Cholera Epidemic of 1873 in the United States.* Government Printing Office, Washington, D. C., 1875.)

demic was in full swing in New York by August and continued until October. At least 3,500 persons died in New York City from the disease within three months. Philadelphia and Baltimore suffered seriously, but Montreal and Quebec were the hardest hit, with very high death rates and a state of complete panic.

Cholera entered New Orleans that same year and caused havoc. It spread up the Mississippi River to meet its counterpart coming west through the Great Lakes and the Ohio Valley. The Black Hawk

War was raging that summer and the toll taken by the disease among American troops was truly heart-rending.

In New Orleans the disease died out in the late fall. During the epidemic, in a city of about 35,000 persons, at least 6,000 died, "showing the frightful loss of one-sixth of the people in about twelve days . . ."[1]

The disease flared up again in New Orleans and in the whole Mississippi Valley in 1833, spreading to the interior towns of Ohio, Tennessee, and Kentucky. A graphic and dramatic description of this terror and devastation is given by Chambers in his chapter, "The 1833 Epidemic in the Blue Grass."[2]

Cholera reappeared in a milder epidemic in the summer of 1834 in New York and Philadelphia. By 1835 it had completely disappeared for reasons that are to us, even today, quite mysterious.

THE EPIDEMIC OF 1849

Cholera invaded all of Europe in 1847 and 1848. The disease came from central Asia, as before, causing more than 1,000,000 deaths in Russia alone. France lost over 150,000 in 1848, and Germany was heavily invaded. In this particular year the heaviest migration to the United States came from Germany. In the fall of 1848, on almost the same date, two ships left for America laden with German immigrants; the "Swanton" with 280 Germans in steerage sailed for New Orleans, the "New York" with 250 immigrants sailed for New York. Both ships became veritable hospitals en route. The disease, however, did not establish itself in New York, for it was held in check by the very cold weather of New Year's Day. It is true that 100 cases had occurred among the quarantined immigrants from the ship, with 50 deaths, but only two native New Yorkers died from the disease. The strict quarantine and frigid temperatures stopped the disease.

The story was very different in New Orleans. Cholera established itself in the city from contact with the "Swanton" passengers, and, although the Board of Health denied the prevalence of the disease, it spread with explosive violence to all parts of the city. Over 4,000 persons died from cholera within a few weeks.

After the purchase of Louisiana from Napoleon, the Mississippi River had become the chief highway and mode of transportation in the immense territories that lay fallow for development to the north

[1] Chambers, J. S.: *The Conquest of Cholera*. The Macmillan Co., New York, 1938, p. 118.
[2] *Ibid.*, pp. 148-79.

and west. A network of railroads was extending from the Atlantic coast to the great river. The river steamboat was at its very height; an appreciation of the tremendous possibilities for development of the West had begun to reach into every village and farm on the Atlantic coast. Then came the thrilling message of the discovery of gold in California and the great 1849 "gold rush" began.

The situation soon became most tragic. Every boat plying the Mississippi carried cholera upstream from New Orleans. The disease spread up the river to all the boom towns on the Mississippi and thence up its tributaries, east and west, to the Ohio and the Missouri. Cholera arrived just in time to meet the great surges of treasure seekers from the eastern states who paused at the rivers to outfit themselves for the perilous journey across the prairies and mountains to the fabulous land of California.

A quotation from the St. Louis papers in July, 1849, expresses a lament that was echoing up and down the river for 2,000 miles:

All worldly matters have now given way in this city to the one absorbing dread of cholera. This terrible destroyer of the human race seems to increase in violence in this city daily, until we can scarcely look at its ravages without a shudder of terror. Already it has carried off over 5,000 of our population and now its blows fall with more fatal and fearful rapidity than ever. To add to our terror medical specifics and medical skill became each day more inefficient and useless to arrest the disease in its progress to fatality. Indeed most of our eminent medical men now declared the disease an outlaw, to which no known rules of treatment can be offered with any certainty of success. Contrary to our first supposition, it seems now to have little or no regard to the classes of society it attacks, as the rich fall with the poor; the temperate and comfortable in life, along with the dissolute, the abandoned or the wretched.[3]

The disease reached California in 1850, and, in Sacramento alone, over 1,000 died of the pestilence in a very short space of time. Cholera had not spread in New York following its first invasion at Christmas time in 1848, but immigrants continued to pour into the city from Europe during the spring and in May the inevitable happened. The disease was introduced by the immigrants. The peak of the infection was reached in July. By September it had disappeared, leaving a record of 5,000 deaths.

Boston was saved from the serious consequences of the pestilence, as it had been in 1832. On receiving warning that cholera prevailed

[3] Chambers J. S.: *op. cit.*, p. 237.

in New York, the mayor and board of aldermen constituted themselves a board of health. The city was divided into districts; each
board member supervised the sanitation of his district. Every yard,
every house, and every stable were given such a cleaning and scrub-
bing as they had never before experienced. Refuse was burned,
privies emptied, and streets cleaned. A special cholera hospital was
prepared and quarantine instituted against infected ports. The disease
appeared, and, all told, 262 cholera patients were admitted to the
special hospital. There were only 162 deaths. It was an enviable
record.

During 1850 and 1851 cholera continued to harass New Orleans
and other cities on the Mississippi. Scattered epidemics occurred in
the interior cities in 1852.[4] By 1853 the disease was dying out in the
interior, but it continued to rage in Europe, for, in November, 1853,
alone, twenty-eight ships bound for New York with immigrants
buried 1,141 victims of cholera while at sea. It was inevitable that
cholera would reinvade the major American ports of entry for European immigrants. However, these attacks were mild and did not
spread widely. The disease did not disappear from this continent
entirely until 1857, after raging with some violence in 1854 at some
of the major ports.

THE EPIDEMIC OF 1866

In 1865 the Mecca pilgrimage again spread cholera into Europe
from central Asia. As before, immigrants carried in steerage brought
the disease from Europe to America. The first infected ship, the "At-
alanta," reached New York on November 2, 1866. Four more infected
ships arrived in New York before the end of the year, but the disease
did not spread, probably because of the cold weather. During the
following year, eighteen cholera ships arrived in New York with 8,491
passengers and crew, among whom 872 persons had died with cholera
en route. In New York that summer there were over 2,000 deaths
from cholera. The disease entered at the port of New Orleans on
July 12 and spread up the Mississippi as in 1849. But the disease was
controlled better than in previous epidemics, since the necessity of
vigorous sanitary measures was understood. The lesson learned by the
Sanitary Commission of the Civil War had been broadcast to all parts
of the country.

[4] *The Cholera Epidemic of 1873 in the United States.* Executive document No. 95.
Part II, "A History of the Travels of Asiatic Cholera." Government Printing Office,
Washington, D. C., 1875, p. 634.

Chambers[5] has estimated that the loss of life in the whole country from cholera during the 1866 invasion must have been over 50,000. He noted that in the epidemic of 1833 a 15 per cent mortality of the total population of an invaded community was not unusual. In 1849 a community mortality seldom exceeded 10 per cent. In 1866 no single invaded community had a higher total mortality than 5 per cent. The epidemic receded in 1867 and disappeared that winter.

THE EPIDEMIC OF 1873

The last American invasion by cholera occurred in 1873. This epidemic has been carefully studied and documented. John M. Woodworth had just been made surgeon general of the United States Marine Hospitals. He took an active part in the control of the epidemic and wrote the introduction to voluminous official reports on the outbreak. In contrast to previous outbreaks, Woodworth and his colleagues now understood full well the importance of sick individuals and their personal effects as being the essential factors in the spread of the disease. He also understood the danger of polluted water and food as a source of infection. He knew that the disease was due to a "specific organic poison" which is found in the alimentary canal of the patient and "is contained in the ejections." Obviously these simple but important facts were of enormous importance in guiding health officials in the formulation of control measures. Cholera was not due to the miasmata, nor to environmental influences such as polluted air, high temperature, and humidity, nor did it come from the sky or from stardust, but was transmitted through fecal discharges of sick patients. To quote Woodworth:

For nothing is more clearly proved by the history of cholera than that epidemics of this dreaded disease can be controlled by *vigorous hygienic measures. The true remedy against cholera is preventive medicine.*

Cholera was prevalent in North Germany, Poland, and Austria from 1870 until 1872. It entered the United States through New Orleans in February, 1873. It entered stealthily and was well established in the interior towns on the Mississippi River before it was finally recognized in New Orleans as true cholera. The whole Ohio Valley was invaded by spring, and many small towns suffered severely. In this epidemic the major tragedies occurred in the rural areas and in the growing villages and small towns of the great interior valley of

5 Chambers, J. S.: *op. cit.,* pp. 285-86.

the Mississippi. The reason was that these villages did not have the same sanitary protection that now prevailed in the cities. The eastern seaboard was largely spared. The details of those local outbreaks, with stories of family disasters and individual self-sacrifice and heroism, are given in the great executive document[6] which has reported the epidemic of 1873. The disease rapidly died out when winter came, and from that time to the present, cholera has not re-invaded America.

As a direct result of this 1873 epidemic, nationwide ship quarantine was instituted under the able direction of Surgeon General John Woodworth. Under the guidance of his administrative talent and careful planning, the modern United States Public Health Service was born. Based on the simple but strong foundation which he built, this small nucleus was to become the great national public health organization that exists today.

[6] *The Cholera Epidemic of 1873 in the United States.*

CHAPTER 11. *A Story of Malaria*

Prop. 1. All right study of epidemics "consists in ascertained facts or phenomena or events, and the whole classified and arranged."

Prop. 3. Our proper conclusion "consists of a rigorous and absolute generalization of these facts, phenomena, wants and relationships, and in nothing else."

Prop. 6. All classification or arrangement depends upon and consists in identity or similarity among themselves of certain groups or phenomena or relationships.

ELISHA BARTLETT, *1847*

Daniel Drake published his great classic on *Principal Diseases of the Interior Valley of North America*[1] in 1850. It was an extraordinary achievement of a remarkable man. He was a true pioneer; a frontier physician of real ability and tremendous energy. He took an active part in the founding of at least three medical colleges. He was an excellent teacher and a superb organizer. He conducted an active clinical practice, yet he also found the time and energy to pursue his major interests, namely, epidemiology and medical ecology.

The data from this book cover the whole drainage area of the Mississippi River and its great tributaries, extending from the Gulf of Mexico into Canada and from the Pittsburgh to the Rocky Mountains. Drake wrote from firsthand experience, for he had investigated practically the entire area, by horseback, oxcart, canoe, and all other means of transportation.

The outstanding conclusion that one draws from Drake's book is that *malaria* was the principal disease of the great interior valleys of North America. Other devastating epidemics might sweep up the rivers and across the plains, but even the worst of them lasted for

---

[1] Drake, Daniel: *Principal Diseases of the Interior Valley of North America.* Winthrop B. Smith & Co., Cincinnati, 1850.

but a few months, and returned at infrequent intervals. Cholera
might cause thousands of deaths in a few weeks' time, and produce
unreasoning panic all up and down the reaches of the Mississippi,
but malaria was omnipresent; every village, every family, every person in the family were victims of chills and fever whenever summer
came. The disease was not limited to the southern states nor to the

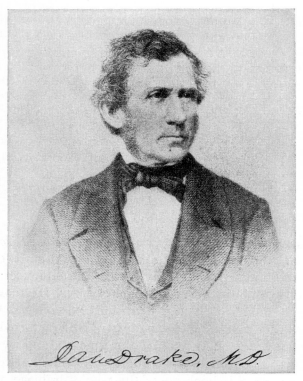

Fig. 12. Daniel Drake, first great malariologist.
(From Juettner, Otto: *Daniel Drake and His Followers.* Harvey Publishing Co., Cincinnati, 1909.)

rural areas. The rapidly growing cities of the North—Cleveland,
Indianapolis, Chicago, Detroit, even towns as far north as Minne-
apolis, Montreal, and Toronto—were heavily infected every summer
and fall with the intermittent fever.

Drake believed that the world in which we live, that is to say, our
environment, has a profound influence upon our health and welfare.
The three important environmental factors are:

1. All that belongs to the earth, e.g., geologic or telluric influence.
2. All that belongs to the atmosphere, e.g., climate and purity or pollution of the air.
3. Whatever pertains to society. This factor includes density of population, intellectual cultivation, recreation, occupation, diet, and other social and physiological influences.

Drake's whole effort in his book was to correlate the major ill-nesses of mankind with unfavorable factors of his environs. This he called the topography of disease.

He noted that malaria became much less prevalent as altitude was gained, either when traveling west toward the Rocky Mountains, or when ascending the Ozarks or the mountains of Kentucky. An alti-tude of 2,000 feet above sea level gave a marked degree of protec-tion. The high prevalence and greater severity of the disease in the river bottoms was, of course, a well-established fact. Drake noted the clear relationship of malaria to ponds, particularly to millponds. He mentioned also a popular opinion of the Pennsylvania mountain area that, where trout abound, ague cannot prevail. (This is true, in America at least.)

In the barrens of Kentucky, Drake found that the autumnal fevers were increasing annually. This he ascribed to the increase of mill-ponds. "Thus while the common, the legitimate influence of settle-ment and cultivation is to abate the frequency and violence of our intermittent and remittent fever, here, as an exception, is a district in which art has, undisguisedly, contributed to their greater preva-lence."[2]

This point is again illustrated by the epidemic of malaria in Wash-ington, Ohio, in 1838. A milldam was erected in 1820, a short dis-tance above the town. This caused an inundation of about 60 acres. When, by June 1, the stream fell too low to admit grinding at the mill, it was the custom of the proprietors to open the floodgates and let the water escape, and thus the health of the village did not suffer during summer and autumn. In 1838 the owners did not release the water until July, and rains did not follow to wash out the silt. In the month of August, the villagers began to sicken with remittent and intermittent fever. Eighty persons in a village of 400 became ill, with eleven deaths. The people who resided to the windward of the pond did not suffer. Those who lived nearest the pond suffered worst. The

[2] Drake, Daniel: *op. cit.,* p. 239.

epidemic was attributed to the effluvia arising from the stagnant pond.

The town of Indianapolis was begun in 1820. The area was covered with trees. By mid-summer of 1821 some 600 persons, miserably housed in tents and cabins, were living in the clearing. The summer was hot and wet, and the luxuriant foliage of the slashed trees underwent rapid decomposition. Malaria in malignant form began in late July. By October practically every person had had severe malaria and seventy-two had died.

Shawneetown, 10 miles below the mouth of the Wabash on the Ohio River, had always been a notoriously "sickly place." In 1838, the state of Illinois employed a number of Irish laborers there, to construct a railroad. It was a sickly year. The town suffered dreadfully, but the strangers fared even worse. All became sick with malaria, and one in seven died. But they dug an immense ditch, 40 feet in depth, which drained all the ponds and swamps in the vicinity of the town. The effect of this measure on health was instantaneous, and has continued ever since.

Drake divided autumnal fever into various categories: remittent, intermittent, malignant remittent and malignant intermittent, protracted, relapsing and vernal intermittents; together with many complications, such as splenitis, enlargement of the liver and the spleen, and so on, but he recognized clearly that all were one disease, due to a specific cause.

His observations on the epidemiology of the disease were most discerning. "It never occurs in epidemic form north of the 44th parallel." The disease extended west 300 miles from the Iowa and Missouri line, fading out as the rainfall of the Great Plains diminished. In the northern area, the disease occurred in the late summer and fall, with relapses in March; however, in the whole southern area, the disease was endemic. As cultivation of the land occurred, the disease tended to abate. This was particularly evident in the Finger Lake region of New York State, and in the region of Rochester, Buffalo, and Toronto.

Malaria was extremely prevalent in Toronto from 1820 to 1850. Nearly half of the diseases treated in the dispensary each autumn were intermittent fever. A regiment arrived in Toronto from England. Promptly a large proportion of the men developed malaria. Another regiment was sent to Toronto from the West Indies. Practically all of these men escaped the disease.

Drake pointed out that the causes of unequal prevalence of malaria may be attributed to:

1. Differences in soil—particularly fermentation of organic matter in the soil.
2. Differences in type of vegetation.
3. Variations in the surface water.
4. Variations in temperature.

He demonstrated that malaria could not exist without fresh-water ponds or other surface water, in conjunction with a suitable temperature.

In effect we may summarize Dr. Drake's theories as follows: ". . . we may, however, assume, that a summer temperature of sixty degrees is necessary to the production of the Fever; and that it will not prevail as an epidemic where the temperature of that season falls below sixty-five; finally, that if the other conditions favoring its production are deficient, it will cease before those reductions of temperature have been reached."

He went on to observe:

Suitable temperature alone is not enough, for the disease will not appear on vessels sailing in the Gulf of Mexico, despite the fact that air, temperature, and relative humidity are favorable. Salt marshes are not dangerous. Surface waters, in which the vegetation is even so much as wetted by sea salt, will not produce fever. Three tentative hypotheses may be presented as to the cause of autumnal fever.

1. The "meteoric hypothesis": This cannot be maintained since neither suitable temperature nor air moisture alone or in combination can produce the disease.
2. The "malarial hypothesis" ("mal-aria"): E.g., air pollution from dead and decaying animal matter and vegetable matter is generally accepted as the cause of the disease. But these conditions often exist without creating fever, and vice versa. Epidemics may even appear in the absence of pollution of the air.
3. The "vegeto-animacular hypothesis": This most closely fits the actual situation. The disease *must* be *due* to a *specific* agent. It must be *organic, living,* and *widely* distributed.

It is true that autumnal fever prevails very unequally in the same locality, in different years. One autumn it may be malignant and epidemic, the next year it may be mild and sporadic. But we must remember that in the vegetable kingdom, a year of great abundance may be followed by an unproductive one. Furthermore, one summer and autumn will be infested by insects far beyond another.

It has often happened that mosquitoes have been absent, from the banks of the middle portions of the Ohio River, for a year, and the next appeared in immense numbers. We have but to suppose insect forms of a parallel size to live under corresponding laws, and the hypothesis now before us offers an explanation of sickly and healthy seasons.[3]

How close he was to the solution of this great mystery! As we follow his clear and logical thinking, we see him utilizing all the epidemiological data that he had collected so carefully, groping through the thousand related, but seemingly contradictory facts, trying so hard to seize upon the one hidden jewel in the mass of detail. We who can see the answer so plainly, long to reach out and help him. If we could only give him a breath of a suggestion. He came so close! Yet half a century was to elapse before Ross was to write his poem of triumph on the day that he discovered the transmission of malaria by the mosquito.

We now know that the *Anopheles quadrimaculatus* mosquito was the important vector of malaria in all the great Mississippi Valley. Its larvae inhabit only fresh water—preferably ponds. It does not thrive in cold climates, and when found in the northern part of the United States it will not appear before July and will disappear with the first frost. Every one of Drake's epidemiological observations was correct. He even made a hypothesis that the transmitter of the infection might be an insect like a mosquito. Why did it not occur to him—"Perhaps after all *it is* transmitted by a mosquito"?

In his summary, Drake made some simple, broad predictions of the future in relation to the diseases of the interior valley of North America. He was an excellent prophet. Every one of his predictions, with the exception of the second, were to come true. Here are his conclusions:

1. Autumnal fever will decrease, and typhus and typhoid fevers will become more prevalent.
2. Gout will occur oftener than at present.
3. The diseases produced by the intemperate use of ardent spirits will diminish.
4. Consumption and scrofula will increase.
5. Apoplexy, palsy, and epilepsy will become more frequent.
6. Diseases of the liver will become less, those of the mucous membranes of the bowels, more prevalent.
7. Lastly, mental alienation will be more frequent.[4]

[3] Drake, Daniel: *op. cit.,* pp. 726-27.
[4] *Ibid.,* p. 701.

The next twenty years were to witness the increase in tuberculosis, and the following half century was to be characterized by a high prevalence of dysentery and typhoid fever. Only after a period of fifty years did the full impact of an increase in the life span of the population finally result in increase of apoplexy, palsy, and "mental alienation." One prediction (No. 2) was erroneous though quite logical—gout has never been a prevalent disease in America.

CHAPTER 12. *Tuberculosis during the First Part*

of the Nineteenth Century

> *I believe that consumption is as amenable to treatment as any*
> *one of our serious constitutional diseases, provided it is diag-*
> *nosed in its incipiency, and the proper hygiene and medical*
> *treatment be resorted to.*

B. F. WYMAN, *1890*

We have no accurate information concerning the prevalence of tuberculosis in the colonies. Frequent references are made in the literature to persons or even whole families that were suffering with consumption; scrofula is frequently mentioned as a common disease of childhood. But these two diseases were not related in the minds of the people, nor was either disease believed to be contagious. Consumption was considered an inherited trait, and since it was so fatal it was regarded as a family stigma, which was to be hidden from view insofar as possible.

From our present knowledge of the epidemiology of the disease, we can well imagine that consumption would not have taken a heavy toll in the scattered families who were the true pioneers and who opened up the forests. As the settlements grew and towns and ports developed, consumption would increase. Beginning in the first quarter of the century, industrialization, which resulted in overcrowding in factory and tenement, would inevitably be followed by an increase in tuberculosis. Many of these factory workers would have little resistance against infection, since they had never been exposed to the disease. A veritable epidemic of tuberculosis might well result.

We have some evidence that tuberculosis presented exactly this sequence of events in America during the fifty to seventy-five years following the Revolutionary War. Rush, who was a keen observer, wrote in 1789:

[Phthisis] is scarcely known by the citizens of the United States, who live in the first stage of civilized life, and who have lately obtained the title of first settlers. . . . It is less common in country places than in cities, and increases in both, with intemperance and sedentary modes of life.[1]

Davis made the following observations:

Close buildings and increased aggregation of population are increasing the prevalence of pulmonary tuberculosis in our country at an alarming rate. . . . In still earlier days, dating back to the early settlements of this country, New England and the Northeastern states were as free from consumptions as are now the much vaunted far-western states and territories. It was immediately consequent upon the change from an agricultural to a manufacturing population that the rapid increase in the death-rate from consumption is apparent in these states.[2]

Hirsch has noted that the extensive immigration and the consequent founding of new towns or the enlargement and overcrowding of old ones in America had a profound influence upon the increase of phthisis in these areas.[3]

We have a few data which indicate that tuberculosis was an important cause of death in America before the industrial era began, but most of these vital records come from the cities, and thus do not indicate the true conditions in the rural areas which made up more than 80 per cent of the total population. For example, the New York Tuberculosis and Health Association[4] has estimated the tuberculosis death rate in New York City in 1804 to have been 6.88 per 1,000 population. The data collected by Hirsch for the pioneer period are as follows:[5]

CITY	PERIOD	DEATH RATE FROM CONSUMPTION PER 1,000 POPULATION
Boston	1811-1840	3.8
New York City	1805-1837	5.3
Philadelphia	1807-1840	5.6

We do not possess accurate records of the prevalence of tuberculosis in the Negro slaves during this period. We do know that the

[1] Rush, Benjamin: "Thoughts upon the Cause and Cure of Pulmonary Consumption," *Medical Inquiries and Observations*, Fourth Edition, Vol. II, p. 37, 1789.

[2] Davis, F. H.: *Tr. Am. M. A.* **29**:149, 1878.

[3] Hirsch, August: *Handbook of Geographical and Historical Pathology*, Vol. III, p 216. London, 1886.

[4] "High Points in Tuberculosis Control in New York City," *Annual Bulletin New York Tuberculosis and Health Association*, 1952.

[5] Hirsch, August: *op. cit.*, p. 175.

Negroes who lived in the northern states had a very high tuberculosis death rate. For those Negroes, both free and slave, who lived in the cities of New York and Philadelphia during the early part of the century, the death rate was as high as 10 to 12 per 1,000 per annum. The prisoners in American jails suffered terribly from consumption. Hirsch[6] estimated that during the period from 1829 to 1845 in the United States, the average annual mortality from tuberculosis for white prisoners was 11.16 per 1,000. He stated that the death rate for Negroes in the Eastern Penitentiary of Pennsylvania for this same period was as high as 40.74 per 1,000 per year.

Scrofula is a tuberculous infection of the lymphatic glands, especially of the neck. It is most frequently acquired from drinking raw milk from tuberculous cows. The disease has almost completely disappeared from the United States, but in pioneer days it was a very common disease, particularly in childhood. The relation of poverty and malnutrition to scrofula was well known, but it was not believed to be contagious. Rather it was thought to be an inheritable trait. In foundling homes, it has been reported that as many as 40 to 50 per cent of the children suffered from this disease, but it was not

[6] Hirsch, August: *op. cit.*, p. 226.

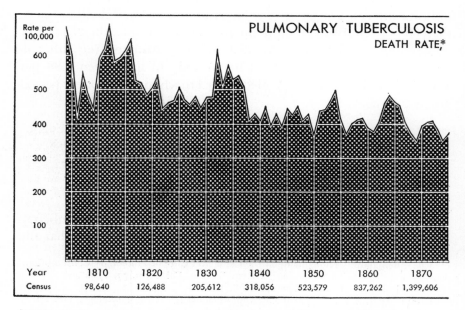

NOTE: Death rates per 100,000 population in expanding area: 1804-1867 (Manhattan, Bronx); 1868-1897 (Manhattan, Bronx, Brooklyn); 1898-1950 (five boroughs of Greater New York).

Fig. 13. Tuberculosis death

regarded with serious concern, since it was seldom fatal. As late as 1885, we find that Hirsch[7] doubted the contagiousness of scrofula. Not only was he sure that it was not related to tuberculosis, but he also did not believe that it was acquired from drinking the milk of scrofulous cows.

Hildreth noted in 1830 that "the diffusion of the malady [scrofula] had kept pace with advancing civilization [in America], proceeding from east to west."[8] In referring to Ohio he said that scrofula is "becoming more frequent" and "will probably continue to increase as the country becomes more highly cultivated and people more luxurious in their habits."

Industrialization and Tuberculosis

The industrialization of the country, which was initiated about 1820, was accompanied by heavy immigration of Irish and Germans, and this resulted in miserable, overcrowded housing conditions in the cities. The rapidly growing factory towns were the worst. The indescribable poverty, ignorance, and filth inevitably produced true

[7] Hirsch, August: *op. cit.*, Vol. II, p. 639, 1885.
[8] Hildreth, Samuel Prescott: "On the Climate and Diseases of Washington County, Ohio," *Am. J. M. Sc.*, 329, February, 1830.

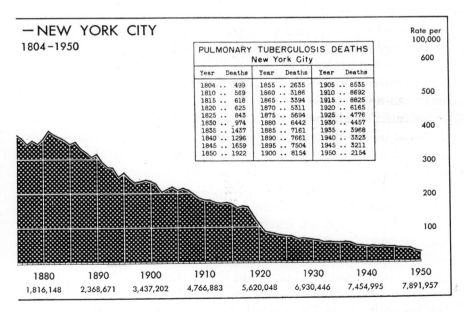

PULMONARY TUBERCULOSIS DEATHS New York City					
Year	Deaths	Year	Deaths	Year	Deaths
1804 ..	499	1855 ..	2635	1905 ..	8535
1810 ..	569	1860 ..	3186	1910 ..	8692
1815 ..	618	1865 ..	3394	1915 ..	8825
1820 ..	625	1870 ..	5311	1920 ..	6165
1825 ..	843	1875 ..	5694	1925 ..	4776
1830 ..	974	1880 ..	6442	1930 ..	4457
1835 ..	1437	1885 ..	7161	1935 ..	3968
1840 ..	1296	1890 ..	7661	1940 ..	3323
1845 ..	1659	1895 ..	7504	1945 ..	3211
1850 ..	1922	1900 ..	8154	1950 ..	2154

─NEW YORK CITY
1804–1950

Rate per 100,000
600
500
400
300
200
100

1880	1890	1900	1910	1920	1930	1940	1950
1,816,148	2,368,671	3,437,202	4,766,883	5,620,048	6,930,446	7,454,995	7,891,957

Compiled from reports of city inspector, the Metropolitan Board of Health, and the Department of Health, City of New York, by G. J. Drolet and A. M. Lowell, New York Tuberculosis and Health Association.

rate, New York City, 1804-1950.

epidemics of tuberculosis. This very general prevalence of the disease reached its climax about 1860.

We have evidence that, as early as 1826, the disease took an enormous toll in the towns. Thacher, in his *American Modern Practice,* may be quoted:

. . . pulmonary consumption constitutes a large proportion of our bills of mortality, and forms one of the crowded avenues to the tomb. It is supposed that about one seventh of all the deaths in Massachusetts, are to be attributed to this fatal disease. . . . [It makes] most deplorable ravages among our youth of both sexes, between the ages of 17 and 27. When hereditary disposition is derived from parents, instances frequently occur of whole families . . . becoming victims in the early periods of life. It seems to be a received opinion that phthisis possesses a contagious nature in a slight degree. There is indeed much reason to apprehend that by sleeping in the same bed with a consumptive patient in the last or ulcerative stage [of the disease], with foetid expectoration, night sweats, and offensive breath, or by being much confined in a close room and imbibing the effluvia from the lungs, the disease may by these means be actually communicated to those who are in [good] health.[9]

In the light of our present knowledge of the epidemiology of tuberculosis, this long and involved sentence is a magnificent example of conservative understatement. How could tuberculosis be avoided when physicians were so strongly indoctrinated with the theories of their medical teachers, in the belief that most diseases, including tuberculosis, are not transmitted from person to person, but acquired through unfavorable environmental factors—particularly bad air?

Shattuck, in his survey of Boston in 1845, gave us a fairly concise estimate of the ravages of consumption in that city. He estimated the population of Boston for each year from 1811 to 1845, and presented a table of the deaths from consumption in that city during this period. He called consumption "the great destroyer of human life," and although he pointed out the inaccuracies of his data and the necessity of careful interpretation of statistical material, nevertheless, "sufficient facts are known to show that from one-fourth to one-seventh of all deaths in the Northern and Middle States, and perhaps in the whole Union, and the civilized world, are caused by consumption." He then stated most prophetically that "this frightful mortality is to be arrested, if at all, by means of *prevention* rather than by cure of the disease after it once becomes seated."[10]

[9] Thacher, James: *American Modern Practice.* Cottons & Barnard, Boston, 1826.
[10] Shattuck, Lemuel: *Census of Boston,* 1845.

We have calculated Shattuck's data on mortality from consumption in Boston from 1811 to 1845, and in Figure 14 have presented a five-year mean for the death rate from tuberculosis of the lungs, per 100,000 population. During this period, Boston grew from a population of 33,787 in 1810 to 114,366 in 1845. (During these same years, the Negro population declined from 4.3 per cent to 1.6 per cent.) As this graph shows, the death rate from consumption certainly was appalling at the beginning of the century. It was cut in

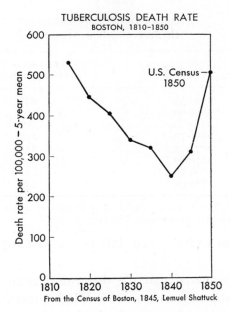

TUBERCULOSIS DEATH RATE
BOSTON, 1810-1850

From the Census of Boston, 1845, Lemuel Shattuck

Fig. 14. Tuberculosis death rate, Boston, 1810-1850.

half by 1840, but then began to increase, and we have good evidence that by 1860 it approximated the death rate of 1810. The worst year that was recorded by Shattuck was 1811. With a population of 34,255, there was a total of 748 deaths, of which 221 were from consumption. The consumption rate fell as low as 265 in 1835, but by 1845 had risen to 374. We have no accurate data on tuberculosis in Boston for the middle portion of the nineteenth century, but a record of the whole story for Massachusetts over a 100-year period indicates clearly that tuberculosis did not decline appreciably as a cause of death in the state until about 1870. (See Figure 31, page 379.) A striking feature of tuberculosis in Massachusetts is that for more than 100 years the death rate in Boston has always been twice as high as the rate for the rest of the state.[11] This phenomenon holds true to the present day.

All the available data from various national sources point to the fact that tuberculosis as a cause of death reached its peak about the middle of the nineteenth century and then leveled off. For example, Rawlings has calculated these rates for Chicago, which was a pioneer city of 30,000 people in 1850.

Table 7

Tuberculosis Death Rate—Chicago*
All Forms—5-Year Mean

YEAR	DEATH RATE PER 100,000 POPULATION
1851-55	250
1856-60	306
1861-65	226
1866-70	248
1871-75	241
1876-80	199
1881-85	202
1886-90	196

* SOURCE: Rawlings, I. D.: *The Rise and Fall of Disease in Illinois.* State Department of Public Health, Springfield, Ill., 1927, p. 388.

Not until 1920 did the rate fall below 100 (97.2) per 100,000 population.

Dubos[12] has estimated that the downward trend in tuberculosis in the United States began about 1860. He has stated that the disease reached a very high peak at the beginning of the industrial revolution when vast numbers of human beings began to move from the rural areas to cities, where crowding, filth, and poor nutrition prevailed.

By the middle of the nineteenth century the more intelligent citizens began to understand the value of pure air, good food, and pure water, and to advocate less promiscuous spitting and other hygienic measures. Many hygienists have claimed that this sanitary awakening turned the tide against tuberculosis. Others think that the chief factor was a steady increase and variety in foodstuffs. Still

[11] Personal communication from Alton S. Pope, director of Division of Tuberculosis, Massachusetts State Department of Public Health, 1950.

[12] Dubos, René, and Dubos, J. P.: *The White Plague.* Little, Brown & Co., Boston, 1952.

others believe that the major factor was a genetic one. The most susceptible of the human strains died of the disease before they produced offspring and thus a naturally immune population was established. It seems most probable that all these factors, and others as well, contributed to this decline in the tuberculosis death rate before the cause of the disease and its mode of transmission were known.

CHAPTER 13. *The Contagiousness of Puerperal Fever*

The state of medicine is an index of civilization of an age and country—one of the best perhaps by which it can be judged.

O. W. HOLMES, *1869*

The first important American epidemiological study on puerperal fever was reported by Oliver Wendell Holmes[1] in an essay that was read before the Boston Society for Medical Improvement, and was published in the *New England Quarterly Journal of Medicine and Surgery* in April, 1843. Only a few copies were struck off. The *Journal* had a small circulation and expired within the year. Nevertheless, the essay was widely quoted and created tremendous opposition on the part of the foremost obstetricians of the day.[2] Holmes was only thirty-four years old at the time. He had an excellent education and was a member of an old Boston family. His appearance was unimpressive, for he was only 5 feet 4 inches in height, thin, with a face that he considered "as a convenience rather than an ornament." His college friends regarded him as frivolous and given to writing poetry. He had only a small practice. Thus, his medical superiors were affronted at the impertinence of this insignificant, inexperienced young physician who presented the thesis that puerperal fever was due, in great part, to the carelessness, ignorance, and negligence of the obstetrician and midwife.

Holmes did not know of the work of Semmelweiss, of Austria, whose results were first published in 1847. But he was able to marshal unmistakable evidence that childbed fever was contagious "and

[1] Holmes, O. W.: "The Contagiousness of Puerperal Fever," *New England Quart. J. Med. & Surg.*, April, 1843. Republished in its entirety with additions in *Medical Essays*, 1861. All students of epidemiology should study this extraordinary essay.

[2] Hodge, Hugh L. (professor of obstetrics at the University of Pennsylvania): "On the Now Contagious Character of Puerperal Fever," lecture delivered October 11, 1852.

was frequently carried from patient to patient by physicians and nurses." Meigs, on the contrary, was sure the disease was due to accident, or Providence, certainly not to contagion.[3]

Holmes made no claim to the originality of his observations or conclusions. The earliest authority that he cites is "Dr. Gordon of

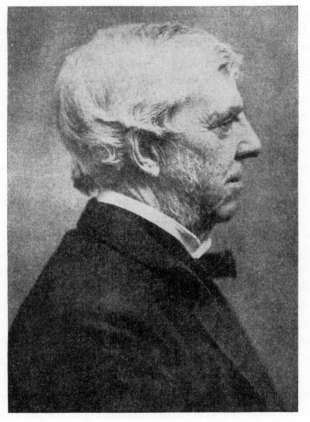

Fig. 15. Oliver Wendell Holmes, epidemiologist of puerperal fever. (Courtesy of Harvard Medical School Library.)

Aberdeen,"[4] who published a treatise on this subject in 1795. Gordon stated that "the disease seized only such women as were visited or delivered by a practitioner, or taken care of by a nurse, who had

[3] Meigs, Charles D. (professor of diseases of women and children, Jefferson Medical College): "On the Nature, Signs and Treatment of Child Bed Fever," letter to his students, 1854.

[4] See "Gordon of Aberdeen" by Herbert Thoms. *Am. J. Obst. & Gynec.*, 15:229, 1928.

previously attended patients affected with the disease. It is a dis-
agreeable declaration for me to mention that I myself was the means
of carrying the infection to a great number of women. . . . I arrived
at that certainty in the matter, that I could venture to foretell what
women would be affected with the disease, upon hearing by what
midwife they were to be delivered. . . ."

Holmes reviewed the literature carefully, citing report after report,
which were made by honest and observing men. The total picture
gave overwhelming evidence that the disease was transmitted directly
by an obstetrician, midwife, or nurse from an infected patient to a
mother in labor.

For example, "a midwife delivered a woman on December 4,
1830, who died soon after with symptoms of puerperal fever. During
the following month this same widwife delivered 30 women, in
different parts of an extensive suburb, of which number 16 caught
the disease and all died. Other midwives connected with the same
charitable institution as the woman already mentioned, were 25 in
number. During this same period they delivered 380 women with
no single case of puerperal fever."

Holmes demonstrated that puerperal sepsis might be acquired
from a physician who had recently attended a case of erysipelas, an
infected amputation, or who had recently performed an autopsy on
an individual who had died from peritonitis, gangrene, or general
sepsis. Holmes cited twenty authors, each of whom had made careful
observations on large numbers of cases, and all of whom had arrived
at the conclusion that childbed fever is contagious. There was no
possibility that the sequence of events could be due to chance variation.

The young physician not only gave the proof of the contagious
nature of puerperal fever, but formulated eight simple rules for prevention of transmission of the disease. These rules are just as serviceable today as they were 100 years ago.

1) A physician holding himself in readiness to attend cases of midwifery should never take any active part in the post-mortem examination
of cases of puerperal fever.

2) If a physician is present at such autopsies, he should use thorough
ablution, change every article of dress, and allow twenty-four hours or
more to elapse before attending to any case of midwifery. It may be well
to extend the same caution to cases of simple peritonitis.

3) Similar precautions should be taken after the autopsy or surgical

treatment of cases of erysipelas, if the physician is obliged to unite such offices with his obstetrical duties, which is in the highest degree inexpedient.

4) On the occurrence of a single case of puerperal fever in his practice, the physician is bound to consider the next female he attends in labor, unless some weeks at least have elapsed, as in danger of being infected by him, and it is his duty to take every precaution to diminish her risk of disease and death.

5) If within a short period two cases of puerperal fever happen close to each other, in the practice of the same physician, the disease not existing or prevailing in the neighborhood, he would do wisely to relinquish his obstetrical practice for at least one month, and endeavor to free himself by every available means from any noxious influence he may carry about with him.

6) The occurrence of three or more closely connected cases, in the practice of one individual, no others existing in the neighborhood, and no other sufficient cause being alleged for the coincidence, is *prima facie* evidence that he is the vehicle of contagion.

7) It is the duty of the physician to take every precaution that the disease shall not be introduced by nurses or other assistants, by making proper inquiries concerning them, and giving timely warning of every suspected source of danger.

8) Whatever indulgence may be granted to those who have heretofore been the ignorant causes of so much misery, the time has come when the existence of a *private pestilence* in the sphere of a single physician should be looked upon, not as a misfortune, but a crime; and in the knowledge of such occurrences the duties of the practitioner to his profession should give way to his paramount obligations to society.[5]

As we have noted, the reaction to Holmes's report, on the part of physicians, was violent. His views were ridiculed and he was subjected to personal abuse and vilification. He refused to retort in kind. "No man makes a quarrel with me, over the counterpane that covers a mother, with her new-born infant at her breast. . . . When facts are numerous, and unquestionable, and unequivocal in their significance, theory must follow them as best it may, keeping time with their step; and not go before them, marching to the sound of its own drum and trumpet."

Holmes made some sage remarks on medical teaching when he referred to the vituperative letters of Dr. Meigs to students, concerning the contagiousness of puerperal fever:

[5] Holmes, O. W.: "The Contagiousness of Puerperal Fever," *Medical Essays*, revised edition. Houghton Mifflin Co., Boston, 1883, pp. 168-69.

In the embryonic stage of professional development, any violent impression of the instructor's mind is apt to be followed by some lasting effect on the mind of the pupil. Some students, from youth, or from want of training, are easily bewildered and confused in any conflict of opinions with which their studies lead them. They are liable to lose sight of the main question, in the collateral issues, and to be run away with by suggestive speculation: they confound belief with evidence, often trusting the first, because it is expressed with energy, and slighting the latter because it is calm and unimpassioned.

Even an impatient or petulant expression which, to a philosopher, would be a mere index of a low state of amiability of the speaker, may pass into the young mind as an element of its future constitution, to injure its temper or to corrupt its judgement.

Oliver Wendell Holmes was not only a philosopher and poet. He must also be ranked as America's first outstanding epidemiologist.

CHAPTER 14. *Typhus Fever, Typhoid Fever, and*

Cerebrospinal Meningitis

> *Every year, thousands of lives are lost that might have been saved, tens of thousands of cases of sickness occur which might have been prevented. A vast amount of unnecessarily impaired health and physical disability exists among those not actually confined by sickness, and means exist within our reach for the mitigation or removal of these evils.*
>
> SHATTUCK REPORT, *1850*

It seems strange to consider together such diverse clinical entities as typhus fever, typhoid fever, and meningococcus meningitis. But in 1825 these three diseases were not differentiated by clinicians. The word "typhus" connotes stupor. This symptom is one of the striking characteristics of all of these diseases. The reports of the "typhus" epidemics of that period are so confused that one cannot be sure which of these three diseases—or perhaps some other disease, such as relapsing fever—is being described under the general term of "typhus fever."

TYPHUS FEVER

This disease is of great antiquity, accompanying wars, famine, and destitution. Epidemics of typhus have always appeared in periods of great distress and turmoil. In North America during the Colonial days the disease was recognized. It was known to occur more commonly in the winter, and it was also understood that it was prevalent among the very poor. As time went by, the period of incubation became known and the immunity that was produced by an initial attack was well established. Fomites, particularly articles of clothing of those who had died of the disease, were considered dangerous. Dark clothing was believed to be worse than light; woolen cloth was

worse than others. Later it was also recognized that the disease occurred in successive occupants of the same building.

Overcrowding, destitution, and undernutrition were believed to
be important secondary factors in typhus fever, but Gerhard[1] in
1836, Bartlett[2] in 1842, and Flint[3] in 1852 all understood the contagiousness of typhus fever, and knew that the spread of the disease
was by intimate contact, not "half-a-yard" through the air.

How close they came to an understanding of the disease! In retrospect, we can see how simple it would have been for them, by de-
ductive reasoning, to arrive at the truth. They needed only to think
of the *one possible factor* that would explain the whole epidemiology
of typhus fever. But more than fifty years were to pass before the
idea dawned on epidemiologists that it is the lowly body louse—
then all-prevalent and ubiquitous—which is the transmitter of the
disease.

It is fairly certain that typhus did not play an important role in
the Revolutionary War, as it has in so many wars in Europe. Washington, during that sad winter at Valley Forge, was certainly vulnerable to typhus fever, but it did not appear. He had enough of sickness
and misery in his troops without having typhus fever to add to the
burden of despair. The disease must have arrived in North America
many times during the Colonial period, but there is no clear-cut
evidence of serious, extensive outbreaks before 1800. The cities were
small, industrialization was in its infancy, and the slums were still
to be.

Miner and Tully[4] in 1823 described the fevers of the Connecticut
Valley. They stated that the region was free from serious epidemics
for a long period following the Revolutionary War. "Many physicians
passed the whole term of their practice and scarcely met an original,
well-marked typhoid disease." A decided change seemed to take place
in 1807. "Typhus, which had disappeared for twenty to thirty years,
now became common in all the Eastern and Middle States."

Tully, in his section of the above-mentioned book, distinguished
"putrid fever," which in all probability was typhoid fever, from

[1] Gerhard, W. W.: "On the Typhus Fever Which Occurred at Philadelphia in the
Spring and Summer of 1836," *Am. J. M. Sc.*, 19:289-322, (Feb.) 1837; 20:289-322, (Aug.)
1837.

[2] Bartlett, Elisha: *The History, Diagnosis and Treatment of Typhoid and Typhus
Fever*. Lea & Blanchard, Philadelphia, 1842.

[3] Flint, Austin: "Relations of Water to the Propagation of Fever," *Reports and Papers
of the American Public Health Association*, 1:164, 1873.

[4] Miner, Thomas, and Tully, William: *Essays on Fevers and Other Medical Subjects*.
E. & H. Clark, Middletown, Conn. 1823.

"jail fever," which he recognized as true typhus fever. Matters were complicated for Miner by the appearance of a malignant fever in Middletown, Connecticut, in 1820, which he correctly surmised was yellow fever.

Gerhard[5] cited an epidemic of typhus fever in Philadelphia in 1836. The disease, however, made no extensive invasion of America until the middle of the nineteenth century. It came from Europe. Toward the end of the Irish potato famine, the disease devastated these unfortunate sufferers in their homeland. Over a million cases occurred in Ireland within a five-year period. Typhus entered our larger ports with the Irish immigrants, and by 1845 was causing serious loss of life in New York, Philadelphia, Baltimore, and other port cities. The terrible conditions under which the poor immigrants lived is vividly described by Stephen Smith[6] of New York in *The City That Was*. His denunciation of the "fever nests" in the slums of New York City led to a sanitary survey of that city in 1865. The report of this survey,[7] in turn, resulted in the concept of adequate health administration and led ultimately to the establishment of our modern municipal health departments. But this is a story for a subsequent chapter.

TYPHOID FEVER

For centuries typhoid fever had been confused with typhus fever as well as with other diseases. M. Louis[8] in France, in 1829, coined the name "typhoid fever" and made the first clear-cut clinical distinction between typhus fever and typhoid fever. He stressed the importance of the intestinal lesion as a cardinal sign of typhoid fever. James Jackson, Jr.,[9] a medical student from Boston, who had studied under Louis in Paris, observed the characteristic lesions of typhoid fever in 1830, but his article was not published in the United States until 1835. Gerhard,[10] in Philadelphia, demonstrated the typical intestinal lesions of typhoid fever in 1835. He had studied an epidemic of the disease in Philadelphia and became the first American physician to recognize typhoid fever as a clinical entity.

[5] Gerhard, W. W.: *op. cit.*

[6] Smith, Stephen: *The City That Was.* Frank Allaben, New York, 1911.

[7] Smith, Stephen, and associates: *Report of the Sanitary Condition of the City of New York.* D. Appleton & Co., New York, 1865.

[8] Louis, M.: *Researches on Typhoid Fever,* 2 vols. Paris, 1829.

[9] Jackson, James, Jr.: *Memoirs of James Jackson, Jr.* Published after his death, Boston, 1835.

[10] Gerhard, W. W.: *op. cit.*

Elisha Bartlett,[11] writing on "American Fevers" in 1842, treated typhus and typhoid fevers as distinct diseases and described very clearly the differences between these two infections. He also noted the immunity that is produced by an attack of typhoid, and mentioned the phenomenon of "family invasion." The contagiousness of typhoid fever became more evident with the industrial development of New England. By 1842 Lowell, Massachusetts, with 22,000 population, was the largest manufacturing city in the nation. The employees averaged from fifteen to thirty years of age, and most of them were new residents: young women who had lived in the villages and had moved to the city to work in the cotton mills. Bartlett described a series of epidemics of typhoid fever that occurred in the girls who worked in these mills. Sometimes the disease was confined to the workers in one mill, sometimes to one workroom, or in some instances to a single boarding house. The only explanation that could be entertained was that the disease was contagious. Bartlett pointed out that typhoid fever occurred essentially in epidemic form; it was more prevalent in the fall and was more likely to occur following a hot, dry summer. He cited Pettenkofer's views that the prevalence of the disease was directly related to the amount of water in the soil. He understood that typhoid fever was transmitted directly from a sick person to a normal healthy contact, but he was not sure of the mode of transmission. The disease, he believed, was acquired through food or drink, and also by inhaling emanations from the stool of the infected patient.

Austin Flint[12] showed that in the North Boston epidemic of 1843, typhoid fever could be transported by a sick person to a locality where the disease was unknown. He did not realize that this particular outbreak was due to contaminated well water, but years later, after reading Budd's[13] classical studies on typhoid fever, he returned to North Boston, and in 1873 published a supplementary report in which he had worked out the water-borne characteristics of the 1843 epidemic. Flint thought that the "fresh evacuations" of the patient were harmless. The poison developed in their putrefaction. Murcherson[14] cited an epidemic of typhoid fever that was described by W. Taylor in 1858, in which milk was incriminated as the infecting agent. Budd's study on the St. John Wood School epidemic was not published in the *Lancet* until 1856, and his views of the water-borne

[11] Bartlett, Elisha: *op. cit.*
[12] Flint, Austin: *op. cit.*
[13] Budd, William: *Lancet*, November 15, 1856.
[14] Murcherson, C.: *The Continued Fevers of Great Britain.* London, 1873.

source of infection in enteric disease were not widely accepted until many years later. The commonest concept was that typhoid fever was due to inhalation of sewer gas. The disease was always a result of decomposition of fetid matter and was not necessarily derived from a specific infection. This was still the opinion of many physicians as late as 1885. Murcherson stated in his *The Continued Fevers of Great Britain* that he did not believe in a specific infective agent, and clinched his argument by saying that typhoid fever often arises "without possible contact with another case." The great obstacle was that no one had developed the concept of a *healthy carrier.*

CEREBROSPINAL MENINGITIS

Meningococcus meningitis was confused with typhus fever and other epidemic diseases during the entire nineteenth century. In 1807 a very serious outbreak of this disease occurred in New England. It was described by Miner[15] as a "Spotted Fever." He believed the epidemic to be a new disease, quite distinct from typhus fever. From his description of the clinical course of the disease, one must conclude that he is describing fulminating cerebrospinal meningitis.

Gallup[16] in 1815 described the "Epidemical Diseases of the State of Vermont." He gives a good description of "Spotted Fever," which undoubtedly was cerebrospinal meningitis.

A committee of the Massachusetts Medical Society, consisting of Drs. Thomas Welch, James Jackson, and John C. Warren,[17] in 1810 made a report "Respecting a Disease Commonly Called Spotted or Petechial Fever" which was then epidemic in various parts of New England. They investigated the disease by questionnaire, a method that in subsequent years was to be used in great profusion by epidemiologists and public health workers. There were seventeen items, the most important of which may be summed up as follows:

1. A history of the onset of the epidemic.
2. Symptoms of the illness and their duration.
3. The effects of exposure, fatigue, and diet upon the disease.
4. The contagiousness of the disease.
5. Age, sex, social class, profession, and temperament of those attacked.
6. Prognosis of the disease.

[15] Miner and Tully: *op. cit.*
[16] Gallup, J. A.: *History of Epidemical Diseases of the State of Vermont,* 1815.
[17] Welch, T.; Jackson, J.; and Warren, J. C.: "Respecting a Disease Commonly Called Spotted or Petechial Fever," a report of the Massachusetts Medical Society, Boston, 1810.

7. Relapses and sequelae.
8. Methods of treatment and their effects.
9. Autopsy findings.
10. Previous appearance of this disease in the community.
11. Usual mortality among "brute animals in the neighborhood."

The committee received replies from the physicians of twelve communities. Analysis of these replies resulted in a fairly complete, composite description by physicians of a severe typhus-like disease. The case fatality rate was not known accurately. At the beginning of the epidemic it was over 50 per cent, but at the end of the epidemic the death rate had fallen to about 10 per cent. From the clinical description of the cases it seems certain that the outbreak was cerebro-spinal meningitis. Certain conclusions were arrived at: (1) the committee did not believe the disease was contagious; (2) they showed that it affected young men and young women chiefly; (3) certain unfavorable environmental factors predisposed to the disease, but did not produce it.

SUMMARY

We may surmise that typhoid fever occurred every fall throughout the United States during the nineteenth century. During the first fifty years it was sporadic or prevailed in small community outbreaks. No widespread epidemics occurred until the cities grew, industry developed, and community-wide water supplies and sewage disposal systems were established. Typhus fever and cerebrospinal meningitis appeared and disappeared in occasional localized epidemics. These three diseases were not generally regarded as infectious but were believed to be due to environmental factors over which the individual or the community had little control. The great epidemic diseases—smallpox, cholera, and yellow fever—were clearly established as pestilential and disastrous; but the "typhus fever" group of diseases were considered inevitable and normal, and thus these outbreaks are buried in the great "undertones" of the causes of illness and death of the nineteenth century.

CHAPTER 15. *General Sanitation*

The United States may be considered as a country in which no legislation exists regulating its sanitary condition.

COMMITTEE ON SANITARY IMPROVEMENT
AMERICAN MEDICAL ASSOCIATION, *1848*

Community sanitation was a matter of primary concern to local boards of health during the first half of the nineteenth century. The general concept prevailed that most disease was produced by accumulations of noisome, bad-smelling, decaying animal or vegetable matter. This miasmatic material arose in the air as an invisible vapor and was carried into the house. Night air was much more dangerous than day air. Sunlight was a great purifier, for it destroyed dangerous miasmata. Human excreta and other human wastes become hazardous because of the accumulation of odoriferous matter in which pestilential material fermented.

Thus the major preoccupation of local boards of health related to those materials and community wastes that caused bad-smelling accumulations of community filth. Slaughterhouses, pigsties, dead horses, dogs and cats, tanneries, rotting fish, or any other accumulation of putrefying matter was of great concern to the local health officer. (A dead whale washed up on the beach was particularly dangerous.)

There was no concept of transmission of infection through water and no realization that food might be contaminated with infectious agents through its handling by persons who were ill with disease. There was no realization that human excreta might contain specific agents of infection. Only smallpox was considered as a true contagion, that is, spread directly from person to person by contact. There was no understanding of the nature of intermediate hosts such as mosquitoes, flies, fleas, and body lice in the transmission of disease. Some believed that disease might be spread through the clothing that had been used by sick people; therefore the clothing and bedding of those who had died of pestilence were frequently burned. Decaying human bodies were considered more dangerous than bodies of dead animals, and thus the proper location of cemeteries and the regulations for proper disposal of human bodies became of serious concern to health departments.

Dr. David Hosack,[1] a New York physician who was prominent during the early part of the nineteenth century, outlined a basic community program in environmental sanitation that illustrates the fact that farsighted men, who are well ahead of their generation in social consciousness, may pave the way for subsequent social developments. In 1820 he made the following recommendations for New York City:

1. Improvement of the municipal water supply.
2. Introduction of a sewage disposal system.
3. Better housing for the poor.
4. Widening of the streets.
5. Substitution of building stone for wood.
6. Suitable construction of wharves and docks.
7. Limitation of burials within the city.

Years were to pass before any of these sanitary recommendations were put into effect, yet Hosack saw the need for them and his ideas were gradually introduced into the life of the community.

The current concepts of the requirements for community sanitation are reviewed for us in a report which was presented by John Bell in 1859 on "The Importance and Economy of Sanitary Measures to Cities."[2] Dr. Bell reviewed the history of municipal sanitation from the time of Egypt and Carthage, down through the medieval period to modern times. It is quite clear from his discussion that the earliest concepts of the causes of plague and pestilence had remained unchanged through the ages. This belief was that the actual sources of infection were not from man himself. People who lived in closely packed cities produced an accumulation of filth. "A compost is formed of all kinds of abominations, [and] this became a per-

[1] Hosack, David: "Observations on the Means of Improving the Medical Policy of the City of New York," discussion in the Hall of the College of Physicians and Surgeons, November 6, 1820.

[2] See *Proceedings and Debates of the Third National Quarantine and Sanitary Convention.* Edward Jones & Co., Printers to Board of Education, New York, 1859, pp. 441-620. This volume also contains John Griscom's "Report on Sewage, Water Supply and Offal" and Henry Clark's "Draft of a Sanitary Code for Cities."

petually sustaining cause not only of periodical fevers but even of plague itself." Thus the hypothesis developed and was maintained for centuries that a clean city must be a healthy city, and a dirty city where filth accumulated was always in potential danger. Sanitation of a city, therefore, should be organized so as to remove all the filthy accumulations of aggregate living. Equal emphasis must be placed on the removal of pigsties and the cleansing of privies. Burial of the dead, washing of the streets, ventilation of buildings, control of slaughterhouses, construction of public wash houses—each of these activities was of equal importance in environmental sanitation and disease prevention. In addition every window must be protected with tight shutters to exclude the night air.

The concept of a specific agent of disease that is transmitted from person to person, directly or indirectly, through various vehicles, did not dawn upon the people until many years later. Disease was due to a putrefaction within the mass of filth, and not to any specific substance introduced by man.

Bell made a series of suggestions to the New York City Board of Councilmen in 1859.[3] All of these recommendations for sanitary betterment and community cleanliness were splendid, and when they were eventually put into effect they did have an influence in the reduction of illness and death in cities. But the real cause of infection was not understood, and thus the direct methods of control were not applied.

Henry G. Clark, city physician for Boston, presented his "Draft of a Sanitary Code for Cities" to the Quarantine and Sanitary Convention in New York in 1859. He had little faith in quarantine as a public health measure but believed strongly in the efficacy of sanitary measures in control of fevers. He insisted that plague was not contagious and he was sure that the same was true for yellow fever and typhus fever. He also stated that it was generally agreed that cholera was not contagious. Smallpox was the one exception, but this disease could be controlled by vaccination without recourse to isolation measures. Thus it seemed logical to Clark to abandon quarantine entirely as a public health procedure. He noted the fact that in the cholera epidemic of Boston in 1849, the hospital on Fort Hill, which was used as a pesthouse, had 641 deaths in four months. Of these fatalities, only 163 were natives, the rest foreigners, chiefly Irish, who were poor, ignorant, and intemperate, and who lived in over-

[3] Bell, John: *Report on the Importance and Economy of Sanitary Measures to Cities,* Document 20, New York Board of Councilmen, 1859.

crowded, dirty, degraded houses. None of those who took care of the sick in the hospital became ill—with two exceptions. This he felt was good evidence that the disease was due solely to filthy and unsanitary living conditions. He emphasized the great dangers of effluvia from burying grounds, and strongly recommended that cemeteries be located in rural and isolated areas.

Thus we learn from these authors and from many other sources that, in pioneer days, human wastes—particularly feces and urine—were not considered as menaces to the public health. Surface defilement of the soil with fecal matter was not thought to be harmful because of the absorbing and deodorizing powers of the earth. Disease supposedly was produced by accumulations of putrid material. In that era, as in many parts of the world even today, the simplest and most common method of disposal of human wastes was upon the surface of the ground. Within a short space of time, these wastes disappeared completely, under the influence of natural forces. There was no arrangement for waste disposal in the pioneer home. The nearby woods or any sheltered place was selected for reasons of modesty and privacy. Since accumulations of filth produced odors, care was taken not to select the same disposal place each time. When villages were established it became impossible to utilize suitable isolated places for feces disposal, and thus the device of a private place or "privy" was evolved. These very convenient little houses were usually placed in the garden at a short distance from the house, and were used by the women and children. The men and boys used the stable, the woods, or other suitable protected places. The privy was not considered a sanitary device but simply a place for quiet, unmolested, decent, and dignified retirement. Since the privy produced an accumulation of filth, with a bad odor, it began to be regarded as a source of possible disease production, and thus the supervision of the cleaning of village privies became one of the major responsibilities of the community board of health. Benjamin Rush in his "Inquiry into the Various Sources of Summer and Autumnal Disease" noted, as his eighth cause, "Privies."

The diarrhea and dysentery are produced oftener than any other form of summer or autumnal disease by the factor of privies. During the Revolutionary War, an American regiment of 600 men was affected with a dysentery from being encamped near a large mass of human feces. The camp was removed and the disease ceased.[4]

[4] Rush, Benjamin: *Medical Inquiries and Observations,* Fourth Edition, Vol. III, p. 110, 1815.

The household "water closet" was invented in 1810, but was not used generally, even in the cities, as a method of disposal for human wastes until well past the middle of the century. Family customs and habits change slowly. Thus, one can find at the present day, in American homes, all the stages in the development of our system of disposal of human wastes. There are still isolated rural areas in the United States where the family utilizes the "handy woods" for feces disposal with no sign of a privy about the place. Many farmers and even villagers still use the next stage of sanitary development, namely, the open-back surface privy. In fact, the sanitary pit-toilet for rural homes was not devised until well into the twentieth century, and the septic tank for rural homes is a recent invention.

WATER SUPPLIES AND SEWAGE DISPOSAL

Community water supplies were provided in a few towns even before 1800; but many years elapsed before the community water system, which piped water into the homes, was used to carry off the household wastes. At first a simple drain beneath the faucet carried the waste waters out to the soil near the house. No indoor toilet was employed. The family used an outdoor privy for feces disposal and did not install a water closet until many years later.

Eventually the towns grew so large that adjacent natural water sources did not suffice and thus economy demanded that water be conducted from afar to meet community necessity not only for the use of households but for manufacturing purposes. The source of this water was almost always a lake or a stream.

From the very outset, it has been a general rule in the United States that the establishment of a community water supply will precede the development of a sewage system by a period of years, ranging from five to fifty. We brought water to the city but provided no facilities for its removal. The cities grew rapidly following the War of 1812, and the development of community systems of water supplies was actively promoted by private companies, particularly in the cities of New York, Boston, and Philadelphia; but few public sanitary sewage systems were constructed in American cities before 1850. Municipal ownership of water supplies and sewage disposal plants was not a common practice in the first part of the nineteenth century. Practically all the early systems were developed by private companies, which were organized for profit. During the period from 1800 to 1817, there were only seventeen community

water supplies in the whole United States. All but one were privately
owned. By 1860, 148 communities had water supplies, some 40 per
cent of which were publicly owned.

The history of the introduction of pure water into the city of
Boston,[5] which was compiled by a "member of the board," is an
interesting historical document that gives, in great detail, the disadvantages of the democratic process in the development of an essential municipal facility. Water in Boston was first supplied by
surface wells, ponds, and brooks. A private water conduit company
brought water to the city from Jamaica Pond in 1795. Thirty years
later the great surgeon, John C. Warren, took an active part in
agitating a plan for a municipally operated water supply. This
matter was debated for years.

Lemuel Shattuck, a member of the city council in 1838, introduced
a resolution approving a plan for supplying Boston with a sufficient
quantity of pure and wholesome water from Long Pond (Cochi-
tuate). The water system was to be constructed and owned by the
city. Careful studies were made of the city's probable future needs,
and finally, in 1846, the state gave Boston the authority to construct
a water supply. Nathan Hale, together with James Baldwin and
Thomas Curtis, were selected as water commissioners. The work was
done with rapidity, and the great public celebration of the completion of the water system was held on September 18, 1848. The procession was probably the most grandiose that Boston had ever seen.
It took two hours to pass a given point. After all the addresses, the
central water gate was opened and the water began to rise. "After a
moment of silence, shouts rent the air, the bells began to ring, can-
nons were fired and rockets streamed across the sky. The scene was
one of intense excitement, which is impossible to describe but which
no one can forget." The average daily consumption during the first
year of operation—1849—was 3,680,000 gallons in a city of about
135,000 people (27 gallons per capita). Twenty years later, daily consumption had risen to 13,000,000 gallons.

So far as I can determine, Lemuel Shattuck, who introduced the
original resolution, was not asked to make an address at the final
celebration, or even to ride in the procession. In fact, his name does
not appear in the final report.

[5] *History of the Introduction of Pure Water into the City of Boston, 1652-1868,*
by a member of the board. Alfred Mudge & Sons, City Printers, Boston, 1868.

The Sanitation of the City of Chicago[6]

The city of Chicago was laid out in 1833 on a site that had been chosen originally by Marquette and Joliet. It was at first a trading post with the Indians. The area was flat and low, with poor sanitary drainage. The city grew rapidly but facilities did not keep pace. The water supply was taken both from Lake Michigan and from shallow wells. Both of these sources of water became heavily contaminated with sewage. From 1833 to 1856 the only drainage of the city was open ditches alongside the streets (except for 3 miles of wooden conduit). The sewage of the city was discharged into the Des Plaines River and into Lake Michigan. "The effect of discharging the contents of sewers into the river was gradually manifested by its increasing discoloration and offensiveness, thus affecting the Lake so that the water supply of the city was more or less complained of." It was noted, furthermore, that in the cholera epidemic of 1849, nearly all who drank water from a shallow well on North LaSalle Street died of cholera. This fact so impressed the people that a tunnel was constructed, by a private company, whereby the city was supplied with Lake Michigan water from a point 2 miles off shore. It proved to be "a very wholesome and satisfactory water" for the city.

It was then realized that, although ample provision for a water supply had been made, there were no proper means for getting rid of the city's wastes and sewage. Since Chicago was built on such flat ground, this resulted in disaster, for sewage accumulated and polluted the whole city. For six years in succession (1849-1855) Chicago suffered from epidemics of severe intestinal infections, chiefly cholera, typhoid fever, and dysentery. This intolerable situation caused community-wide agitation which resulted, in 1856, in the creation of a sewage commission. This commission was effective from the very date of its inception.

The crude death rate for Chicago from 1843 to 1856 averaged 37.9 per 1,000 population per annum. The average death rate per annum for the four years following the sanitary improvement of the city fell to 24.7 per 1,000 population. The citizens believed—and they were probably right—that the major part of this saving of life was due to more adequate provision for sewage disposal.

[6] Data on Chicago collected from: Cheesborough, E. S.: "The Drainage and Sewage of Chicago," *Tr. Am. Pub. Health A.*, 4:18, 1877; Rauch, J. N.: *Sanitary Problems of Chicago*, Report Illinois State Board of Health, p. 94, 1879.

MILK SANITATION

Milk sanitation, down through the first half of the nineteenth century, can be discussed in a few paragraphs. North,[7] in his review of this subject in *A Half Century of Public Health,* has stated that between 1839 and 1879 he could find only thirteen articles in the scientific or medical literature upon the subject of milk. It was known that a certain disease called "milk sickness" could be transmitted through milk. This disease is due to a poisonous alkaloid from a plant that is eaten by cattle when pastures are scanty. The alkaloid is excreted in the cows' milk.[8] No one believed that epidemic disease could be spread through milk, although a few communities made regulations forbidding the sale of watered or adulterated milk and fraudulent milk products.

In 1854, a Mr. Hartley[9] read an essay on "Milk as an Article of Human Sustenance" to the New York Association for Improving the Conditions of the Poor. He presented a certificate signed by fifty-eight New York physicians, who affirmed that "milk of cows, fed chiefly on distillery slops, is extremely detrimental to health, especially of young children, as it not only contains little nutriment for the purposes of food, but appears to possess unhealthy and injurious properties, owing in part to the confinement of the cows, the bad air which they consequently have to breathe, as well as the unnatural and pernicious slop on which they feed."

This is the earliest reference that I have encountered in American literature on milk sanitation.

PRESERVATION OF FOOD

Food preservation has been widely practiced by individual farmers and housewives from early Colonial days. Although the bacteriological principles were not understood, experience had shown that salt, spices, nitre, and many other substances preserved food from spoilage. (See "Diet of the Early American," Chapter 17.)

The Indians taught the pioneers the great value of drying food. The canning[10] of food was introduced as early as 1821 by William Underwood.

---

[7] North, Charles E.: "Milk and Its Relation to Public Health," *A Half Century of Public Health.* American Public Health Association, New York, 1921, p. 236.

[8] Some authors have stated that Abraham Lincoln's mother died from milk sickness.

[9] See *Eleventh Annual Report of the New York Association for Improving the Condition of the Poor,* 1854.

[10] The word "can" is derived from canister. This was a handmade vessel, manufactured from tin, to package tea.

He applied the "Appert Method" which was developed in France in 1810. At first glass containers were used. It was believed that if all the air was removed from the container, the food would not spoil. Canning remained a household procedure and did not develop into a great national industry until the end of the nineteenth century.

FRAUDULENT FOODS

A great deal of fraud was practiced in the food industry throughout the nineteenth century. Animals that had died of some illness, particularly of hog cholera, were sold as food. Often the farmer would discover that the animal was sick and thus he would slaughter it before it died. Sausage meat was heavily adulterated, chalk and water were added to milk, apples and potatoes were "deaconed,"[11] sand was added to corn meal, and chalk was added to flour. All these procedures were considered shrewd but more or less legitimate business practices, and certainly were of no concern to the health department. When local public health laboratories were finally established in the last part of the nineteenth century, their major activities for years related to the discovery and prosecution of merchants who were selling adulterated or fraudulent foods to the people. There was no inspection of food handling, of restaurants, or of meat preparation establishments by the public health authorities. In fact, practically all the health department regulations of the nineteenth century are concerned with disposal of wastes and relate to community "housekeeping" and community cleanliness.

[11] "Deaconing" was an accepted term which meant placing the small wormy apples on the bottom of the barrel with a few rows of fine apples on top.

CHAPTER 16. *Industrial Hygiene*

COLONIAL DAYS TO THE TWENTIETH CENTURY

The protection of the health of the industrial worker is not an individual question. It is a social question demanding social regulation. The prevention of occupational diseases is essentially a function of government.

JOHN B. ANDREWS, *1916*

The entire early history of industrial hygiene in America, before the year 1900, can be summarized in a few pages. The earliest reference that we have discovered which is concerned with diseases related to occupation is found in the voluminous correspondence of the Colonies' great citizen, Benjamin Franklin. In his letter to Benjamin Vaughan in 1786 he wrote:

The first Thing I remember of this kind was a general Discourse in Boston, when I was a Boy of A complaint from North Carolina against New England Rum, that it poison'd their People, giving them the Dry Bellyach, with Loss of the Use of their Limbs. The Distilleries being examin'd on the Occasion, it was found that several of them used leaden Still-heads and Worms, and the Physicians were of Opinion, that the Mischief was occasioned by the Use of Lead. The Legislature of the Massachusetts thereupon pass'd an Act, prohibiting under severe Penalties the Use of such Still-heads and Worms thereafter. Inclos'd I send you a Copy of the Acct. taken from my printed Law-book.

In 1724, being in London, I went to work in the Printing-House of Mr. Palmer, Bartholomew Close, as a Compositor. I there found a Practice, I had never seen before, of drying a Case of Types (which are wet in Distribution) by placing it sloping before the fire. I found this had the Additional Advantage when the Types were not only dry'd but heated, of being comfortable to the Hands working over them in cold weather. I therefore sometimes heated my case when the Types did not want drying. But an old Workman, observing it, advis'd me not to do so, telling me I might lose the use of my Hands by it, as two of our Companions had nearly done, one of whom that us'd to earn his Guinea a Week, could not then make more than ten shillings, and the other, who had the Dangles but seven and six-pence. This, with a kind of obscure Pain, that I had sometimes felt, as it were in the Bones of my Hand when working over the Types made very hot, induced me to omit the practice. But talking afterwards with Mr. James, a Letter-founder in the same Close, and asking him if his People, who work'd over the little Furnaces of melted Metal, were not subject to that Disorder; he made light of any danger from the effluvia, but ascribed it to the Particles of the Metal swallow'd with their Food by slovenly Workmen, who went to their Meals after handling the Metal, without well washing their Fingers, so that some of the Metalline Particles were taken off by their Bread and eaten with it. This appeared to have some Reason in it. But the Pain I had experienc'd made me still afraid of those Effluvia.

When I was in Paris with Sir John Pringle in 1767, he visited *La Charité,* a Hospital particularly famous for the Cure of that Malady, and brought from thence a Pamphlet containing a List of the Names of Persons, specifying their Professions or Trades, who had been cured there. I had the Curiosity to examine that List, and found that all the Patients were of Trades, that, some way or other, use or work in Lead, such as Plumbers, Glaziers, Painters, etc., excepting only two kinds, Stonecutters and Soldiers. These I could not reconcile to my Notion, that Lead was the cause of that Disorder. But on my mentioning this Difficulty to a Physician of that Hospital, he inform'd me that the Stonecutters are continually using melted Lead to fix the Ends of Iron Balustrades in Stone; and that the Soldiers had been employ'd by Painters, as Labourers, in Grinding of Colours.

You will see, that the Opinion of this mischievous Effect from Lead is at least above Sixty Years old; and you will observe with Concern how long a useful Truth may be known and exist, before it is generally received and practic'd on.[1]

There were no factories, in the modern sense, during Colonial days. Water-power mills were found in every community and were usually family affairs. The factory system began in 1767, with the invention, by Hargreaves, of the spinning jenny. Watt's invention of the steam engine in 1785 resulted in the development of textile factories, construction of mill villages, concentration of population, exploitation of child labor, and seventy-two hours of work a week. The steam engine required the development of coal mines, which

[1] Pepper, William: "Medical Side of Dr. Franklin," *Univ. Pennsylvania M. Bull.,* Vol. 23, 1910.

involved long hours of work and even more dangerous and unhealthful living and working conditions within the coal mines. Here, too, child labor was exploited. The first cotton spinning mill in America was established in Rhode Island by Samuel Slater in 1800. New England soon became the national center of the textile industry. By 1831 there were over 800 textile mills in the United States, with 57,460 employees. Fifty years later this number had grown to 172,544 employees with a reduction of the number of mills to 756.

During these fifty years, industrial hygiene did not materialize as a science. The authorities, in a few states, were concerned with such primary matters as the curtailment of long hours of work, the abatement of the dark and dismal working conditions in the mills, and the disgraceful exploitation of child labor. There was no system of accident prevention and no methods were instituted for protection or promotion of the health of workers.

Southwood Smith of England concerned himself actively with the welfare of the poor (see page 241). As a result of his reports, the Factory Act of Parliament was passed in 1833. This act prohibited employment in factories of children under eight years of age. Children older than eight could work not more than six hours a day, and all employed children were required to attend school at least three hours a day. Gradually the English child labor laws were introduced into the various American states. Pennsylvania inaugurated child labor laws in 1848. The New York legislature, in February, 1849, passed a law that "no child shall be employed in any factory or work shop who shall not have attained the age of ten years and be able to read and write. No child shall, under any circumstances, work more than ten hours a day." When the Civil War began in 1860, most of the industrial states had passed some form of child labor law.

During the first half of the nineteenth century, American industrial development was promoted for the benefit of the factory owner with little concern for the comfort, welfare, and health of the worker or his family. Wages and standards of living of the factory workers were very low. The crude death rate and the infant mortality rate in factory towns were far above the average for the country as a whole. Tuberculosis took a heavy toll among the millworkers and their families. As we have noted on a previous page (see page 164) typhoid fever occurred in epidemic waves in the unsanitary dwellings of the New England factory girls. The nutrition of the millworker and his family was miserably inadequate. Horace Greeley was addressing the factory workers when he coined his famous slogan: "Go West, young man, and grow up with the country." He knew full well the hopeless plight of the mill hands and was encouraging them to break the bonds of industrial enslavement and leave the factory towns for the wide open spaces of the far West.

Conditions in the cotton mills of Lowell, Massachusetts, were so notorious in 1841 that the *Boston Times* and the *Boston Quarterly Review* attacked the millowners for their negligence. Elisha Bartlett,[2] who had studied an epidemic of typhoid fever among the factory girls in Lowell in 1835, replied with a strong "vindication of the character and conditions of the females employed in the Lowell mills."

CONTROL OF INDUSTRIAL HAZARDS

Industrial hygiene had its birth in Ramazzini's *De morbis artificum diatriba* in 1700. He called due attention to the influence of occupation upon health, but his work had little impact upon English-speaking countries. Thackrah[3] in 1831 wrote the first English work on the influence of trades upon health. He investigated brass poisoning and diseases due to dusts, and also made careful observations on special trade hazards.

Shoemakers, it is well known, are placed in a very bad posture,—a posture second only to that of tailors. The abdominal viscera, and especially the stomach and liver, are compressed. Lads put to this employ often suffer so much from headache and general indisposition that they are obliged to leave it; and men who have been able to bear it for years, lose appetite and strength.

Sir Humphry Davy invented the safety lamp for coal miners in 1816, and Tanquerel des Planches (1809-1862) made studies of lead poisoning, but the various publications upon these subjects had no concrete effect in promoting the health of the workers in American factories and mines. There was no system of factory inspection for the detection of industrial hazards, and there were no laws that were concerned with amelioration of unsatisfactory working conditions. In 1852 Massachusetts passed a law regulating safety devices for steam boilers, and in 1877 a bill was introduced in the Massachusetts legislature concerning dust removal in the textile mills. At the same

[2] Bartlett, Elisha: *Treatise on Typhoid Fever.* Lea & Blanchard, Philadelphia, 1842.
[3] Thackrah, Turner, C.: *The Effects of Arts, Trades, etc., on Health.* First American Edition, Philadelphia, 1831.

time, regulations were made compelling the use of safeguards for industrial machinery, for fire protection, and also for proper lighting, heating, and ventilation of the mills. Finally, in 1888 general factory inspection was introduced in Massachusetts. Other states, even those with an active industrial development, did not keep pace with Massachusetts in health protection for the industrial laborer.

A. H. Smith[4] carried out his classical experiments on *caisson disease* in 1873, but the full benefits of his observations on the physiological effects of increased atmospheric pressure were not translated into industrial health promotion practices for many years to come. Not until the end of the nineteenth century do we encounter real progress in the promotion of industrial hygiene in America.

[4] Smith, A. H.: Prize Essay, Alumni Association of the College of Physicians and Surgeons of New York. Printed by *Brooklyn Eagle,* 1873.

CHAPTER 17. *The Diet of the Early American*

The conditions of perfect health, either public or personal, are seldom or never attained, though attainable.

SHATTUCK REPORT, *1850*

The American food pattern of the first half of the nineteenth century was, by all modern standards, far from adequate. It is true that we were an agricultural people and that an abundance of nutritious food was available, including fresh fruit and vegetables of all types during the summer season, but the farm hands would not eat the "rabbit fodder." They wanted "hearty food."

The standard diet consisted of meat, salt pork, corn meal, hominy, beans, whole wheat bread, and hot biscuits, with vegetables in season. Molasses was used for sweetening in the South, maple sugar was utilized in the North. Lard was the source of fat. Meat consumption in 1830 was 178 pounds per capita annually. One hundred years later it was 125 pounds. Fruit was banned, particularly for children, since fresh fruits and some fresh vegetables as well (cucumbers, sweet corn, and tomatoes, for example) were supposed to produce "cholera morbus" and bloody diarrhea of young children. Root vegetables, such as turnips, beets, and potatoes were acceptable, but all other fresh vegetables were regarded as "fodder." Milk and butter were seasonable, even on the farm. The only fresh fruits that could be stored were apples and pears, and these did not keep throughout the winter. In many areas green corn and watermelons were considered a hazard, since they "produced malaria."

Refrigeration was devised by a Maryland farmer, Thomas Moore, in 1803, but did not come into general use until the invention of the ice cutter by Nathaniel Wyath. (Although invented in 1827, this tool was not generally utilized until after 1840.)

Alcohol was widely used as a food, chiefly in distilled form. Intemperance was very common and was related, in part at least, to an insufficient and poorly balanced food supply. Charles Dickens found us to be a nation of dyspeptics, addicted to alcohol and chewing tobacco, with supplements of corn bread, salt pork, and beans.

The food of the city dweller, particularly the factory worker, was always close to a famine ration. Milk was of extremely poor quality, and was scarce and expensive. The cows which furnished milk to city children were often very badly cared for, fed with brewery waste, and often (we now know) riddled with bovine tuberculosis.

The regular diet of the factory worker's family consisted of bread, potatoes, and molasses, with meat or fish once a week. Only three pints of milk a week per family were available. Horace Greeley as early as 1837 emphasized the fact that city children were a prey to famine, and in 1850 he issued his clarion call advising young men to go West—to accept the great opportunity, and above all things, to avoid the cities, with their dangers of hunger, want, and exposure to disease.

The tomato had been introduced as a food and medicine by Dr. Siccary, a Portuguese Jew, in the early 1700's. Thomas Jefferson stated that Siccary was the person, who, against great opposition, had insisted upon the medicinal value of tomatoes. Siccary believed that if a person were to eat a sufficient abundance of tomatoes, he should never die. In order to prove his theory, he himself ate abundantly of this vegetable and lived to a ripe old age. But the tomato was not generally accepted as a food, and in many communities it was regarded as poisonous and very dangerous. This tradition prevailed in many rural areas throughout the nineteenth century.

The whites had learned from the Indians their very practical methods of drying meat and some fruits. The preserving of fish and meat by salt was a common practice. But the principles of food preservation and storage that were to revolutionize the American dietary during the twentieth century were all undreamed of by our forefathers.

A rough idea of popular concepts relating to diet may be obtained from the discussions on food that are found in the household textbooks on medical and hygienic care which adorned the mantel over the fireplace of nearly every pioneer home. Wallis in his book on preventive medicine[1] in 1793 extols the importance of fat as a solid food:

[1] Wallis, George: *The Art of Preventing Disease and Restoring Health.* London, 1793.

In some countries, men are not allowed fit for service, or get hired, without, they can bolt bacon; that is, swallow it unmasticated, cut into pieces about an inch and an half square, and this in tolerable quantities. This is done in order that they may attend closely to their labour, without spending any time in taking nourishment for their necessary support; for bacon being fat, and hardened by salt in its curing will be a long time in its undigested state by means the craving of the appetite are kept off, the strength supported.

Buchan wrote a very popular book on domestic medicine[2] which was a household necessity for half a century and which went through many editions. It has a lengthy section entitled "Observations on Diet, Particularly that of the Common People."

He begins with a discussion of bread, which he notes should not be eaten in too great quantities, even though it is the staff of life. He insists that white bread from finely milled flour, though most elegant, is least nutritious. Peas and beans are substitutes for bread as well as butter, but the latter should not be eaten in too great quantities. Root vegetables such as potatoes and turnips are a fairly satisfactory substitute for bread, but carrots are a poor food. Little mention is made of fresh leafy vegetables and fruits. Meat of all types is considered an essential of diet and is to be eaten twice a day. Buchan advocates the utilization of milk but states that "people despise this wholesome and nourishing food because it is cheap, and they devour with greediness flesh and fermented liquors, while milk is deemed fit only for their hogs."

Scurvy was not clearly recognized as a dietary deficiency disease even as late as 1835, despite the clear-cut experiments of James Lind in 1747 on the prevention of scurvy on board ships. It was generally believed that a monotonous diet of salt meat produced scurvy, and Buchan recognized that the disease could be cured by the consumption of fresh fruits and salads. He mentioned specifically oranges, apples, watercress, lettuce, dandelions, parsley, and a decoction of the tips of the spruce tree.

Rickets was a weakness of childhood which was due to diseased parents, to want of care, and to living in damp small houses, where the air was confined. It was a disease of the poor and ignorant who lived in the newly created city slums. Buchan states that "when the mother is too indolent to carry her child abroad into the open

[2] Buchan, William: *A Treatise on the Prevention and Cure of Disease,* 22nd Edition. Robert Campbell & Co., Philadelphia, 1842.

air it will hardly escape the disease." The cure for rickets was wholesome food, open dry air, and sufficient exercise. Not for many years do we find a reference to the specific value of cod liver oil as a remedy for rickets. "Medicines are of little avail [in rickets]. The disease may often be cured by the nurse, but seldom by the physician."

Gout was well understood to be a disease which was due primarily to continuous indiscretions in diet. The consumption of an abundance of "heavy red meats," of sauces and meat gravies, and the drinking of heavy wines were considered to be the cause of gouty attacks. In contrast to scurvy and rickets, it was an elegant disease, an affliction of the rich and elderly.

Dunglinson[3] was the first professor of hygiene in an American medical college. His book on the *Elements of Hygiene* gives an interesting classification of foods as follows:

1. Fibrine—flesh and blood of adult animals.
2. Albumen—eggs, nerves, brain.
3. Gelatine—veal, certain fish, calves' feet.
4. Fats and oils.
5. Cheese, milk, and other caseous foods.
6. Starches.
7. Mucilaginous foods—carrots, turnips, beets.
8. Sugar and all other sweet foods.
9. Acid foods—apples and other fruits. Tomatoes are mentioned in this list.

He notes that there is a great prejudice against fruits as suitable food, particularly since people have believed that they produce cholera. He believes that this prejudice is due to the fact that "fruits arrive at maturity [at a season] when gastric and intestinal derangements are common, and being often eaten, especially by children, in an unripe state and in undue quantity their use has been esteemed hazardous."

It is interesting that this prejudice continued in America for more than 100 years, for in the first part of the twentieth century in the rural areas, the term "cholera morbus" was still used to designate a summer diarrhea of sudden onset in small children. In many areas even now—1955—summer diarrhea is believed to be due to the

[3] Dunglinson, Robley: *Elements of Hygiene*. Carey, Lea & Blanchard, Philadelphia, 1835.

consumption of green corn, watermelon, cucumbers, tomatoes, and other fresh fruits or vegetables.

Dunglinson makes some comments on *dental caries* that have a most modern ring:

> It is not a matter of facility to explain why teeth became carious. . . . Various causes of an extraneous character . . . have been assigned. [The] excessive use of sugar has been invoked, but . . . this has been a convenient sort of bugbear to children, to prevent them from indulging in an expensive article of diet, [for] sugar could only act by the acid contained in it. But when teeth are removed from the body they require a powerful chemical agent to destroy them.
>
> . . . persons of unhealthy habit, and of particular districts, are infinitely more liable to dental caries than others. [This indicates that, if there is no internal disposition to caries, the tooth may remain sound for life.][4]

Beaumont's[5] studies in 1833 on the physiology of digestion were carried out on Alexis St. Martin, the French-Canadian *voyageur*. These observations had a profound influence upon the medical concepts of that day relating to digestion of food. Dunglinson, as early as 1835, included the results of these studies in his lectures to students and in his text on hygiene.

Ira Warren,[6] whose *Household Physician* was published in 1860, quotes extensively from Beaumont's studies and also reviews the work of Baron Liebig on food analysis. In this text on domestic medicine, Warren selects milk as the standard food element. He then compares the amount of nitrogen in various foods with the amount contained in milk. Food is divided into two main groups, namely, the nitrogenized or azotized, which produce flesh and blood, and the non-azotized, which produce heat and energy. Due emphasis is placed upon the value of salts, particularly lime, iron, sulphur, phosphorus, and sodium. Warren divides foods into four categories—(1) fatty, (2) starchy and saccharin, (3) albuminous, and (4) gelatinous. He emphasizes the fact that meat is not an essential—for indeed "the majority of mankind eat no flesh at all." He felt that the average American ate too much meat and he deplored the prevalent idea that a man should eat freely of meat at least twice a day. The importance of beans and corn as staple items of food is brought out, as well as

---

[4] Dunglinson, Robley: *op. cit.*, pp. 331-32.
[5] Beaumont, William: *Experiments and Observations on the Gastric Juice.* F. P. Allen, Plattsburg, 1833.
[6] Warren, Ira: *The Household Physician,* Sixth Edition, 1860.

the value of potatoes and cabbage. Turnips, carrots, beets, and parsnips are considered to be poor in nutritious qualities, but should be served to please the palate and to furnish variety. In city markets, however, Warren states that these foods were so expensive that they did not furnish an economical diet. Fruits are not classified at all by Warren.

Warren had no concept of food deficiency diseases except scurvy. This disease could be cured by fresh fruit and vegetables and was caused by eating too much salt pork and beef. The idea that a proper diet would *prevent* scurvy was not fully acceptable even as late as 1860. One dietary change, however, was beginning to emerge at that time. "Milk is supplied by nature to be our first and *best food.*"

It is difficult for us of the present generation to remember that practically all the basic studies in nutrition have been carried out since the beginning of the present century. The modern period may be said to have begun with the work of Eijkman, who discovered in the East Indies in 1897 the importance of rice polishings in the prevention and cure of beriberi. The very term "vitamin" was not coined by Casimir Funk until 1912.

PRESERVATION OF FOOD

This one factor of extraordinary dietary improvement, namely, preservation of food, has been, perhaps, the most important single influence in the prevention of illness and promotion of the abundant health of the American people. The results have been achieved not alone through the efforts of dietitians and public health educators. Departments of agriculture and agronomy, fisheries, the meat packers —in fact, all the types of industry that have been engaged in the production, packaging, storage, and preservation of food have, by co-ordinated efforts, worked a miracle. They have made the diet of the average American highly nutritious, relatively inexpensive, and adequate for all his needs. All this has been accomplished within the past 100 years.

We often deplore the raucous and sometimes venal methods that are used by food producers in promoting their special products. But it must be confessed that these health education measures have been tremendously effective, and, on the whole, of great benefit in the promotion of the health of the American people.

CHAPTER 18. *The Medical Care of Slaves*[1]

Measures for prevention will effect infinitely more than remedies for the cure of disease.

SHATTUCK REPORT, *1850*

Negro slaves were first brought to the Virginia colony in 1619. Their value soon became evident because of their resistance to malaria and yellow fever, and because of their ability to work in warm climates. The slaves were carefully selected, particularly in relation to nutrition, teeth, eyes, pulse, lung capacity, posture, voice, and exercise tests. The traffic in slaves increased steadily until the prohibition of slave importation became effective nearly 200 years later.

The transportation of slaves was poorly planned. Unsanitary conditions often prevailed on board ship, and epidemics occurred frequently. After arrival, the slaves were carefully seasoned, and were not worked too hard at first. They brought malaria with them, but they were relatively immune to its ravages. The adults were almost completely immune to yellow fever.

During the first four years after arrival, the mortality rate of slaves was high—even up to 30 per cent. The introduction of new slaves into a plantation frequently produced epidemics. When the importation of slaves was prohibited in 1808, the native-born slaves became very valuable property, and were given excellent care. Usually, the plantation had a contract with a physician to provide medical and dental attention, including all necessary preventive services.

The slaves were given comfortable houses, suitable recreation, good food, and adequate clothing. Some of the larger plantations maintained a hospital with practical nurses in attendance. House cleanliness as well as bodily cleanliness was required; and the rules

[1] Much of the information in this chapter was secured from Miss Marshall's report. Marshall, Mary Louise: "Medical Care of Slaves," *Medical Library Association Bulletin*, 26:115, 1938.

provided for regular hours of work and rest. At childbirth a midwife was provided, and the mother rested for four weeks after the birth of the baby. The mother was then given light work. She nursed the child for twelve months, and during this period was required to perform only three-fifths of a day's work. A field-work mother was allowed to return from the field to her quarters three times a day for forty-five minutes to nurse her baby, during the first eight months of its life. Then she came twice a day. A pregnant mother was put on the "sucklers' gang" at the fifth month. The day nurseries were in charge of one of the older women.

In the smaller and more remote plantations, the overseer was the doctor. He had a family doctor book and a large box of home remedies. For years, Ewell's[2] *Planter's and Mariner's Medical Companion* was the standard text for planters in promoting the health of slaves.

Ewell's recommendations were quite practical. He insisted on cleanliness for the slaves, both personally and in their household; good quarters, fresh air, three changes of clothing, and a plantation hospital for the sick.

The principal diseases of slaves were smallpox, cholera, measles, pneumonia, pleurisy, diphtheria, and helminthiasis. Tetanus in infancy was troublesome, and consumption took a heavy toll. As we have noted, the Negroes were relatively resistant to malaria and highly resistant to yellow fever. Ewell discussed the dangers of effluvia rising from the marshes in early autumn, and the necessity of avoidance by the slaves of "moist cold." He had a high confidence in the specificity of various remedies that he recommended in his text. "What numbers of infant slaves have died miserably of lock jaw and of cholera morbus for lack of a vial of laudanum!" Ewell was a strong advocate of smallpox vaccination for slaves. He discussed in detail the value of good diet and exercise in the fresh country air as the treatment for rickets. He also recommended raw and fresh vegetables of all types in the treatment of scurvy.

Consumption was a serious problem. He believed in exercise in dry country air, when not carried to the point of fatigue. Long rides

[2] Ewell, James: *Planter's and Mariner's Medical Companion.* John Bioren, Philadelphia, 1807. Ewell describes the last illness of George Washington in some detail. The old general became ill after a severe exposure to rain and snow on December 13, 1799, when riding out to inspect one of his farms. He developed a high fever, and from the description of symptoms, developed a typical streptococcus "septic sore throat," with all its characteristic manifestations. Ewell's description does not suggest that Washington's last illness was diphtheria, as is so often stated.

on horseback were recommended as an effectual mode of exercise, if one avoided the night air and the intense heat of midday. Patients were to ride only a few miles at first, then gradually increase the duration as they gained in strength.

The care of slaves became so well organized during the early part of the nineteenth century that the expectation of life of a twenty-year-old male slave was only one and a half years less than that of his master.[3] After the slaves were freed in 1862, however, indices of morbidity and mortality of the Negroes increased steadily and at times precipitously, for social and economic reasons that are now clearly understood. Even though nearly a century has passed since Lincoln freed the slaves, nevertheless the morbidity and mortality rates for most of the important diseases in America, including maternal and infant mortality, still are higher for Negroes than for whites.

[3] Hoffman, F. S.: *Race Traits and Indices.* American Economic Association, 1896.

CHAPTER 19. *Health Education*

*Knowledge has for its only just and lasting foundation a rigid,
impartial and inflexible requisition of the truth.*

JACOB BIGELOW, *1835*

Periodicals

A unique feature of the pioneer period was the introduction of the
health education journals. The first of these was the *Medical and
Agricultural Register,* established in 1806 and edited by Daniel
Adams.[1] In the initial number, the editor pointed out that "news,
politics, theology, literature, natural history and the fine arts have
each their periodicals, while *health and agriculture,* subjects which
one way or another come home to every man's business and bosom,
have been in a measure neglected. . . . This periodical has for its
object the widest diffusion, and the greatest possible extent of the
knowledge of the best means of preserving the health, and promoting
the agriculture of a growing and extensive country."

This first volume contained much valuable information concerning
management of crops and dairy herds; care of swine and chickens.
It gave useful hints on personal hygiene, and discussed the means of
distinguishing a physician from a quack. Consumption was a topic
of great concern. Why was the disease on the increase, and why was
it more fatal to females than to males? Epidemiological discussions of
malignant angina, smallpox, and typhus fever were included in the
text, with emphasis on the necessity for better vital statistics.

Dr. Beddows of Deerfield, Massachusetts, who had tried an unusual
method for the treatment of consumption, wrote as follows: "Residence in a stable with cows: This appeared at first to check the
disorder, and strong hopes were entertained that it might effect a
cure, but these hopes have nearly vanished, and it is feared that this

[1] Adams, Daniel: *Medical and Agricultural Register for the Years 1806-1807.* Manning
& Loring, Boston.

will add one more to the methods of unsuccessful experiments of this mode of treatment."

This little journal soon expired.

The *Journal of Health*[2] was established in 1830 by an association of physicians. Its motto was, "Health—the poor man's riches, the rich man's bliss." It was published for four years. The articles were devoted almost entirely to personal hygiene, including diet, recreation, temperance, and mental hygiene. There were a few epidemiological discussions, but little or no mention was made of public health practice. Much of the practical advice in hygiene was excellent. Some of it was absurd. Industrial hygiene emerged in a well-conceived article concerning "trades producing consumption," since stone quarriers and masons at that period—about 1830—were well known to be particularly subject to tuberculosis. In the last issue, August, 1833, the editors informed their readers that the *Journal* was suspending because, despite a large circulation, subscribers had not paid their "arrearages." In this final letter we learn for the first time that the editors were Dr. John Bell and Dr. Francis Condie, both distinguished physicians of this period.

W. W. Hall's[3] *Journal of Health* was begun in 1854. His motto was "Health is Duty." This lively little journal was concerned almost entirely with personal hygiene, and much of the advice and information was excellent. Mental hygiene was frequently discussed: "Whom to Marry?"; "The Children of the Rich"; "Cholera Phobia"; "Mind and Health"; "The Philosophy and Art of Happiness." One can be sure that many readers were disappointed when the Hall journal was suspended after a short period.

Domestic Medicine: Health Guidance Texts for Home Use

A most significant medical institution of the early 1800's was the textbook of "popular" medicine. These were published in great numbers, and some of the best-known texts, such as that of Dr. William Buchan,[4] went through many editions (more than twenty). These books were to be found in every home. They shared the prominent place on the mantelpiece which was reserved for the family

[2] *Journal of Health,* conducted by an association of physicians, Vol. I. Philadelphia, 1830.

[3] Hall, W. W.: *Hall's Journal of Health,* Vol. I, January, 1854. Henry D. Price, New York.

[4] Buchan, William: *Domestic Medicine,* or *A Treatise on the Prevention and Cure of Disease* (orig. English Edition). Adapted to the climate and diseases of America by Isaac Cathrall. Robert Campbell & Co., Philadelphia, 1797.

Bible and *Pilgrim's Progress.* The people lived in scattered farm-houses, often snowed in during the winter. Physicians were inaccessible and expensive, and were not called except in great emergencies. Every plantation owner, every ship captain, in fact every farmer and farmer's wife, was a rough-and-ready physician, and the medicine chest was a family fixture.

Many of these family medicine books were written by prominent physicians and contained wise advice. One of the best was by James Thacher,[5] the distinguished practitioner of Boston. All emphasized preventive medicine.

Buchan was an English author, but there were many American republications of his text. Sometimes one suspects these were appropriated without copyright. The 1816 American edition of Buchan[6] is called *Every Man His Own Doctor,* or *A Treatise on the Prevention and Cure of Diseases.* It also contained an appendix, which was described as a "Complete Treatise on the Art of Farriery."

The book that was most popular with sea captains, and also with southern planters who owned Negro slaves, was *The Planter's and Mariner's Medical Companion* by Dr. James Ewell,[7] a physician of Savannah. This book was published in 1807, and dedicated to President Thomas Jefferson. It was an excellent guide to prevention and cure of disease—practical, sensible, and effectively written.

The first popular text that the author has encountered, which was devoted solely to preventive medicine, was *The Art of Preventing Diseases and Restoring Health* by Dr. George Wallis of London, published for the first time in New York in 1794. This book contained chapters on food and nutrition, on home nursing, and on personal and mental hygiene, as well as an extensive discussion of communicable diseases and their control.

The first American text on preventive medicine that we have found is *Means of Preserving Health and Prevention of Disease* by Shadrack Ricketson, a New York physician. This book was published in 1806. It was largely concerned with personal hygiene and particularly with diet. In 1835 Dr. Robley Dunglinson, professor of hygiene and jurisprudence at the University of Maryland, published *Elements of Hygiene.* Insofar as the author knows, this was the first American

---

[5] Thacher, James: *American Modern Practice,* or *A Simple Method of Prevention and Cure of Diseases.* Cottons & Barnard, Boston, 1826, 796 pp.

[6] Published by N. Whiting, New Haven, 1816.

[7] Ewell, James: *Planter's and Mariner's Medical Companion.* John Bioren, Philadelphia, 1807.

text that was written for medical students in the field of hygiene and preventive medicine. It was essentially a series of lectures on personal hygiene that Dr. Dunglinson gave to his medical students at Maryland University. Thus we may consider him the first professor of preventive medicine in the medical colleges of America.

Newspapers

The newspapers and weekly periodicals of the pioneer period were, to be charitable, not an effective force in sound health education of the people. The advertisements for patent medicines of great variety were accepted without question as to the validity of their extraordinary claims of universal benefit to all mankind. Quackery abounded, and the quacks had no difficulty in presenting their claims to the people through the daily papers if they paid advertising rates for this publicity.

The people were, in general, quite gullible and innocent about most matters relating to personal hygiene and to preventive medicine, as well as to proper therapy in time of illness. The education that they received in those matters through the newspapers was almost universally biased and often willfully false.

Itinerant Quacks

Each spring the itinerant "Indian medicine man" gathered together his group of vaudeville entertainers, and assembled his gaudy equipage and a suitable supply of sovereign remedies. He toured the rural areas, first attracting a crowd by pulling teeth without charge. After lively and raucous entertainment by his vaudeville troupe, he then settled down to the serious business of the evening. For he had for sale—at only half its original price—

Marvelous Electro See, gentlemen, a remedy which is derived from the revealed art and deepest medical secrets of the American Indian, and is compounded according to the most recently discovered knowledge of modern European science. It cures backache, toothache, headache, stomachache, liver disease and female complaint. It strengthens the weakness of men, removes worms of children, regulates the bowels and, in, fact, it cures all the aches and pains to which the human flesh is heir.[8]

Most of these "health educators" were unmitigated rascals who preyed, without conscience, upon the gullible public, but some of the

[8] This harangue was memorized by the author when, as a boy of ten, he listened to the lectures of the Indian medicine man as he stood on the tailboard of his gaily painted covered wagon.

quacks were quite sincere, and treated the people with generosity and high purpose. The greatest of them all was Samuel Thomson, who, after many vicissitudes, finally founded the "Thomsonian System of Medical Care." Eventually his influence spread from the most remote log cabin in the wilderness right to the steps of the White House in Washington. He developed the first prepayment plan in America for medical care for the whole family. His story is so interesting and so representative of the times that we have given a short summary of his life and works in the following chapter.

CHAPTER 20. *An Early Prepayment Plan for Medical Care*[1]

THE THOMSONIAN SYSTEM OF BOTANICAL MEDICINE

It is readily admitted by most distinguished men in the profession that there is no art or science so little understood and miserably conducted as that of Medicine.

SAMUEL THOMSON, *1832*

Samuel Thomson, born in 1769 in New Hampshire, developed a "Botanic System" of medical care during the early part of the nineteenth century which swept the whole nation and which endured for many years. Furthermore, he developed a plan, on a local community voluntary basis, for prepayment of medical care, with formation of "Friendly Societies" in each community. These groups provided for exchange of home nursing care, interchange of therapeutic information, and also exchange of actual remedies.

Thomson had little use for the practicing physician. He was frank to admit that he had had no formal medical training. "The way to become a fashionable physician," he notes, "is to spend three years reading physic, then receive a degree and diploma from some medical society; the time is spent in learning Latin names of different preparations, with names, colors and symptoms of all kinds of diseases, and a sufficient knowledge of the nature of medicine to know how much poison can be given without causing death."

He objected strenuously to the medical practice then current of treating disease by bleeding, by blistering, and by administering mercury, arsenic, nitre, antimony, opium, and other poisons. He also

---

[1] This chapter reproduces excerpts from a paper by the author originally published in the *Journal of the History of Medicine.* Copyright Spring 1951 by the *Journal* and used by its permission.

objected to the system of practice then employed "because people
are kept ignorant of everything of importance in medicine, by its
being kept in a dead language [Latin]."[2]

Thomson believed that radical surgery, particularly amputations
of infected legs and hands, was a pernicious procedure, and he had

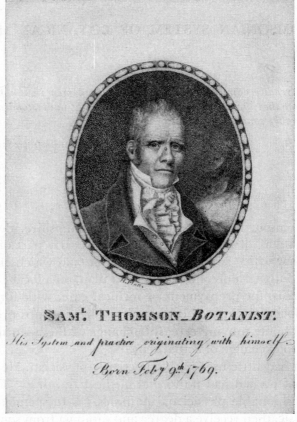

SAM. THOMSON—*BOTANIST.*

His System and practice originating with himself.

Born Feby 9th 1769.

Fig. 16. Samuel Thomson, superb quack and ex-
ponent of prepayment for medical care. (From
Thomson, S.: *New Guide to Health,* or *Botanic Family
Physician.* J. Howe, Boston, 1822.)

little faith in the use of caustics for cancer of the face and the breast.
His method of treatment was based, for the most part, on the use of
"simples such as would promote digestion and aid nature." The
"system" consisted of numbered secret botanical prescriptions. Num-

[2] Thomson, Samuel, *New Guide to Health,* 1822. Printed for the author and sold
by him.

ber *one* was an emetic herb to clear the stomach. Number *two* was a drug to aid digestion. Number *three* was intended to act as a purge, in order to clean the bowels of mortification, and so forth. As time went on, higher numbers up to seven or eight were established. He was a firm believer in the value of sweating, which was produced by steam baths and hot applications.

"Doctor" Thomson had no medical degree, nor did he receive any formal medical training. He learned medicine the hard way, through trial and error, in the bitter school of personal experience. He was a farmer's son, who had had to work very hard while still a small boy. Thus he took a great dislike to farm work. Dr. Kitteridge, a community root-and-herb doctor, treated this farm boy when he was nineteen years old for a seriously infected ax wound of his leg with excellent results. The young man decided to take up the profession of herb doctoring seriously, and began treating his neighbors with herbs and roots that he gathered in the woods. He effected remarkable cures. Often persons who were given up as hopeless cases by their physicians would come to him as a last resort, and would recover after he had administered his secret remedies.

As he became more successful, he aroused the jealousy of physicians. A Dr. French was a redoubtable enemy who made life miserable for young Thomson and finally had him thrown into jail and tried for willful murder of some six persons. Thomson's friends and patients came to his aid and he was vindicated and released from prison. The next year Dr. French was himself in jail for robbing a graveyard of a dead body which he had sold for $60.

Samuel Thomson possessed great energy and complete self-confidence. He was physician, nurse, midwife, and pharmacist—gathering, preparing, and administering his special remedies. He traveled the country over and often was in danger of his life. He soon demonstrated that he had a genius for organization. First he developed his system of treatment, then went to Washington, just after the city had been burned by the British in 1813, and secured a patent on his various secret prescriptions. All the drugs that he used were plants, roots, and herbs. Number *one* was his great standby, for it was a very strong and effective "puke." He also developed a system of massage, and used steam and hot baths most effectively. At first he sold "rights" to individuals in the various communities. These "rights" gave a family the privilege of using his method of treatment. Finally he evolved "The Friendly Botanical Society" with chapters in each

town. Every family which purchased a "right" became a member of
the Society, and thus was entitled not only to the medicines, "but all
the privileges of free intercourse with any one who has bought a
right; to converse, to receive, and to give instructions in sickness,
when called upon by another member."

The Thomsonian system spread throughout the New England
states, then down into New York, and west into Ohio and the hinter-
land. Thomson and his followers had great difficulties with physicians, and he also had trouble collecting his fees and commissions
from his widely scattered agents, but he possessed the secrets of the
several prescriptions and was able to reap a harvest through the sale
of medicines. This grew to such a business that he speaks of purchasing Cayenne pepper from Madagascar in 3-ton lots.[3]

The Thomsonian system finally became so popular that the
Friendly Societies were established "in all of the States and in Canada," and many reputable physicians gave up the use of heavy metals,

---

[3] Thomson in 1822, published a *New Guide to Health,* or *Botanic Family Physician,*
in which he gives some of the secrets of his method of treatment and discusses the
nature of the numbered prescriptions.

"Number 1 is intended to Cleanse the Stomach, overpower the Cold and promote a
free perspiration." It was the tincture or dry powder of an emetic herb, *Lobelia
inflata.* He discovered the properties of this plant, by chance, as a small boy.

Number 2 was intended to retain the vital heat of the system. The basis of this
prescription was Cayenne, or capsicum. He gave very large doses—up to a teaspoon of
the powder taken in sweetened hot water.

Number 3 was intended "to scour the Stomach and Bowels, and remove Cancer."
Many herbs and roots were utilized: bayberry, white pond lily root, hemlock bark,
marsh rosemary root, sumach bark, leaves, berries, and the like.

Number 4 was "Bitters to correct the Bile and restore Digestion." A great many
different plants were used for this prescription: balmony, poplar bark, golden seal
root, and so on.

Number 5 was a "Syrup for the Dysentery to strengthen the Stomach and Bowels."

Number 6 was "Rheumatic Drops to remove pain and prevent mortification." The
essential of Number 6 was the meat of peach stones, or wild cherry stones. A cordial
was made of the seeds, with hot water, loaf sugar, and brandy. Gum myrrh and spirit
of turpentine were used in this prescription. *Good brandy* was an important ingredient.
In addition many accessory vegetable compounds were utilized, such as a nerve powder
of dried lady-slippers, spearmint, peppermint, pennyroyal, hoarhound, tanzy, camomile,
and so forth.

Thomson gives sage advice concerning methods of home treatment, with specific
directions for the family medicine chest and general directions in curing or preventing
disease.

A stock of medicine for a family for one year, "which will enable them to cure
any disease, with which a family of common size may be afflicted" was as follows:

1 oz of the emetic herb (Lobelia powder)
2 oz of Cayenne
1-2 lb of bayberry root bark
1 lb of poplar bark
1 lb of ginger
1 pt of rheumatic drops.

bleeding, and blistering, employing instead botanical remedies more or less in accord with the Thomsonian system. In order to combat Thomson, the Medical Society of New York State was able to get a bill passed in the legislature in 1820, depriving all but physicians of the right to practice medicine as well as the right to administer drugs. The Pennsylvania legislature passed a similar law, but Governor Schultz "put a stop to it, for which he is entitled to great praise." (Thomson had treated Governor Schultz's family free of charge.)

The medical profession was Thomson's worst enemy and it found him a formidable antagonist. His description of a family physician during a community epidemic, of fairly obvious typhoid fever, must have caused many a physician to grit his teeth in ineffective rage.

A child is taken with the belly-ache. The family doctor is sent for, who pronounces its disorder to be worms, gives calomel and jalap to destroy them, which reduces the child very much. The next visit, bleeds it, to lay the fever, then gives it a fever powder composed to nitre, opium and camphor, once in two hours. The patient now lays in a stupid, senseless posture, with crimson spots on the cheeks, denoting putrefaction. The doctor is again sent for in haste, who now pronounces it to be the putrid fever. The bleeding is repeated, and the fever powders continued. The nerves become convulsed, and the doctor is again sent for, who pronounces the disorder to be the putrid nervous fever, and that it has become contagious; the child dies, the family, worn out with fatigue, and being much alarmed, begin to become sick, and by the time the corpse of the child is interred, are all down with the disorder. The doctor now has much employ, the neighbours are called in to watch, the putrefaction runs high; the neighbours, one after another take the disorder, and return home sick; the doctor is called, business gains rapidly in consequence of the same treatment, until the fever has gone through the whole village. All thank the doctor for his incessant attention and kindness; and he boasts of wonderful success, having lost but fifty out of one hundred and fifty! His bill is paid with the greatest satisfaction. By this time the doctor can build his house without sitting down "to count the cost."

What is the cause of all this village sickness? A child was taken with the bellyache; and had no doctor been known, the mother, with one gill of pepper and milk, could have cured the child, and saved all this slaughter of the scourge of a family doctor.

Thomson's "Proposals for a Revolution in the Practice of Medicine" has a most modern and familiar ring. It contains a particularly valuable suggestion: that the Society member who insists that he is ill, and demands medical attention in order to get full value of his prepayment policy, shall be compelled to take the full course of treatment—including Number one, the very efficient "puke."

THOMSON'S PROPOSALS FOR A REVOLUTION IN THE PRACTICE OF MEDICINE

People have paid doctors for being sick, for about four thousand years. Let them now turn about, and pay for their health, which is much more reasonable. Let the doctor enter into contract with the head of a family, to keep the family in health, for a certain sum, for each member of the family, for one year; conditioned that for each day's sickness in the family, by any member thereof, the doctor shall forfeit twenty-five cents, to be deducted from the sum agreed upon. Hence all the account there is to be kept, is, the number of days of sickness there is in the family, in order to know what amount there is to be deducted from the sum agreed upon. And to prevent any imposition on the doctor, by the family, anyone saying: 'I am sick,' to save twenty-five cents; the doctor must be called, and they must go through a *regular course of medicine,* or else not have any allowance made for their sickness. But if they comply, the doctor must not only attend them for nothing, finding his own medicine, but also pay them twenty-five cents for every day they are sick; to be deducted at the end of the year, from his salary.

As Thomson so sagely remarks: "Were this plan generally adopted it would save nine tenths of the sickness of our country."

Sam Thomson was the greatest *quack* that America ever produced. He was a most remarkable man, with many admirable qualities and progressive ideas. How the doctors must have hated him! But he had a profound influence in modification of the drastic therapy of the day and was largely responsible for the early legislation in many states requiring that all practitioners of medicine shall possess a state license which is secured only after demonstration of at least a minimum of medical knowledge and professional competence.

CHAPTER 21. *Child Health*

Business of being a baby must be classified as an extra-hazardous occupation.

S. W. NEWMAYER, *1911*

Children fared quite well during the Colonial period. Families were large and lived for the most part on farms. Here children played an important part in the economy and welfare of the family. A large family was a great asset. Family planning, so much in vogue at the present time, was not a question of limitation of family size, since the larger the family the greater the family prosperity. In 1810 the average married woman had eight children, not counting miscarriages and stillbirths. The infant death rate was high—how high we do not know, as no accurate data are available—but we do know that the maternal mortality rate was at least six or seven times as high as in 1950. Many of the old cemeteries of the eighteenth century have a major headstone, with the name of the head of the family, who lived to a ripe old age. Surrounding this stone, one finds satellite stones of three or four wives, who had died in succession, from childbirth or allied causes. Often, too, each mother is surrounded by her satellites of infant grave markers.

Bolduan has made an estimate of the infant mortality in New York City from 1810 to 1940. At the beginning of the nineteenth century the rate was 120 per 1,000 live births. This rate increased to a peak of 230 by 1870, with a steady decline thereafter to about 120 at the end of the century. (See Fig. 17.)

The industrial advances of the early nineteenth century proved to be a great detriment to children. The demand for child labor made a large family even more desirable, for children could be put to work in the mills at an early age. Certain restrictions were placed eventually on exploitation of child labor, but these laws, by their very implication, now sound like barbarism. In Rhode Island, for ex-

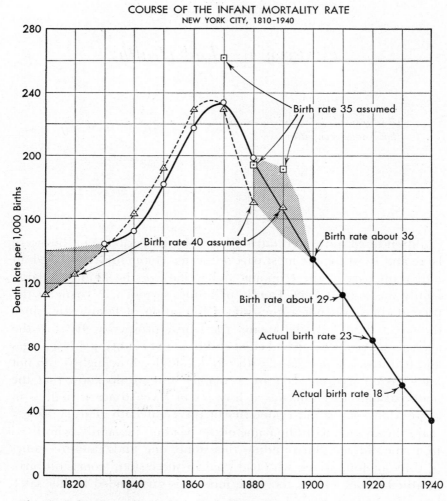

Fig. 17. Infant mortality in New York City, 1810-1940. The rates are per 1,000 live births. Small circles indicate the rate based on estimates of births arrived at from the census population under five. (From Bolduan, C. F.: "The Public Health of New York City," *Bull. New York Acad. Med.*, 19:437, [June] 1943.)

ample, when cotton mills were first developed, children from seven to twelve years of age were utilized, so that, in 1831, one-half of the employees of textile mills in Rhode Island were *young children*. In 1835 in the textile mills of Pennsylvania, one of every five hands employed was a child under twelve years of age. The average working week was seventy-two hours, with a day's work often lasting twelve to fourteen hours. Massachusetts passed the first child labor law, which required that no child under fifteen could be employed in a factory unless he had attended school at least three months of the preceding year. Exploitation of children became so serious that in 1842 Massachusetts passed a law providing for a ten-hour working day for children under fourteen years. In 1845 Connecticut prohibited employment in factories of children under ten, and in 1849 Pennsylvania not only prohibited children under thirteen years from working in textile mills, but also passed a law prohibiting children under fourteen from working more than ten hours a day. These regulations could not withstand the pressure of both industry and of parents as well, for it was often the parents who insisted that the mills employ their young children in order to develop these sources of family revenue. Even as late as 1888, Massachusetts passed a regulation prohibiting children under thirteen years from working in manufacturing establishments during school hours. New York passed a compulsory school law in 1852, and many states soon followed suit. By 1874 New York required fourteen weeks of schooling each year, and other states followed this leadership, but again this type of law was not enforced in many states. Even today, in many New England textile towns, one finds old employees who started to work in the factory before their tenth birthday, with little or no education beyond the fourth grade. As van Eigen has pointed out, "before 1900 the American child had no real friend or public defender." The National Child Labor Committee was not founded until 1904, and even in 1910[1] over 2,000,000 young American children were employed in gainful occupations.

It is impossible to secure an accurate appraisal of the ill effects of bad housing and the long hours of factory labor on the growing child. We know full well that these conditions should not be permitted, but we find it hard to produce direct evidence that premature death, disability, and disease are brought about by these conditions.

Death rates by age groups for the period 1800 to 1850 are not very reliable. We do have evidence that during this era many more children died between the ages of five to fifteen years than die at present. These deaths were due for the most part to infectious diseases, particularly scarlet fever and diphtheria. Tuberculosis, for reasons that we do not understand, has always spared the children in the age group of five to fifteen years. But the specific mortality

[1] Kober, G. M.: "History of Industrial Hygiene and Its Effects on Public Health," *A Half Century of Public Health*. American Public Health Association, New York, 1921, pp. 361-411.

rates in childhood are crude indices of bad social conditions. The misery due to malnutrition, to overwork, to physical exhaustion, and to lack of play and opportunity for spontaneous self-expression cannot be measured in terms of morbidity and mortality rates. We are sure that the children who lived in the rural areas in the United States during the nineteenth century had a severe, disciplined, and hard life, but on the whole they enjoyed a healthy and wholesome existence. The children who were reared in the cities, and particularly in the factory towns, had a miserable, overworked, undernourished, and impoverished life of hardship, unhappiness, frequent illness, and premature death.

The high prevalence of the contagious diseases of childhood during the nineteenth century has been forgotten, since practically all of these diseases have now been brought under control. We can obtain some estimate of the effects of the most important of these infections by means of an analysis of the mortality statistics of the national census of 1850.[2]

Table 8
Proportion of Deaths of Children in 1850*

AGE GROUP	NUMBERS	PER CENT OF TOTAL POPULATION	PER CENT OF TOTAL DEATHS
Under 1 year	629,466	2.7	16.8
1- 4 years inclusive	2,868,327	12.3	21.2
5- 9 ” ”	3,241,268	13.9	6.7
10-19 ” ”	5,420,421	23.3	8.7

* SOURCE: From *Mortality Statistics of the Census of 1850,* Washington, D. C., 1855.

The total population of the nation was 23,191,876. Table 8 gives the proportionate distribution of children in America in 1850, together with the percentage of the total deaths of the children during that year.

The devastating destruction of little children during that year is revealed in this table. Infants under one year comprised less than 3 per cent of the population but provided 16.8 per cent of the deaths. This was more than six times the general death rate. Children from one to four inclusive suffered from twice the general death rate. The group from five to nine years of age inclusive enjoyed a relative immunity from serious illness. They made up 14 per cent of the population, with 6.7 per cent of total deaths.

[2] De Bow, J. D. B.: *Mortality Statistics of the Census of 1850.* The Seventh Census, Washington, D. C., 1855.

"Zymotic" diseases were the primary cause of this very high death rate of children under five years of age. This category included fevers in general; measles, smallpox, influenza, and most of the intestinal infections, such as cholera, dysentery, cholera infantum, typhoid fever, cholera morbus, and so on. Other important infections were "whooping cough," scarlet fever, and diphtheria. The list of zymotic diseases did not, however, include pneumonia, tuberculosis, or convulsions.[3]

Table 9

Deaths of Young Children from "Zymotic" Diseases in 1850*

AGE	TOTAL DEATHS	PER CENT OF TOTAL DEATHS	DEATHS FROM ZYMOTIC DISEASES	PER CENT OF TOTAL DEATHS FROM ZYMOTIC DISEASES	DEATH RATE PER 1,000 LIVING IN AGE GROUP	DEATH RATE FROM ZYMOTIC DISEASES PER 1,000 LIVING IN AGE GROUP
Under 1 year	54,265	16.8	20,064	15.2	86.2	32.0
1-4 incl.	68,713	21.2	37,637	28.6	23.8	13.1
5-9 incl.	21,721	6.7	12,278	9.3	4.1	2.1

* SOURCE: From *Mortality Statistics of the Census of 1850*, Washington, D. C., 1855.

Table 9 clearly shows the great severity of infectious diseases in little children. Over 28 per cent of all deaths in America from the acute infections, excluding tuberculosis and pneumonia, occurred in the age group one to four years. Deaths in infants and children under five years comprised nearly one-half of the total infectious disease fatality of the nation. After the age of five years a child enjoyed a relative immunity from acute contagious diseases.

Another method of expressing these facts is that in 1850 thirty-two of every 1,000 babies under one year of age in the nation died of acute infection. Thirteen of every 1,000 children from one to four years of age inclusive died from these same causes.

We have prepared a summary of the ten leading causes of death for each age group in childhood and youth for the census year 1850 (see Table 10). Many causes of death are not known, and some of the diagnostic categories are not too clearly defined, but the general picture is most illuminating.

[3] Our present epidemiological knowledge compels us to the conclusion that hookworm disease was an important cause of illness and death among the children of all the southern states during the pioneer period. This infection was introduced by the Negro slaves from Africa. Negro children were relatively immune to the effects of this parasite, but white children suffered severely. The epidemiology of this disease was worked out in the United States by Stiles in the early part of the twentieth century.

Table 10

The Ten Important Causes of Death in Childhood—1850*

CHILDREN UNDER 1 YEAR: TOTAL NUMBER, 629,466		CHILDREN 1-4 YEARS INCLUSIVE: TOTAL NUMBER, 2,868,327	
CAUSE OF DEATH	TOTAL DEATHS	CAUSE OF DEATH	TOTAL DEATHS
1. Croup	4,728	1. Dysentery	8,164
2. Dysentery	3,311	2. Scarlet fever	5,156
3. Convulsions	2,824	3. Croup	4,934
4. Whooping cough	2,113	4. Cholera	4,283
5. Pneumonia	2,042	5. Fever	3,633
6. Cholera infantum	1,842	6. Whooping cough	2,659
7. Fever	1,719	7. Pneumonia	2,528
8. Cholera	1,417	8. Cephalitis	2,066
9. Consumption	1,294	9. Worms	2,049
10. Scarlet fever	989	10. Convulsions	2,036

CHILDREN 5-9 YEARS INCLUSIVE: TOTAL NUMBER, 3,241,268		CHILDREN AND YOUTHS 10-19 YEARS INCLUSIVE: TOTAL NUMBER, 5,420,421	
CAUSE OF DEATH	TOTAL DEATHS	CAUSE OF DEATH	TOTAL DEATHS
1. Scarlet fever	2,344	1. Consumption	3,479
2. Cholera	2,308	2. Cholera	3,090
3. Dysentery	2,172	3. Fever	2,804
4. Fever	1,741	4. Typhoid fever	2,668
5. Typhoid fever	1,112	5. Dysentery	1,439
6. Croup	846	6. Pneumonia	1,209
7. Dropsy	724	7. Dropsy	972
8. Cephalitis	715	8. Accident	807
9. Pneumonia	674	9. Cephalitis	798
10. Consumption	614	10. Scarlet fever	784

* SOURCE: From *Mortality Statistics of the Census of 1850*, Washington, D. C., 1855.

Diphtheria and scarlet fever played a very important role as causes of death in young children. The intestinal infections, particularly diarrheal diseases of infancy, were probably the leading causes of death in children under five years, since cholera infantum, cholera morbus, dysentery, convulsions, teething, and worms, as well as many of the deaths from fever, belong in this one category.

Tuberculosis was an important cause of death in infants. This disease dropped in importance for the next fifteen years and then became the *leading cause* of death in youth.

The most striking thing about this analysis is that practically every important cause of death in childhood in 1850 was from an acute infection. An exception to this rule was accidents in youth (ten to nineteen years). Of the 807 accidental deaths during this year, 693 were of boys. (This does not include drownings, which totaled 531—over 400 of which were of boys.)

The picture has entirely changed in 100 years. We now have a much more accurate and complete record of the causes of death in childhood. Thus the whole picture of prevalence of infectious diseases in childhood can now be brought into clear focus. We can be sure of one fact. Every single one of the ten important causes of illness and death in infancy and early childhood in 1850 has been wiped out. The slate is clean. Childhood has become a period of abundant health and of preparation for a full and satisfactory adult life, free from invalidism and from the scars of the early acute infections. This astounding achievement is one of the great triumphs of sanitation and of public health. Not only the saving of life has been achieved, but life has been spared to be lived more fully and abundantly.

CHAPTER 22. *Mental Health Promotion*

> *No country has yet been ruined by expenses incurred in protecting the public health.*
>
> H. P. WALCOTT, *1886*

The first step that a community must take in promotion of mental health is a plan for suitable care of the mentally ill. Furthermore, it is axiomatic that the stage of development of a community plan for care of mental disease is an excellent index of the social development of a people. The more intelligent and adequate the provision for care of mental illness, the more advanced is the degree of civilization of the community. Thus an analysis of our system of care of mental illness is, in a sense, an appraisal of the social development of America.

We have noted in our discussion of medical care in the colonies that the earliest hospitals in America made some provision for care of the insane. This was true in Philadelphia in 1752, in New York in 1792, and Baltimore in 1797. Virginia was the first state (colony) to make provision for care of mental illness—in Williamsburg. This institution was called the Eastern State Hospital for the Insane, and was chartered in 1768. In Philadelphia a special institution for mental disease was established by the Quakers in 1818, "where the insane might be regarded as men and brothers." The New York Legislature in 1821 appropriated $12,500 a year for fifty years for the maintenance of Bloomingdale Asylum, and that same year, John McLain of Boston left $100,000 as an endowment for an asylum for the insane that was given his name. Hartford Retreat in Connecticut was established in 1824, and the Massachusetts State Insane Hospital at Worcester was built in 1830.

But these few institutions were quite unable to meet the hospitalization requirements for the insane of the entire nation. At this critical period, there appeared a great crusader for the development of governmental institutions for care of the insane. This crusader was a remarkable woman, in fact, one of the greatest women that America has ever produced. Her name was Dorothea Dix. Almost single-handed, she awoke the whole nation to a great need, and by her indomitable will and tremendous energy, she succeeded in establishing state institutions for mental diseases throughout the land.

Dorothea Dix was born in Hamden, Maine, in 1802. Her childhood was haphazard and difficult. Self-taught, she became a school-

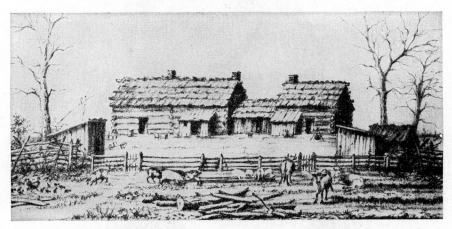

Fig. 18. First building in Indiana to be designated as an insane sylum (about 1840). (From Rice, Thurman B.: "The Origin and Development of the City Hospital," *Monthly Bull. Indiana State Board of Health,* April, 1947. Courtesy of the Indiana State Library.)

teacher at fourteen years of age. Later she became a governess in the home of W. E. Channing in Boston. He had tuberculosis, and in 1830 took his whole family, including Miss Dix, to St. Croix in the West Indies. This voyage was intended to improve his health. It resulted in the infection of his children's tutor. Miss Dix became ill with tuberculosis while in St. Croix. She was presumably infected in the home of her employer, and the disease was to harass her until her death. In 1836 she went to England for her health, and remained for a year in order that she might miss the rigorous New England winter. She then returned to Boston and took theological training. She was assigned in 1841 as a Sunday school teacher to a class of twenty women in the East Cambridge House of Correction. It was there that she found insane women confined with criminals, crowded into filthy cells, neglected, and maltreated. She secured the assistance of Dr. S. G. Howe and Charles Sumner and began her campaign. Miss Dix visited almshouses and jails; everywhere she found the insane in "cages, closets, cellars, stalls and pens, chained, naked, beaten with rods, lashed into obedience."

Horace Mann joined her crusade, as did John G. Palfry. Despite

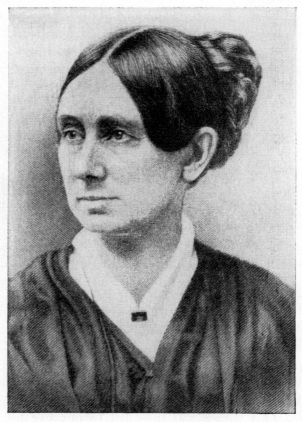

Fig. 19. Dorothea Dix, founder of mental hygiene in America. (From Tiffany, Francis: *The Life of Dorothea Lynde Dix.* Houghton Mifflin Co., Boston, 1891.)

strong opposition, she obtained legislative action in Massachusetts for a program for adequate state care of mental disease.

She then went to Rhode Island and secured a single gift of $40,000 from a wealthy man, Cyrus Butler, for a hospital for the insane in that state. In 1845 she was active in New Jersey, and finally secured funds for the great state institution for mental diseases at Trenton, which she called her "first-born" child. The state held her in great esteem, and it was here in this institution, in an apartment given her by the trustees, that she died forty-five years later.

After her triumph in New Jersey, Miss Dix moved into the South and West. She became a famous person. In three years she traveled over 10,000 miles by every imaginable means of conveyance. She was ill almost constantly, for she became heavily infected with malaria, and the pulmonary hemorrhages from tuberculosis were always recurring. Despite her handicaps, she visited 18 penitentiaries, 300 county jails, and over 500 almshouses during the years 1842 to 1845. Her personality was overwhelming; she was an old maid, an invalid, and a New England schoolmistress, without personal beauty or attraction. Yet she possessed a burning zeal for a great cause, and she swept the whole nation with her enthusiasm. The upshot was that more than 20 state institutions for the care of the insane were established as a direct result of her efforts.

In 1848 she began her plans for a nationwide, federally aided program for care of mental disease. She had strong support, so effective, indeed, that her bill providing for a land grant of 12,225,000 acres for federal aid to mental hospitals throughout the land *passed both houses of Congress.* To her great disappointment, in fact to her almost complete despair, the bill was vetoed by President Franklin Pierce. It was the great defeat of her life, and broke her heart and spirit. When the Civil War began in 1860, Miss Dix was nearly sixty years of age. She took an active part in the organization of nursing care for wounded northern troops. She was made superintendent of all women nurses, and was decorated by Secretary Stanton, but she never was able to establish herself in this new field. She was a promoter—not an organizer—and was signally unsuccessful in her administrative Civil War work. It was a mistake for her to attempt this new endeavor, for her life work already had been accomplished.

President Pierce was accused of all sorts of political chicanery because of his action in vetoing the federal land grant bill for the care of the insane, but his reasons were sound, and his veto was a conscientious one. He said, "I do not believe that the Federal Government should assume a responsibility at this time, which might lead to the Federal Government taking charge of all the poor of all the states. The fountains of charity will be dried up at the base, and the several states, instead of bestowing their own resources on the wants of their people, may themselves become the humble suppliants for the bounty of the Federal Government, thus reversing their true relation to this union."

Nearly a century was to pass before the fears of President Pierce were actually to become a reality.

BIBLIOGRAPHY

Greenbie, M. G.: "Dorothea Dix," *Lincoln's Daughters of Mercy*. G. P. Putnam's Sons, New York, 1944.

Psychiatric Milestone, A. Bloomingdale Hospital Centenary, privately printed, New York Hospital, 1921.

Tiffany, Francis: *Life of Dorothea Lynde Dix*. Riverside Press, Cambridge, Mass., 1891.

CHAPTER 23. *Vital Statistics*

The registration of vital statistics is the firm basis on which the whole structure of sanitary science and practice must rest.

CHARLES V. CHAPIN, *1901*

The collection and the recording of vital data have become an essential and integral part of public health practice and of our social structure. The methods that are employed and the results that may be secured are so well understood, and are so valuable to the state and to the individual, that we find it difficult to imagine any community existing without this essential facility. Yet it was not always so. In fact, an accurate and reasonably complete recording of such basic data as births and deaths has been secured for the whole United States only within the past twenty-five years.

THE COLONIAL PERIOD

We made no mention of vital statistics in our discussion of the Colonial period because the recording of vital data was not accepted as a governmental function at that time. Rather it was a function of the church. Accurate records of deaths were kept by each of the churches, although the actual causes of death were not often given. Births were not recorded except by the individual's family, but baptisms were, and since most babies were baptized during the first year of life, a limited amount of information in these matters may be obtained from the old church records.[1]

In 1753 *Gentleman's Magazine* of London[2] published an account

[1] Ernest Caulfield's superb study in 1939 of the throat distempers of New England from 1735 to 1740 was based almost entirely on old church records. (Caulfield, Ernest: *True History of the Terrible Epidemic Vulgarly Called the Throat Distemper, Which Occurred in His Majesty's New England Colonies between the Years 1735 and 1740.* Published for the Beaumont Medical Club by *Yale Journal of Biology and Medicine,* New Haven, 1939.)

[2] *Gentleman's Magazine:* Edited by Sylvanus Urban and printed by E. Cave at St. John's Gate, London, 1753, Sept., p. 413.

of the "Burials of Boston, New England, from the year 1701 to 1752 and the christenings from 1731 to 1752." Their table gives us no base line for our calculation of rates, for we do not know the population of the city. Nevertheless, the data are most informative. The devastating effects of smallpox epidemics are clearly brought out in their tables. For example, during the smallpox year of 1721, there

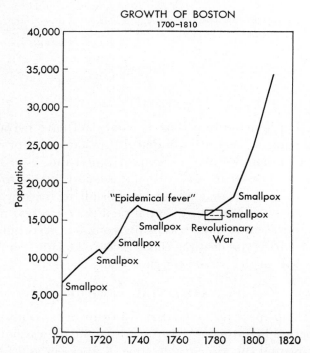

Fig. 20. The growth of Boston was very slow during the entire Colonial period. From 1740 through the Revolutionary War there was no increase in population. Smallpox played an important role in this growth curve.

were 1,102 deaths in the town in an estimated population of 11,000. In 1752 Boston had a population of about 16,000; of these 7,669 had smallpox with 569 deaths from the disease. The total deaths for that year nearly equaled the total for 1721, for 1,009 persons were buried during that twelvemonth (in 1752).

During those years when no great epidemics occurred, the crude death rate averaged about 35 to 40 deaths per 1,000 population. The article noted that burials exceeded baptisms by 1,534 over a twenty-one-year period. But this does not mean of course that deaths actually exceeded births. It is much more probable that deaths were recorded better than births and also that many infants died before they were baptized.

It is quite difficult to obtain an accurate estimate of the population during the Colonial period, for the census was taken for the purpose of allocation of taxes and thus was a gross underestimation. For example, the tax census of Boston in 1742 gave a total of 16,382 persons, omitting 110 in the almshouse and 36 in the workhouse. It included 1,200 widows, "a great number so poor that they could not be taxed. Several persons besides were gone to Cuba and several sons and apprentices were designedly overlooked to ease the quota of Boston from the Tax." We have obtained rough estimates of the population of Boston covering the entire period of the eighteenth century. These data come from a variety of sources, chief of which is Shattuck's 1845 *Census*.[3] They are presented in Figure 20. They show clearly that Boston remained almost stationary in size for half a century, e.g., from 1740 to 1790. Only after the establishment of the Union did the town begin its growth. Boston's growth was quite typical of the major cities of the other colonies. Even as late as 1790, the largest cities of the nation were:

New York	49,401
Philadelphia	28,522
Boston	18,320
Baltimore	13,503

The earliest American life table was prepared by Edward Wigglesworth[4] in 1789. His table is based on 4,983 deaths of which 1,942, or 39.2 per cent, occurred during the first five years of life. A summary of this table follows:

Expectation of life at birth						28.15 years
"	"	"	"	5	years	40.87 "
"	"	"	"	20	"	34.21 "
"	"	"	"	50	"	21.16 "
"	"	"	"	65	"	12.43 "

[3] Shattuck, Lemuel: *Census of Boston*, pp. 3-4, 1845.
[4] Wigglesworth, Edward D. P.: "A Table Shewing the Probability of the Duration, Decrement and Expectation of Life, in the States of Massachusetts and New Hampshire, 1789." See interesting discussion by Hoffman, F. L.: "American Mortality Progress during the Past Half Century," *A Half Century of Public Health*. American Public Health Association, New York, 1921, p. 94.

BILLS OF MORTALITY

The earliest vital statistics which were issued in the United States were the *Bills of Mortality for Portsmouth, New Hampshire.* These were assembled by Dr. Lyman Spalding.[5] Dr. Nathan Smith, who founded Dartmouth Medical College, had been impressed by the studiousness of Lyman Spalding as a boy in Cornish, New Hampshire, and he had aided the youth in securing an education. Spalding practiced in Portsmouth, and in 1801 was active in the control of small-pox by means of the new vaccination technique. He originated his *Bills of Mortality for Portsmouth* in 1801 in order to increase public interest in tuberculosis as an important cause of death, and also in order to establish the average of longevity for purposes of life insurance and of annuities. They were published for a ten-year period.

THE CENSUS[6]

The first census of the United States was undertaken in 1790, and a census has been conducted each ten years thereafter. The first six censuses were simply an enumeration of the people in the various communities. The first census of 1790 was provided for by the Constitution so that "representation and direct taxes shall be apportioned among the several States which may be included within this Union, according to their respective numbers." Thus the provision for authorizing a decennial census was embodied in the Constitution for political purposes solely, and with no thought of providing for any systematic collection of statistical data beyond the political necessities of the government. There was no thought of providing a basis for collection of mortality data, nor of furnishing material for the purpose of protecting the public health. Indeed, as Wilbur has emphasized, "Public health was entirely without the purview of the fathers of the republic and lay unrevealed in the womb of the future."

The United States was the first nation to provide for a regular political enumeration of its inhabitants. But Wilbur was quite correct when, in 1911, he said:

The establishment of a regular census of the population and registration of vital statistics are the first steps taken in placing a country upon a

[5] Spalding, Lyman: *Bills of Mortality for Portsmouth, New Hampshire,* for A.D. 1801-1811.

[6] Wilbur, Cressy L.: "The Census and the Public Health Movement," *Ann. Am. Acad. Polit. & Social Sc.,* **37**:286, 1911.

plane of modern civilization. While the United States led the world in respect to census of the population, we still rank with the most unprogressive and semicivilized countries as concerns the registration of births and deaths.[7]

It was not until the first modern registration law for the collection of vital statistics was passed by England and Wales in 1836 that the concept began to develop that one of the chief functions of the state is the protection of the lives of the people from the dangerous enemies of disease.

The census of 1850[8] was the first evidence of an American concept that due attention should be given by the federal government to the recording and the analysis of causes of death. The data from this census are presented in some detail in an earlier chapter (see Chapter 9, "The Period of Great Epidemics"). Since 1850 each decennial census has become more complete, more accurate, and more effective. These reports are now among the most valuable of all government documents. Their publication is eagerly awaited, and the results are very widely used for the great benefit of all the people.

As we have already noted, the only enumeration of births, deaths, and marriages during the Colonial period was the records of the church. The cemeteries were always in close proximity to the church and so the death records were kept quite accurately; but there was no exact record of the *causes* of death.

Accurate municipal death records were begun in New York in 1804. These were followed by the publication of mortality statistics by the city of Boston in 1813, Philadelphia in 1825, and Baltimore in 1836. Births were recorded very poorly. In fact it was not until 1891 that the annual number of recorded births in New York City exceeded the number of recorded deaths.

The American Statistical Society was organized in 1839 under the active stimulation of Lemuel Shattuck. Undoubtedly this association received its impetus from the work of William Farr, the great vital statistician of England. As a direct result of the formation of the American Statistical Society in Boston, the state of Massachusetts in 1842 passed a law initiating state-wide registration of vital data. The registration law of New York was passed in April, 1848. Connecticut and New Jersey both adopted similar laws that same year.

[7] Wilbur, Cressy L.: *op. cit.*

[8] De Bow, J. D. B.: *Mortality Statistics of the Census of 1850.* The Seventh Census, Washington, D. C., 1855. Dr. Edward Jarvis was of great assistance in formulating this report and in classifying the causes of death.

In 1847, at the first meeting of the American Medical Association, Dr. John Griscom of New York suggested the appointment of a committee to study better methods of recording births, deaths, and marriages. He also proposed a standard nomenclature for causes of death. This committee was formed, and in 1848 Griscom made a short report[9] urging all physicians to call this matter to the attention of their state legislatures. This effort was so effective that eight states, between 1850 and 1860, made provision for registration of vital statistics. Unfortunately, the intense political excitement and the resultant Civil War, beginning in 1861, "utterly dissipated all interest in these matters and the cause of registration was set back at least twenty years, for it was not until the 70's that attention began to be given again to the subject of public health."[10]

The founder of accurate recording of vital statistics in the United States was undoubtedly Lemuel Shattuck, and the cornerstone is the *Census of Boston,* which was compiled in 1845. This document is of such great importance in the whole field of public health in America that we must give it special consideration.

The Census of Boston of 1845[11]

The report of the census of the city of Boston[12] in 1845 was a precursor of Shattuck's more famous report of 1850, but in many ways it is equally important, for in it one can obtain a very clear picture of the economic and social conditions of that day.

The nation was in a period of vigorous growth. Immigration[13] from Europe was at flood tide. From 1790 to 1810, some 6,000 persons came to America each year from Europe, but this flow was completely stopped by the war with Britain in 1812. Laws regulating immigration were passed in 1819, but during the subsequent ten years only 150,000 persons entered the United States. Then came the political persecutions in Germany and the potato famine in Ireland. These initiated the avalanche. Over 4,000,000 persons came from Europe to America from 1819 to 1855. Of these, 1,700,000 were Irish, and 1,200,000 were Germans. In 1848 alone, 230,000 entered our borders. The peak was reached in 1854 with a total of 400,000. Males out-

[9] See *Tr. Am. M. A.,* Baltimore meeting, 1848.

[10] Wilbur, Cressy L.: *op. cit.*

[11] Smillie, W. G.: Excerpts from "Lemuel Shattuck—Still a Prophet; Lemuel Shattuck—America's Great Public Health Pioneer," *Am. J. Pub. Health,* **39:**135, 1945. Reproduced by permission.

[12] Shattuck, Lemuel: *Census of Boston,* 1845.

[13] Bromwell, W. J.: *History of Immigration to the United States.* Redfield, 1856.

numbered females 2 to 1. More than half of the immigrants were between fifteen and thirty years of age. Laborers made up the largest quota, with very few skilled workers, and almost no professionally trained people.

Industrialization of the Atlantic seaboard had begun, and the textile factories of New England absorbed large numbers of these immigrants. There were no child labor laws. Children went to work in the factories at eight years of age, and the working day was twelve hours or more.

Housing laws were nonexistent. There were no departments of health in the modern sense; when epidemics occurred, a special board of physicians was selected to deal with the immediate situation. Isolation, quarantine, and even the reporting of communicable disease was opposed because "(a) these regulations interfered with private rights, and (b) they were injurious to business." It was generally held that a disease such as scarlet fever, which was highly prevalent and severe, "occurs under no fixed laws, and seems inclined to abide with us."

The nation was young, vigorous, boisterous, callous, exuberant, with all the virtues and all the faults of a gangling adolescent, who has outgrown his clothes, broken away from his parents, and has awkwardly tried out his strength. He is uncertain and insecure, but bursting to demonstrate his great importance to the whole world.

Massachusetts was one of the more conservative and settled sections of the nation, but foremost in the coming industrial revolution. It must also be remembered that it was largely New England men who gave the impetus and leadership to the western expansion.

As we have noted, the Shattuck report of 1845 on the census of the city of Boston gives us an accurate picture of the mode of life and the state of civilization in the nation as a whole.

From the report of 1845, we have compiled certain simple vital data which are comparable with similar data for the Boston of 1945, just a century later.

The city had grown sevenfold. The distribution by age groups of the population in 1845 and 1945 is shown in Figure 21. The graph shows that the city, once composed of young, vigorous men, was now staid, and well past middle age. The Boston of 1845 was not only made up of young people, but they had large families. Males greatly outnumbered females; most of these young men were recent immigrants from Ireland. The birth rate was very high with a correspondingly high death rate and a shocking infant mortality rate. The maternal mortality rate was a tragedy. In the slums of the city, Shattuck says the birth rate was over 60 per 1,000 population, and the infant death rate was estimated to be between 300 and 400. In the immigrant section, he estimated that one mother in 37 died from childbirth.

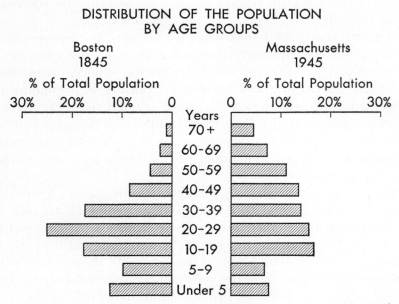

DISTRIBUTION OF THE POPULATION BY AGE GROUPS

Fig. 21. Distribution of the population by age groups. This graph shows preponderance of the younger age groups in the population a century ago. Data for 1845 from Lemuel Shattuck's *Census of Boston*. Data for 1945 from the Massachusetts State Board of Health's annual report. (Compilation from Smillie, W. G.: "Lemuel Shattuck—Still a Prophet," *Am. J. Pub. Health*, **39:**135, [Feb.] 1949.)

We have tabulated the important causes of death in 1845 and, insofar as possible, have compared them with similar causes of death in Boston in 1945 (see Figure 22). The striking features of this chart are:

1. The high prevalence of communicable diseases.
2. The heavy toll in 1845 from tuberculosis.
3. The seriousness of scarlet fever.
4. The absence of degenerative diseases as leading causes of death.

The terminology of 1845 is somewhat obscure. The term "diseases of the bowels" includes for the most part typhoid fever and bacillary dysentery, but excludes inflammation of the bowels (appendicitis).

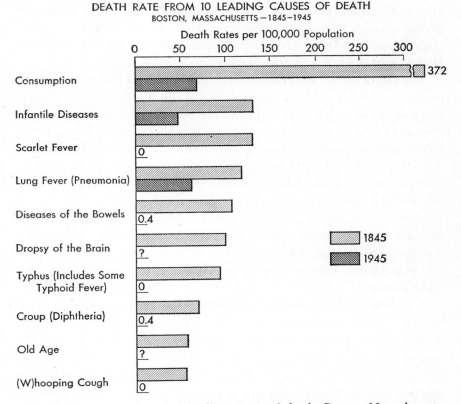

DEATH RATE FROM 10 LEADING CAUSES OF DEATH
BOSTON, MASSACHUSETTS — 1845–1945

Fig. 22. Death rate from ten leading causes of death, Boston, Massachusetts, 1845-1945. This graph shows an almost entire disappearance in 1945 of the important causes of death 100 years ago. Data from Lemuel Shattuck's *Census of Boston,* 1845, and the Massachusetts State Board of Health's annual report, 1945. (Compilation from Smillie, W. G.: "Lemuel Shattuck—Still a Prophet," *Am. J. Pub. Health,* 39:135, [Feb.] 1949.)

Dropsy of the brain or hydrocephalus, which is given as an important cause of death, is described by Thacher[14] as "a very serious disease of childhood, commencing suddenly, and terminating fatally in a very few days. Such is the ambiguity of its symptoms that it is difficult to determine what are its real characteristics. The indis-

[14] Thacher, James: *American Modern Practice,* or *A Simple Method of Prevention and Cure of Diseases.* Cottons & Barnard, Boston, 1826.

position of the child is sometimes attributed to teething or to a disordered state of the bowels. Frequently it resembles the common febrile complaints of childhood."

This disease dropped out of the nomenclature within a few years. It was like the "hives," which was frequently given as a cause of illness even as late as our own generation. If the child had a fever with a rash, it was the "hives";[15] without a rash, it was "inward hives." If the child died, it had "the bold hives."

The physicians of the community were not interested in preventive medicine, but confined themselves to the treatment of disease. Doctors were numerous. In the classification of occupations in Shattucks's *Census of Boston* of 1845, there were 680 persons in the city of 114,000 population whose occupation "contributed to health." This list included, of course, some auxiliary professions, such as sextons, undertakers, botanic medicine dealers, leechers (fifteen— all women), and one electrician. But there were 236 bona fide doctors, 169 druggists, and 57 dentists. Ninety women were classified as nurses, all of course with practical training only. Ten of the doctors were women. Thus, the medical profession, in proportion to the population, outnumbered the physicians of Boston today. But what doctors!

It must be remembered that there were few restrictions on medical practice. Physicians were trained by studying with another doctor as praeceptor. Formal medical training consisted of a four months' course of lectures. With a few exceptions, the medical colleges were not under university auspices. A few leading doctors in any community would simply organize a medical school, give a series of lectures, and divide the fees. The American Medical Association was founded in 1847. Its original purpose was primarily to raise the educational and ethical standards of the medical profession, and to curb, in some degree, the disgraceful practices of badly trained, grossly unqualified physicians.

Medical research in all of America was practically nonexistent.[16] The American Association for the Advancement of Science was founded in 1848. But it was made up largely of geologists, with almost no physicians in its membership. (It is true that John Collins Warren, a surgeon of Boston, in 1837 had attended a meeting of the recently founded British Association for the Advancement of Science

---

[15] Rush states that "hives" was derived from "heaves," e.g., difficult and labored respiration due to laryngeal diphtheria.

[16] Wilbur, Cressy L.: *op. cit.*

in London and, on his return, agitated for a similar society in America, but to no avail.)

Shryock[17] states that in 1840 "medical research had not permeated even the best medical centers. The schools remained didactic, clinical teaching barely existed, and pathological investigation was sporadic." Samuel Jackson, commenting favorably upon the intensive medical research in Germany, added indignantly, "Not one man is now conducting similar studies in the United States."

Furthermore, scientific research was not fashionable. The commercial spirit pervaded the whole nation. Money was the goal of every man. It was the only criterion of success. The physician's only means of support was clinical practice, and there was little or no prestige in research. Those who might engage in clinical investigation as a primary pursuit were regarded by their fellows with scorn and suspicion, or at best as hare-brained eccentrics.

The average income of physicians was estimated in 1845 to be about $800 per annum, of which $600 was net profit. But a dollar in 1845 had greater purchasing power than a century later.

Jarvis,[18] a physician, wrote a series of articles in the *Atlantic Monthly* in 1869 on the "Increase in Human Life." He pointed out that a good mechanic in 1821 worked a full day to earn the equivalent of a bushel of wheat, whereas in 1861 he could earn a bushel of wheat in one-half day. By 1955 a skilled artisan could earn the equivalent of a bushel of wheat in about forty-eight minutes of an eight-hour day. Thus in 1848, as in 1955, the wages per hour of a skilled laborer were greater than the hourly rate of average annual income of a practicing physician.

Hospitals were for the poor. The Boston Dispensary had served for many years as a public clinic for the sick poor, and the Massachusetts General Hospital, in 1848 as in 1955, was one of the leading philanthropic hospitals of the nation. The concept was just emerging that the community is directly responsible for providing a municipal hospital for care of the sick poor, and a proposal had been advanced for establishment of the present Boston City Hospital. Treatment of mental disease had not been widely recognized as an official state responsibility.

In brief, the city of Boston in 1845, representing the more cultured portions of the United States, had no concept of community responsibility for the promotion of the public health.

[17] Shryock, R. H.: *American Medical Research*. The Commonwealth Fund, New York, 1947.
[18] Jarvis, Edward: "The Increase of Human Life," *Atlantic Monthly*, 1869.

CHAPTER 24. *The American Medical Association*[1]

THE PIONEER DAYS

A large amount of scientific work cannot justly be expected of the medical profession in a new country.

E. H. CLARK ET AL., *1876*

The American Medical Association was formed in 1847 as a nation-wide attempt to promote standards of medical education and to improve medical ethics.

At the end of the eighteenth century there were approximately 4,000 physicians practicing in the United States. About one in ten was a graduate of a well-qualified medical college. The remainder had received their training under the praeceptor system, often in a most haphazard manner.

An attempt was made to establish standards for medical practitioners in 1807. State medical societies were formed; these societies appointed "censors" who examined candidates for licenses to practice. A certificate of competence was given to successful candidates. The medical societies, beginning with the Medical Society of the County of New York and the Medical Society of Maryland, then established "proprietary" medical schools. Previously all American medical colleges had been established as an integral part of a university. Now proprietary medical schools, following the examples of New York and Maryland, began to sprout like mushrooms all over the nation. These schools, which were sponsored by local medical societies, shortened the lecture terms of training and eliminated preliminary educational requirements. Professorial chairs were sold to the highest bidder. The schools that offered a medical diploma with expenditure of the least amount of time and money attracted the largest student body.

[1] See Fishbein, Morris: *History of the American Medical Association, 1847 to 1947.* W. B. Saunders Co., Philadelphia and London, 1947.

During the period of 1830 to 1840 the number of medical schools in the nation doubled. The training consisted of two courses of lectures of sixteen weeks each (in the better schools), with variable periods of training under a praeceptor. The nation was expanding rapidly and a pioneer spirit prevailed, with little tendency to curtail individual initiative by restrictive legislation; .but it soon became apparent that the situation had become intolerable.

Attempts were made in 1835, without success, to call a convention of delegates from all the medical colleges. In 1839, in order to put some restrictions on the medical schools, another conference was planned, but it was not held. Finally on May 5, 1846, Dr. Nathan Smith Davis succeeded in calling a national convention of physicians in New York. As might have been anticipated, less than a third of the medical schools were represented by delegates. Nevertheless, an organization was formed which was called the "American Medical Association."

Dr. Davis presented a resolution calling for:

1. A longer course of instruction for medical students (six months a year for two years instead of four months.)
2. Sequence and grading in the curriculum.
3. Separation of teaching from licensing power.
4. Suitable preliminary preparation to be a requirement for entrance to a medical college.

The opposition to the association's program by existing medical colleges was very strong, and the association had a most stormy and tenuous existence during its early years.

Public health was an integral and important part of the association's program from the outset. Dr. John H. Griscom introduced a resolution, at its first meeting, that a committee be appointed to study the most efficient methods of registration of births, marriages, and deaths.

At the 1848 meeting a communication was sent from the Medical Department of the National Institute in Washington, D. C., and signed by Dr. James Wynne and Dr. John M. Thomas. These men informed the association that the National Institute had appointed a committee in 1845 to inquire into the "Sanitary Conditions of the United States." This committee had sent out questionnaires to physicians, but Dr. Wynne reported, rather pathetically, that two prominent causes retarded the work of the committee:

1. General apathy in the minds of medical men on the subject of hygiene.
2. The favorable opinion of everyone of the healthiness of his own particular locality.[2]

The committee quoted Dr. Southwood Smith's *First Report on the Committee on Large Towns* (England): . . . "no one will deny that deficient ventilation, improper drainage, accumulation of filth and scanty supply of water are predisposing causes to disease, and when conjoined, cannot fail to produce a high mortality."

The Memorandum of the National Institute recommended to the American Medical Association that:

1. A Permanent Committee on Hygiene be appointed in the association.
2. The various states should be urged to establish uniform systems for registration of births, deaths, and marriages.

This Memorandum was accepted and a committee established.

At this meeting of the American Medical Association in 1848, the first public health papers were presented. Two subjects were discussed:

The danger of coffee and tea in the diet of persons under the age of puberty.

The influence of the substitution of tea and coffee on the health of the laboring classes.

That same year the Committee on Practical Medicine discussed current epidemics, particularly typhus in the recently arrived immigrants. The cleanliness and good personal hygiene of the German immigrants were compared with the filth, carelessness, and ignorance of the Irish, and the correlation of filth and prevalence of typhus fever was noted. There was an interesting discussion of the differential diagnosis between typhoid and typhus fever; and epidemics of smallpox, dysentery, and measles were noted as important factors in the death toll of the immigrants.

The 1849 meeting of the association reported an epidemic of "angina." It was also stated that typhoid fever had raged during the year. Several epidemics of dysentery were mentioned. The analysis of

[2] A century later, their public health descendants who sent out comparable questionnaires on the sanitary condition of the various communities in the United States encountered exactly the same two "prominent retarding" factors.

the sanitary condition of several of the important cities was presented that year.

Daniel Drake received great acclaim at the meeting of 1850 for the publication of his extraordinarily comprehensive volume, *The Diseases of the Interior Valley of North America.* It was truly a great book and to this day remains a classic in medical ecology (see Chapter 11).

Nathan Davis spoke on the nutrition of childhood at the 1854 annual meeting. He emphasized the great value of pure and abundant milk, particularly for children, and demonstrated a specimen of "dried" milk. This is one of the earliest of all medical papers in American literature on child health promotion.

As one reviews the minutes of the annual meetings of the American Medical Association during its first two decades, it becomes quite clear that the life of the organization was a hazardous one, and its influence and leadership were most ineffective. Only a small fraction of the total roll of the medical profession was represented in its membership. Every effort was made to destroy it. The association's most bitter and violent opponent was the New York State Medical Society, with other local and state societies doing their best to break the national society. The ideals and stated purpose of the American Medical Association were to improve the quality of licensure throughout the land and to promote better medical teaching. This platform was a direct threat to powerful, well-entrenched, vested medical interests that were scattered throughout the nation. During the first quarter century of its existence, the association made such powerful enemies, and had so few adherents, that the general impression was created that even as late as 1870 it was "an utter and complete failure." It was not until the beginning of the twentieth century that the American Medical Association began to occupy its preeminent place as a representative medical institution in the social structure of America. Throughout its history it has been vitally interested in the promotion of the public health, and has been instrumental in initiating many of the reforms in the whole broad field of public health administration.

CHAPTER 25. *Sanitary Surveys*

Of removable causes of disease, the chief is uncleanliness.

JOHN SIMON, *1876*

In recent years the *sanitary survey* has become a most effective tool for the appraisal of existing public health facilities. More important still, it serves as an aid in planning for the existing activities and in initiating new health organizations and facilities. The sanitary survey is generally considered to be a modern innovation of public health practice, but it is not new. In fact, sanitary surveys were begun in America at least 150 years ago.

One of the earliest sanitary surveys of an American community was made in 1806 in New York by a citizens' committee.[1] John Pintard, Wynant van Zant, and Edward Miller made this report. Their recommendations were simple but sound. They reviewed the existing sanitary facilities of New York and recommended:

1. An ample supply of pure, potable water.
2. Construction of common sewers.
3. Drainage of low marshlands.
4. Construction of a masonry wall along the waterfront.
5. Proper interment of dead bodies within the city.
6. Planting of trees and healthy vegetables.
7. Prohibition of habitation in damp cellars.
8. Prohibition of the use of houses where "malignant fever" had occurred.
9. Provision for increased accommodations at Bellevue Hospital.
10. Erection of a private hospital for people of means.
11. Regulation of and quarantine of vessels from southern ports during July, August, and September.

---

[1] *Report of Citizens' Committee on the Sanitary Conditions of New York City* by John Pintard, Wynant van Zant, and Edward Miller, January 20, 1806.

The population of New York City in 1805 was estimated at 75,770, and it was increasing more rapidly than in any other city on the coast.

If the recommendations of this sensible public health report had been carried into effect, they would have resulted in an enormous saving of life, as well as the prevention of much serious illness during the coming years. For the most part the recommendations were ignored, and the improvements that were suggested were not initiated for many years to come.

The National Institute in Washington, which was a distinguished scientific body, had a medical department. In 1845 this department organized a hygiene committee. For several years this committee attempted unsuccessfully to make surveys of the nation's health. When the American Medical Association was founded in 1847, the National Institute requested that the association establish a hygiene committee. A Memorial,[2] signed by James Wynne and John M. Thomas, was addressed to the founders of the American Medical Association. These men suggested that a hygiene committee of the association, if formed, should make every effort toward the establishment by the various states of a uniform system for the registration of births, deaths, and marriages. The memorandum also indicated the importance of making studies of existing sanitary conditions in selected communities. It stated:

The United States may be considered as a country in which no legislation exists, regulating its sanitary condition. The densely populated cities present the greatest complication of sanitary evils.

The National Institute indulges in the hope that under the auspices of the American Medical Association, the sanitary condition of the nation may be fully developed, human life prolonged, and the desolations of disease curtailed.

This hope was more than realized, for the American Medical Association took an active part in health promotion during the following years and was one of the strong forces in securing better methods for recording of vital data and in promotion of the public health.

The Hygiene Committee of the American Medical Association was formed in 1848, and during the following year it conducted an active campaign to secure sanitary surveys in various parts of the nation. The very next year we find, in the second volume of the

[2] "Memorial to the American Medical Association from the National Institute of Washington," *Tr. Am. M. A.,* Baltimore, 1848.

Transactions of the American Medical Association,[3] the report of this committee on these matters. At this meeting, which was held in Boston, there were reports on the sanitary conditions of Concord, New Hampshire; Portland, Maine; Philadelphia; Boston; Baltimore; Charleston, South Carolina; New Orleans; Louisville; and Cincinnati.

The data that were collected were simple but important and fairly uniform:

1. Population.
2. Prevalence of disease.
3. Drainage.
4. Street cleaning.
5. Ventilation in densely populated zones; in houses and in overcrowded tenements.
6. Sanitation of schools.
7. Hospitals and dispensaries.
8. Source of the town's water supply.
9. Effective municipal regulations relating to the above subjects.

The physicians who made the reports had little valid information concerning the prevalence of disease, but each attempted to show that his community was more healthy than others and relatively free from hazards. Even the physicians from New Orleans, a city with a very high death rate, felt that "their City [was] fair, and free from undue illness." We now have every reason to believe that this appraisal was heavily weighted by local pride and patriotism.

One of the best of the early community surveys was made in 1845 by John H. Griscom[4] of New York. He pointed out that the crude death rate per annum in New York in 1810 was one death per 46.5 persons. At the time of his report the rate had risen to one death per 27 persons. The fundamental cause of the increase was a high infant death rate in the slums of the city. Twenty per cent of the total mortality occurred in infants under one year of age. Dr. Griscom outlined certain objectives of public health which were good foundation stones for future workers:

[3] See *Transactions of the American Medical Association*, Vol. II, Boston, 1849. The early *Transactions of the American Medical Association* contain a wealth of information concerning the existing health organizations in various parts of the nation. Vol. VIII is of particular interest.

[4] Griscom, John H.: *The Sanitary Condition of the Laboring Population of New York City*. Harper & Co., New York, 1845. (Note the influence of Chadwick in the title.)

1. There is an immense amount of sickness, physical disability and premature mortality among the poorer classes.
2. These conditions are unnecessary, being, to a great degree, removable.
3. These physical evils are productive of moral evils of great magnitudes and numbers which if considered only from a pecuniary point of view, should arouse the government and individuals to the best means for their relief and prevention.
4. The objectives of public health are to suggest means for alleviating these evils and preventing these menaces to a great extent.

The Shattuck report, which was published in 1850, was initiated as a sanitary survey of the state of Massachusetts. Shattuck took this opportunity to formulate a program of adequate health service for the state and to develop his philosophy of public health, but in reality the state legislature had appropriated and designated the funds "to prepare and report to the next General Court, a plan for a Sanitary Survey of the State."[5] The appendix of this famous report does contain sanitary surveys of Franklin County and of the towns of Lawrence, Attleborough, Plympton, and Lynn, and the early part of the report contains some information on the sanitary conditions of Boston. The report itself, although it is not a sanitary survey, is of such fundamental importance that it will be reviewed in detail in a subsequent chapter (see Chapter 27).

The American Public Health Association has developed the sanitary survey to a high degree of efficiency. The traditions of this association, in the initiation of sanitary survey schedules, are based on a report[6] of a committee that was appointed at the first meeting of the association. John S. Billings was chairman. This report by Dr. Billings presented at the outset the sanitary survey schedules that had been first drawn up by the Hygiene Committee of the American Medical Association in 1848. He noted that the state medical societies undertook to collect the data that were required for these reports, but they were quite unsuccessful. He emphasized the point that "a comprehensive sanitary survey of a state probably will never be accomplished by a state medical society." The Billings committee presented a list of schedules which are given below. If

[5] *Report of a General Plan for the Promotion of Public and Personal Health* by the Commissioners appointed under a Resolve of the Legislature of Massachusetts, Boston, 1850.

[6] "Report of Committee on the Plan for a Systematic Sanitary Survey of the United States," *Reports and Papers of the American Public Health Association for the Years 1874 and 1875*, Vol. 2, p. 41.

the data were carefully collected, these schedules might serve today as an excellent outline for a community-wide sanitary survey.

SANITARY SURVEY SCHEDULES[7]

1875

Location, population, and climate
Topography
Water supply
Drainage and sewerage
Streets and public grounds
Habitations
Gas and lighting
Garbage and excreta
Markets
Slaughterhouses
Manufactories and trades
Public schools
Hospitals and public charities
Police and prisons
Fire protection
Cemeteries
Public health regulations
Registration of births and deaths and statistics of disease
Quarantine

THE PRACTICING PHYSICIAN AND COMMUNITY SURVEYS: AN EARLY CONCEPT

Dr. Edward Jarvis, an eminent Boston physician once said (in about 1845): "Our education [as physicians] has made our calling exclusively a curative and not a conservative one, and the business of our responsible lives has confined us to it. Our thoughts are devoted to, our interests are concerned in, and our employments are connected solely with, sickness, debility or injury—with diminution of life in some of its forms. But with health, with fullness of unalloyed, unimpaired life, we professionally have nothing to do."[8]

It is quite true that throughout the nineteenth century and down through the early part of the twentieth, the dictum of Jarvis held firm. Physicians showed little concern for the public health. For the

[7] Prepared under the direction of the American Public Health Association, 1875. See Vol. 2, p. 44, *Reports and Papers* of that association.

[8] Jarvis, Edward: *Communications*, Massachusetts Medical Society, Vol. VIII, p. 1, 1847.

most part, a physician who took an active part in public health matters—and particularly a doctor who became a health officer of his community or even a school physician—was regarded by his colleagues as a peculiar person, probably a failure in practice, or an idealist without proper perspective. Only very recently has it been considered at all respectable for a physician to associate himself with public health affairs. Thus it is most refreshing to learn that, even before the middle of the nineteenth century, some of the more far-sighted physicians had begun to appreciate the fact that the physician has a specific community responsibility in health promotion.

Dr. John Fisher[9] in 1848 made a most interesting and important address to the Massachusetts Medical Society. He pointed out the fact that when the Society was chartered in 1781, it assumed an obligation to promote the *public health,* "which is essential to the happiness of society."

He also pointed out that the members of the society had been remiss in this matter. Physicians had devoted themselves entirely to the study of the cure of disease, and had done nothing to determine the agents which produce disease; in other words, to study their prevention. He stressed the interesting fact that American physicians were not in a position to rival their European brothers in a study of the pathology or the treatment of disease, but a newly settled country such as America offered an ideal situation to study the *causes* of disease. "We have ceased to believe that diseases come from mysterious causes, from a capricious Providence or represent the judgments of Heaven, and acknowledge that they have their origin in the influence of the elements, in constitutions and habits, and in the use we make of our organs and functions."

He suggested that a general form be prepared by the Massachusetts Medical Society on which could be compiled essential statistical data that would be furnished by the members. These data would be related to deaths, as correlated with certain environmental factors. For example, the topography and physical characteristics of every district and town should be recorded, with elevation, type of soil, drainage, wind exposure, and so on. The character and habits of the people in relation to disease prevalence should be noted. The domestic and social conditions of the family, and the intelligence and degree of education of parents should be recorded also.

[9] Fisher, John: *Transactions of the Massachusetts Medical Society,* 1848.

Dr. Fisher cited certain data which relate to occupation and its influence on the death rates. He presented the following table:

Table 11

The Average Age of Death in Certain Trades in 1847*

	NUMBER OF MEN	AGE AT DEATH (YEARS)
Blacksmiths	35	39
Carpenters	99	48
Shoemakers	118	48
Farmers	703	65

* SOURCE: *Tr. Massachusetts M. Soc.*, 1848.

He showed that poverty bore a direct relationship to the life span. The average length of life in a family in different occupations, including father, mother, and the children was:

1. Laborers, fishermen, journeymen, mechanics, and factory workers: twenty-seven years, five months.
2. Merchants, capitalists, salaried and professional men: thirty-three years, two months.
3. Farmers who owned and cultivated their land: forty-five years, eight months.

This is a most original and advanced concept of the influence of social and environmental factors on illness. More advanced still was Dr. Fisher's suggestion that the practicing physician should not only observe these matters but record them for purposes of statistical compilation and analysis. This concept was a great credit to its author and to the group that he addressed.

The reporting of births and deaths by physicians was soon to become a general practice in Massachusetts, but the reporting of occupational disease was postponed for over half a century. The inclusion of social and economic data on the death certificates was not initiated for years to come. But the seed was sown, even though it would not germinate for many a season.

CHAPTER 26. *The Awakening of Public Health in Europe*

ITS INFLUENCE UPON AMERICA

Persistence in sanitary reform in spite of absence of epidemics is the only test of the enlightenment of the reformer.

STANFORD E. CHAILLÉ, *1829*

GERMANY

Johann Peter Frank (1745-1821) is the true founder of modern public health in Europe. He was a man with great independence of thought. Early in his medical career he became imbued with the idea that the state has a definite responsibility for the promotion of the health of its citizens. His ideas are contained in *A Complete System of Police Medicine,* which was published in a series of volumes between 1779 and 1817. This monumental task covered every phase of man's life. Frank's concepts were far ahead of his time. He was interested in general sanitation, as well as housing and municipal planning. He realized the importance of sewage disposal and a pure water supply. He also considered in his text the whole broad field of child hygiene, school health, and nutrition. He gave particular attention to the composition of school lunches. His interest in hospital organization was profound and his discussions on the subject of comprehensive medical care, as well as personal hygiene and environmental sanitation, are quite in line with our present thinking.

Frank had little influence beyond Germany and Austria. Great Britain did not feel the impact of his advanced social concepts except in a most indirect way. Certainly the physicians of North America were unaware of his existence. Apparently those of our countrymen who were interested in the social and economic developments of America did not read German.

FRANCE

France, at the beginning of the nineteenth century, organized a very interesting system of health administration, which has extended its influence down to the present day. The key to this organization was a semiofficial body called the Council of Health, *Conseil de Salubrité*. The first council was organized in Paris in 1802. The members of the council were appointed by the government for a term of years, and the position, though it carried no pay, was considered to be one of great honor. The council acted purely in an advisory capacity. It was held in high esteem and its decisions had almost the force of law. The duty of the council was to study the problems that were assigned to it by government. A careful investigation was made of each question and a report was prepared, with suitable recommendations as to the action that should be taken. The administrative body then carried those recommendations into effect. The Paris Council made annual reports from 1803 to 1828. After some delay, a general report was published covering the years 1828 to 1839, and in 1847 another general report was issued covering the years 1840 to 1845.

This plan of organization was extended to the whole of the country. France was divided into 86 departments, which were subdivided into 363 *arrondissements*. Each of the latter had a council of public health, which was made up of from seven to fourteen persons. Each member was selected by the prefect for four years. In the provinces, the position was also one of great honor, and carried no salary. This type of health organization had much to recommend it, but was not adopted by Great Britain, nor the United States.

GREAT BRITAIN

England, although traditionally our enemy and oppressor, continued to have the closest bonds of common interest with North America, despite differences in political policy and despite a mutual lack of understanding, with resultant continuous minor frictions which sometimes threatened to break into open and serious quarrels. But American culture was basically English, notwithstanding the enormous migration of Germans during the early part of the nineteenth century, and despite our long and close political friendship with France. One of the chief reasons that we looked to, and depended upon, England for our cultural advancement was that we used the same language and thus could read the books and current literature of that country. In retrospect, it now becomes quite clear that the social and scientific advances in the United States during the nineteenth century were derived, in great part at least, from English sources.

Public health administration in England in 1800 was primitive and fragmentary. For the most part it consisted of boards of health which were selected from time to time for the purpose of controlling epidemics.

Fevers, as such, were not dealt with preventively, only epidemics. Each epidemic was a tragedy. When it was played out, all properties were dispersed and the stage left unfurnished. The usual course of events was first the occurrence of an epidemic with its rapid extension; then public excitement; public meetings, followed by the appointment of a "Fever Committee" or "a Board of Health." Then came the collection of funds, a rushing about for sites for temporary hospitals, attendants for home care, the organization of a staff of fumigators, etc. Then, in due time, the disease began to decline, the pesthouses were pulled down, and the nurses, doctors and attendants who had not been buried were paid off. A report by the Board of Health or the Committee was made of receipts and disbursements, and then the Board of Health ceased to function. The play was over.[1]

The initial steps in the formation of a sound public health service were taken through a fortuitous circumstance, namely, the intellectual curiosity of a young law student.

Edwin Chadwick (1800-1890)

Chadwick, a young student in London, was preparing to become a barrister. In his casual reading he encountered a report by the government actuary which stated that, in spite of improvement of the conditions of life in the middle class in England, there had occurred no corresponding improvement in life expectation of this group. Chadwick did not believe this statement and, more or less for his own intellectual amusement, he made suitable mathematical calculations, which proved that the actuary was wrong. Chadwick published his results in 1828 in the *Westminster Review*. His article was entitled "Essay on the Means of Insurance against Casualties of Sickness, Decrepitude and Mortality." This little essay has been called the "foundation of sanitary science" in England. The reason

---

[1] Russell, James: *Evolution of Sanitary Administration in Glasgow,* 1905.

that this study is of such fundamental importance is that it stimulated Chadwick to take an interest in measures which might be used for control of disease and death.

In 1829 Chadwick published an article in the *London Review* on "Preventive Police." This concept undoubtedly was derived from Johann Frank of Germany. That same year Chadwick wrote a review of "The Public Charities of France."

This latter article was read by England's great philosopher and sociologist, Jeremy Bentham, who was then eighty-two years old. He asked Chadwick to live in his home and to give him assistance with *The Administrative Code*. When Bentham died, he left Chadwick a legacy. This chain of circumstances launched the young barrister on his great career as founder of modern public health in Great Britain. In addition it may also be said that he initiated public health in America, for the simple reason that Shattuck derived a great deal of his inspiration from Chadwick and his associates.

Chadwick was appointed Poor Law Commissioner in 1832 and was selected as a member of a Commission on Factory Inspection in 1833. Here began his first conflict with vested interests, since he tried to secure more favorable working hours for factory workers and particularly for children who labored in the textile mills and the collieries.

The Poor Law was passed in 1835, and, though it had great imperfections, it "saved the nation from social disaster."

The Birth and Death Registration Act, in which Chadwick was much interested, was passed in 1836, and at this time Dr. William Farr was appointed Compiler of Abstracts. This was a most fortunate selection, as will soon become apparent.

In 1842 Chadwick published his great classic, *General Report on the Sanitary Condition of the Labouring Population of Great Britain.*

This remarkable volume first considered the prevalence of epidemic, endemic, and contagious diseases among the laboring people. Chadwick was able to show that the poor people of Great Britain suffered from disease and disability to a much greater degree than the well-to-do. His conclusion was that the abject misery of the working people was due in great part to the unsanitary environment in which they dwelt. In that period of scientific thought, disease was believed to be due to miasmata and to bad odors of any and all types. Thus, very serious consideration was given to street cleaning, to drainage, and to disposal of human and manufacturing wastes, as well as debris from pigsties and other animal refuse. Housing for the poor was a matter of great importance. The report covered the whole question of overcrowding of the poor and of ventilation requirements for bedrooms, workshops, and the like.

Chadwick buttressed his arguments with a careful study of vital statistics, and he calculated the life span of various social groups. He showed the actual cost to the nation of the neglect of sanitation measures, and he proved beyond question that preventive medicine raises the standards of health of the people. He brought out the important point that the employer of labor can play a critical role in promoting the health of his employees, and outlined suitable legislation for a well-balanced health service. It is a great book.

Chadwick was quite aggressive as a member of the Poor Law Board and made many antagonists. He was not a tactful man. He had a direct and outspoken manner and a burning zeal for social reform, together with a great desire to get things accomplished. These are splendid qualities, but they did not always win him complete accord and sympathy.

The Poor Law Board was dissolved in 1844 and the first true Board of Health was established in 1848, with three commissioners, namely, Lord Carlysle, Lord Shaftesbury, and Mr. Chadwick. The following year Dr. Southwood Smith, the great epidemiologist, was appointed as a medical adviser. The board lasted only five years. Chadwick was, in fact, the Board of Health. He was accused of being most forceful and dictatorial. He made thousands of enemies, particularly among vested interests. He had no conciliation in his make-up and no compromise—so that he became the "best-abused" man in all England. He was retired at the age of fifty-four with a government pension of 1,000 pounds. But his work was done, and so well done, and his theories were so sound, that his co-workers were able to carry on from the point where he left off, without serious setback.

William Farr (1807-1883)

As we have already indicated, William Farr was another of the "giants that walked the land" in the development of public health in England. His parents were very poor, and he was adopted by a village philanthropist, Mr. Pryce. The young Farr began his medical practice in 1833. He wrote a series of lectures on public health which he called the science of "hygiology," but could obtain no opportunity to deliver them to students. They were finally published in the *Lancet* in 1835. His ability as a medical writer led to his appointment as joint editor of the *British Annals of Medicine* in 1837, and this same year he wrote an important treatise on "Methods for Determining the Duration of Diseases at Every Period of their Progress."

When the Birth and Death Registration Act was passed in 1838, he was the logical person to be selected as Compiler of Abstracts of the Registrar General's Office. The first annual report was published in 1841.

One must give complete credit to Dr. Farr as the founder of Great Britain's national system of vital statistics. He dwelt continually upon the necessity for (1) exactness of diagnosis of causes of death and (2) precision in nomenclature. He became the foremost expert of the whole world in vital statistics. He traveled to all parts of Europe and was widely recognized as an author and speaker. But he never became Registrar General. When his superior, Major Graham, retired from the Registrar General's Office in 1880, Farr, though quite old, expected that he would be given the appointment, at least for a few years. He was not selected, and in great disappointment, he resigned his office and retired.

John Simon (1816-1904)

Chadwick was the great pioneer of public health in England, but John Simon was the administrator who carried those early concepts of Chadwick into execution.

Simon was brilliant almost to the point of precocious genius. He came from a wealthy family and had every educational advantage. He was made a Fellow of the Royal Society at twenty-nine years of age. In 1847 he published an article, "On the Aims and Philosophic Method of Pathological Research," in which he pointed out the great significance to society of the science of preventive medicine. In 1848 he became Medical Officer of Health of London. In this capacity he demonstrated great administrative talent.

As we have already noted, the Board of Health was established in 1848, and this board, which was, in its essence, Chadwick, came to an end in 1854. It was terminated largely because the House of Commons became so irritated by Chadwick's masterful and uncompromising policies that it refused to continue his work. Simon, for one, fully recognized Chadwick's contributions to English public health, for he says in his *English Sanitary Institutions:*

Mr. Chadwick, beyond any man of his time, knew what large fresh additions of human misery were accruing day by day under the almost universal prevalence of sanitary neglect, and the indignation he was entitled to feel at the spectacle of so much needless human suffering is not an ignoble excuse for such signs of over-eagerness as he may have shown.

But Simon was a tactful man and an excellent administrator. He carried on where Chadwick left off. He continued his labors as Medical Officer of Health from 1855 to 1872.

He was one of the founders of the Epidemiological Society in 1850. In 1856 he issued reports on the epidemics of cholera of 1848 and 1853 and showed the relation of the disease to polluted water supplies. He was able to prove that those communities with the best water supply had the least cholera. In 1857 he wrote the "History and Practice of Vaccination" and in 1858 he wrote the "Sanitary State of the People of England." He made an industrial hygiene report in 1862, giving special consideration to the dangers of lead, mercury, arsenic, and phosphorus to the industrial workers. His survey of hospitals was completed in 1863 and the article on "Housing of the Poor" in 1864.

When the decision came to amalgamate the Health Department with the Poor Law Board in 1871, Sir John Simon was made Chief Medical Officer. He realized all the pitfalls of this type of organization and was sure that the government was taking a retrograde step. As he had anticipated, the Medical Department was placed in a subordinate position under the Poor Law staff. Funds for public health were cut, and opportunities were lost to develop an efficient public health service. He became embittered and disillusioned, retiring from the service in 1876.

Southwood Smith (1788-1861)

Smith was the fourth man of outstanding stature in the foundation of British public health. He has received less acclaim than his fellows, but in many ways he was the most farsighted of all. He was an epidemiologist.

In 1830, as a physician in the London Fever Hospital, he called public attention to bad environment as an important cause in the production of fevers. He investigated working conditions of factory

laborers in 1832, and, as a result, a regulation requiring factory inspection was passed. Southwood Smith made his report on "Physical
Causes of Sickness and Mortality" in 1838, and that same year he
made a report on "Prevalence of Fever in Twenty Metropolitan
Parishes." In 1840 he was appointed as a member of a commission to
inquire into employment of children of the poorer classes in mines
and collieries, as well as in other various branches of trade. He made
a report in 1841 on the "Physical Aspects of Child Labor" and in
1842 on the "Moral Aspects of Child Labor." An abridged combined report was issued in 1843. When the National Board of Health
was founded in 1848, three commissioners were selected, two lords
and a barrister. Obviously, medical advice was needed to enable
the board to function properly. The most logical choice was Southwood Smith. He was appointed and served with great distinction.

His whole philosophy of life was condensed in his Edinburgh
lecture of 1855 on "The Common Nature of Epidemics."[2] In many
of its aspects this lecture had the characteristics of an address of a
public health leader of 1955—100 years later.

His thesis was that "epidemics are under our own control; we
may promote their spread; we may prevent it. We may secure ourselves from them. We have done so. We have banished the most
formidable."

Then, almost as though he were paraphrasing an address of one
of his colleagues-to-be of 1955, he summarized the achievements of
his generation. They were truly phenomenal.

He emphasized the disappearance of plague, greatest destroyer
of all, and then pointed out the practical disappearance of typhus
from London. Remittent fever, which killed both James I and Oliver
Cromwell, had gone from London. "Though it still exists in fenny
and marshy places, no single case of Ague has occurred in our Fever
Hospital since 1825." There had been a marked reduction in "Pneumonia, Peripneumonia and Rheumatic Fever" as causes of illness
and death.

The mortality rates for England and Wales were compared with
the rates for London. The great city, notorious as a pesthole of
filth, iniquity, plague, and death, had grown, through the years, to a
relative state of salubrity (see Table 12).

[2] This lecture together with other writings and official reports are contained in one
small volume. *The Common Nature of Epidemics,* by Southwood Smith, M.D.,
published in Philadelphia by J. B. Lippincott Co. in 1866. The subsequent references
in this chapter are taken from this book.

Table 12

Mortality in England and Wales, Compared with the City of London*
Rate per Annum

YEAR	ENGLAND AND WALES		LONDON	
	RATIO	PER 1,000 POPULATION	RATIO	PER 1,000 POPULATION
1700	1-39	25.6	1-25	40.0
1750	1-40	25.0	1-21	47.6
1801	1-44	22.7	1-35	28.5
1810	1-49	20.2	1-38	26.3
1830	1-58	17.2	1-45	22.2

* SOURCE: Smith, Southwood: *op. cit.*, p. 52.

He compared the life expectation of those living in the best localities with those living in the worst. "Of the children born in the best part of a town one-fifth die before they attain the fifth year; of the children born in the worst, one-half die before they attain their fifth year."

A survey of Surrey, with excellent environmental conditions, showed a life expectation at birth of fifty-three years, whereas in Liverpool it was twenty-six years. Another method of expressing the same situation may be presented from his figures[3] in the following striking way:

	NUMBER OF BABIES BORN	NUMBER LIVING		
		10 YRS. LATER	50 YRS. LATER	70 YRS. LATER
Surrey	100,000	75,423	52,000	28,878
Liverpool	100,000	48,211	25,875	8,373

Southwood Smith believed that public health is a manifestation of civilization, and proceeded to define what he meant by civilization. It was a good, comfortable definition that perhaps only an Englishman could make. Despite its limitations, it has the ring of sincerity and of complete and solid assurance.

In the eyes of Southwood Smith, the essential elements of civilization are:

1. A sovereign authority.
2. Laws incorruptibly administered.
3. Physical comfort generally diffused.

[3] *Ibid.*, pp. 55-56.

4. Intellectual development and activity generally diffused.
5. A recognition of the fundamental principles of religion and morality.

Without the first two he believed there is no security of life or property. "They are the base of the pyramid of a civilized society."

He then outlined a plan for the practical application of the advantages of civilization to the poor people of the community. His program of community sanitation is an excellent one.

1. Subsoil drainage of the building site.
2. Free admission of light and air to each inhabited room.
3. Abolition of cesspools, involving complete and adequate house drainage.
4. Abundant water supply, and immediate removal by it of all refuse which it can hold in suspension.
5. Means of removal of house refuse.

These few requirements were to him the essentials of a healthy environment for satisfactory home and community life. The concluding words of his lecture are so sincere and fine that they must be given in their entirety.

Lastly, we see the first step that must be taken to elevate the people: nay, even to bring them within the pale of the civilization already attained. We must improve their sanitary condition. Until this is done, no civilizing influence can touch them. The schoolmaster will labour in vain; the minister of religion will labour in vain; neither can make any progress in the fulfilment of their mission in a den of filth. Moral purity is incompatible with bodily impurity. Moral degradation is indissolubly united with physical squalor. The depression and discomfort of the hovel produce and foster obtuseness of mind, hardness of heart, selfish and sensual indulgence, violence, and crime. It is the Home that makes the man; it is the home that educates the family. It is the distinction and the curse of Barbarism that it is without a home; it is the distinction and the blessing of Civilization that it prepares a home in which Christianity may abide, and guide, and govern.[4]

The four men, Chadwick, Farr, Simon, and Southwood Smith, had a profound influence upon the development of public health and preventive medicine in the United States. Not one of the four ever visited America. In their writings not one of them gave this

[4] Smith, Southwood: *op. cit.,* p. 60.

country more than casual attention. They were completely preoccupied with the special tasks that they were called upon to perform. Their devotion was for England and for her dependencies. But their publications were read widely in America and their ideas gained acceptance and support.

From his own reports, we learn that Lemuel Shattuck derived a great deal of his inspiration from these four men. Certainly he followed their procedures in making his preliminary sanitary surveys and in the compilation of his famous reports. All unknown to themselves, the founders of modern public health in Great Britain were, at the same time, initiating an equally valuable health service across the Atlantic in the faraway, formerly rebellious, and notoriously uncultured colony of America.

The author is greatly indebted to M. E. M. Walker, author of *Pioneers of Public Health*, published by The Macmillan Company, New York, in 1930 for authentic biographical information concerning Drs. Chadwick, Farr, and Simon. For additional references, the reader is referred to the bibliography that follows.

BIBLIOGRAPHY

Chadwick, Edwin: *General Report on the Sanitary Condition of the Labouring Population of Great Britain,* from the Poor Law Commissioners. W. Clowes & Sons, London, 1842.

————: *Sanitary Inquiry Report,* supplement to *Interment in Towns.* W. Clowes & Sons, London, 1843.

Newman, Sir George: *The Rise of Preventive Medicine.* Oxford University Press, London, 1932.

Quarantine Act of 1825. London.

Report of the Sanitary Commission of Massachusetts, 1849 (the "Shattuck Report"). Dutton & Wentworth, Boston, 1850.

Smith, Joseph Mather: *The Etiology and Philosophy of Epidemics.* J. and J. Harper, 1824.

Smith, Southwood: *The Common Nature of Epidemics.* J. B. Lippincott Co., Philadelphia, 1866.

CHAPTER 27. *The Shattuck Report*

> *It is the duty of the State to extend over the people its guardian care, that those who cannot or will not protect themselves, may nevertheless be protected; and that those who can and desire to do it, may have the means of doing it more easily. This right and authority should be exercised by wise laws, wisely administered; and when this is neglected the State should be held answerable for the consequences of this neglect.*
>
> LEMUEL SHATTUCK, *1850*

The cornerstone of the splendid edifice of public health of the nation was laid in 1850 with the publication of the *Report of the Sanitary Commission of Massachusetts,* commonly called the "Shattuck Report."[1]

Lemuel Shattuck[2] was born in Ashby, Massachusetts, in 1793, and died in Boston in 1859. His parents were farmers. He had a very limited formal education, but through self-education he qualified himself as a schoolteacher and went West to the frontier town of Detroit about 1818 to teach in the district schools. He became interested at once in community welfare.

He organized there, in the fastness of that great wilderness, the first Sunday school in the state of Michigan, and was its superintendent for four years. He returned to the East, married, and settled in Concord. Here he ran a general store for some ten years.

As a member of the school committee in Concord, he reorganized the public school system of the town, and was active in the community affairs.

In 1833 he moved to Boston and entered the book-publishing and book-selling business. He became a member of the city council and

---

[1] *Report of the Sanitary Commission of Massachusetts—1849,* by the Commissioners appointed under a Resolve of the Legislature of Massachusetts. Dutton & Wentworth, Boston, 1850. Reprinted 1948 by the Harvard University Press.

[2] Walker, M. E. M.: *Pioneers of Public Health.* The Macmillan Co., New York, 1930.

took an important part in the long controversy over the introduction of pure water into the city.

Shattuck's interest in vital statistics was aroused through his initial interest in genealogy. He attempted to collect accurate data for the history of his own family, and in 1835 he wrote a *History of the Town of Concord*. Finding great confusion and inadequacy in the church records of births and deaths, he began a personal and almost solitary campaign to obtain the official recording of vital data in Massachusetts. In 1842 he was successful in securing the passage of an act for a registration system of vital statistics for Massachusetts, which became a model for all other states. Since there was no state board of health, the act provided that the returns should be made to the secretary of state. This plan remained in effect in Massachusetts for over 100 years.

The report of the census of the city of Boston[3] in 1845 was a precursor of his more famous report of 1850, but in many ways it is equally important, for in it one can obtain a very clear picture of the economic and social conditions of that day.

As we have noted in Chapter 23, the city of Boston, which in 1845 represented the more cultured portions of the United States, had no concept of community responsibility for the promotion of the public health. There was no permanent local or state department of health. Communicable disease took an enormous toll, particularly in the early decades of life. There was no real understanding of the epidemiology of infectious diseases, and methods of control were primitive and ineffectual. Official registration of vital data had just been introduced, but reporting of contagion was not established. Physicians were poorly trained, with no interest whatever in public health or preventive medicine. Medical research, in fact all scientific research, was nonexistent. Some attempts were made to provide for the general sanitation of the city under official auspices, but the relation of the basic factors in environmental sanitation to prevention of illness was poorly understood.

It was in this completely inhospitable environment that Shattuck compiled his report of 1850. He was actively opposed by physicians, as well as by his peers in the legislature. Bowditch noted[4] (in 1876), "I remember Mr. Shattuck well. Calm in his perfect confidence in

[3] Shattuck, Lemuel: *Census of Boston* (Report to the Committee of the City Council), 1845.

[4] Bowditch, Henry I.: "Public Hygiene in America," *Proc. Internat. M. Cong.*, Philadelphia, 1876.

the future of preventive medicine to check disease, he walked almost alone the streets of his [native] city, not only unsustained by the medical profession but considered by most of them an offense for his earnest advocacy of what seemed to the majority of physicians to be out of a layman's sphere, and withal of trifling moment, compared with the importance of our usual routine of practice. The public, ignorant of hygiene, treated him no better."

One can readily discern the source of Shattuck's stimulus. He was an omnivorous reader, and his interest in vital statistics led him inevitably to study the pioneer activities of another layman, Chadwick of London, the founder of sanitary science in England. Chadwick published his famous *General Report on the Sanitary Condition of the Labouring Population of Great Britain* in 1842. Shattuck was familiar also with the work of the great British vital statistician, William Farr, and drew many of his ideas and much of his inspiration from Southwood Smith and John Simon. The list of books which Shattuck recommended for sanitary libraries and which is appended to the 1850 report, shows clearly that he was quite familiar with the advances in sanitary knowledge that had occurred during the recent years in Europe, and particularly in France, Germany, and England. From these sources of information and methods of procedure, he drew the inspiration to write the *Report of the Sanitary Commission of Massachusetts.*

He secured the assignment to write this report by devious measures. Shattuck in 1847 was a member of the Boston City Council and had been selected to represent the city in the state legislature. The American Statistical Society, of which Shattuck was a member, suggested to the state of Massachusetts in 1848 that a "Sanitary Commission" be appointed "to prepare and report to the next General Court a plan for a sanitary survey of the state, embracing a statement of such facts and suggestions as they think proper." This wording is, fairly obviously, Shattuck's own. The proposal was accepted, and a commission of three was appointed by the governor: one Whig, one Democrat, and one Free-Soiler. They were Lemuel Shattuck of Boston, Nathaniel P. Banks of Waltham, and Jehiel Abbott of Westfield. Shattuck was chairman. One can be quite certain that Shattuck arranged for the original suggestion, engineered the committee appointment, and had his outline of the survey all prepared and the report partially written long before authorization was secured. Of Mr. Banks and Mr. Abbott we know little, either before or after the report was written. Apparently, they played no part whatever in the organization or formulation of the survey, though they are listed as joint authors and are, in theory at least, equally responsible with Shattuck for the ideas that it contains. This is the setting and these are the events that led to the writing of the Shattuck report.[5]

This famous document is made up of four parts:

    I. The Sanitary Movement Abroad.
    II. The Sanitary Movement at Home.
    III. Plan for a Sanitary Survey of the State.
    IV. Reasons for Approving the Plan Recommended.

I. *The Sanitary Movement Abroad*

The initial section of the report is an excellent summary of the development of the sanitary movement in Europe, particularly in France, Germany, and England. We must draw the conclusion from this section that Shattuck had followed the activities of Chadwick and Southwood Smith closely, and that he drew a great deal of inspiration from their work. (See Chapter 26, pages 237, 241.)

II. *The Sanitary Movement at Home*

Part Two is devoted to a report on the development of public health in Massachusetts from earliest Colonial days. A brief discussion of all Massachusetts laws relating to sanitation is presented.

In the appendix Shattuck has included a complete list of the titles of all health acts from 1692 to 1848, together with the details of the Health Act of 1797, which authorized the establishment of local boards of health.

The physicians of Massachusetts, the medical schools, medical literature, and the occurrence of epidemics in the state are presented. We learn of the prevalence of malaria in New England and of the importance of millponds as a source of this infection.

A careful presentation of the vital statistics of the state is made, with a list of causes of death in Massachusetts over a period of seven years—1842-1848 inclusive.

The zymotic or epidemic diseases receive special consideration, since Shattuck felt that "the extent that these diseases prevail is the great index of the public health." He emphasizes the fact that consumption is the leading cause of death, and makes a penetrating

[5] The present tense is used throughout this chapter since the Shattuck report is still a living document.

In this year, also, a very malignant dysentery and bilious fever appeared in Sheffield. It was confined principally to a section of the town not over one and a half miles in diameter,— in the vicinity of a pond known as Hubbard's Pond,—containing about 100 families, or 600 inhabitants. Of these, over 300 were sick, and 44 died ; 12 adults, and 32 children. Among 150 who lived near the pond, on the southeasterly side, less than 10 escaped. Of those on the westerly side, about 50 were affected.

The cause of this remarkable sickness, and others of similar character, which that town suffered in other years, was attributed to this pond. A dam was built at the outlet, and, at times of high water, a large tract of land was overflowed. In dry seasons the water was drawn off, and large quantities of decomposing vegetable matter were exposed to the action of the sun, which produced a poisonous exhalation, or *malaria,* which affected nearly all who inhaled it. The accompanying cut will show the situation of this pond.[1]

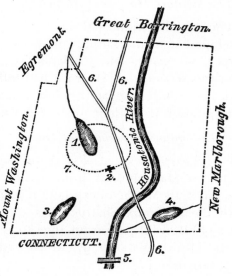

1. Hubbard's Pond, the principal source of malaria. 2. Meetinghouse. 3. Bush's Pond. 4. Ashley's. 5. Dam across the river in Connecticut. 6. Roads. 7. Dotted line showing the space occupied by the endemic of 1796, and within which space it has occurred sporadically since.

Fig. 23. A facsimile of page 72 of the Shattuck report of 1850 discussing the epidemiology of malaria. (Published by Dutton & Wentworth, Boston, 1850.)

analysis of the epidemiology of tuberculosis. He presents some very interesting data of the mortality from tuberculosis in urban and rural areas, as well as comparative data for various American and foreign cities. He realized, far in advance of his time, that if this disease is "ever to be ameliorated or eradicated, it can only be done by prevention, and not by cure. Its onset and development may be prevented."

The increase in sickness in Massachusetts that had occurred because of industrial development and urbanization was apparent to Shattuck, although its full impact was not to be measured for many years to come. The average age of all who died in Boston from 1810 to 1820 was 27.85 years. During the years 1840 to 1845, the average age at death was 21.43 years, a loss of 6.42 years. Comparable data for New York and Philadelphia showed a similar loss of ground.

Thus Shattuck felt that the need for the establishment of an effective public health service had become a matter of paramount importance.

III. Plan for a Sanitary Survey of the State

The body of the report consists of fifty recommendations which present in detail a suitable organization for a state and local health service. Shattuck was authorized to make a sanitary survey of Massachusetts, but what he did, in reality, was to use the authorization for this survey as a framework, under which he built a solid foundation of health organization. It now seems quite clear that he had thought out the whole plan in advance, and had formulated most of its details before the sanitary survey plan was initiated or even authorized.

As Winslow[6] has emphasized: "Of the fifty recommendations— all at the time new and untried principles or policies—careful analysis shows that no less than thirty-six are now universally accepted practices, not only in Massachusetts but throughout the Union." The provisions contained in these thirty-six recommendations are as follows:

A sound basis of public health administration is outlined, including an over-all state health law.

A state board of health (whose membership should include two physicians, a counselor at law, a chemist or "natural philosopher,"

---

[6] Winslow, C.-E. A.: "Lemuel Shattuck—Still a Prophet; the Message of Lemuel Shattuck for 1948," *Am. J. Pub. Health,* **39**:156, 1949.

a civil engineer, and two other persons) with a paid secretary is recommended.

Shattuck envisages a local board of health in each town, with a secretary who is required to make an annual written report; and he urges special sanitary surveys of particular cities, towns, and localities.

Recommendations are specific and detailed with regard to vital statistics, including a decennial state census, uniform nomenclature for causes of death and disease, and collection of data with regard to locality, age, race, sex, occupation, housing, and economic status of the population.

In the field of environmental sanitation, Shattuck emphasizes the control of nuisances endangering human life or health (including specifically the smoke nuisance); the supervision of the construction of new dwellings, factories, or other buildings, and the mitigation of sanitary evils arising from overcrowded lodginghouses and cellar-dwellings; the sanitation of schoolhouses; and exact observation of "the effect of mill-ponds and other collections or streams of water, and of their rise and fall, upon the health of the neighbouring inhabitants" (a sound basis for the study of the epidemiology of malaria).

Specific recommendations provide for control of the sale and use of unwholesome, spurious, or adulterated articles designed for food, drink, or medicine, with special reference to patent medicines and other nostrums and secret remedies.

In the area of communicable disease control, every town should be required to provide periodic vaccination against smallpox; and three recommendations deal with maritime quarantine and the protection of the health of passengers and merchant seamen.

In other recommendations, the report lays the groundwork of programs for "parents and others to whom the care of those in infancy and childhood is intrusted" to "understand and discharge their duties so that a good foundation may be laid for vigorous manhood and old age" and to take measures "to ascertain the amount of sickness suffered among the scholars who attend the public schools, and other seminaries of learning."

There is a farsighted recommendation in the report which suggests that "institutions be formed to educate and qualify females to be nurses of the sick." We must recall that in 1848 Florence Nightingale had not yet established her pioneer training school in England, and that this astounding Boston book-seller based his recommendations on his knowledge of Pastor Fliedner's school at

Kaiserswerth, from which the "Lady with the Lamp" drew her own inspiration.

One of the most interesting of Shattuck's recommendations is No. XLV.

We recommend *that persons be specially educated in sanitary science, as preventive advisers as well as curative advisers.*

The great object of sanitary science is to teach people the causes of disease,—how to remove or avoid these causes,—how to prevent disease, how to live without being sick,—how to increase the vital force,—how to avoid premature decay. And one of the most useful reforms which could be introduced into the present constitution of society would be, that the advice of the physician should be sought for and *paid for* while in health, to keep the patient well; and not, as now, while in sickness, to cure disease, which might in most cases have been avoided or prevented. And this practice, we understand, exists to some extent in some civilized countries. Three existing reasons, however, now occur to us, which we fear will prevent or obstruct, at least for a considerable period, the introduction into our country of this useful reform. One reason is, that persons who are well generally think that they have no need of a physician;— another, that if advice is sought for or given at such times, it is not generally considered worth paying for;—and a third, that there are few persons educated in sanitary science, and capable of giving good sanitary advice. These are fatal errors, and should be corrected, for they have cost thousands of lives. *Sanitary professorships* should be established in all our colleges and medical schools, and filled by competent teachers. The science of preserving health and preventing disease should be taught as one of the most important sciences. It would be useful to all, and to the student in curative medicine as well as to others.

In this one paragraph is condensed the development of the teaching of preventive medicine and public health in America for the next 100 years. More than 70 years were to elapse before universities even began the establishment of special departments for graduate training in public health, and the first full-time professor of preventive medicine in a medical college was not appointed until 1909 (Milton J. Rosenau at Harvard).

We feel sure that Shattuck obtained the inspiration for this remarkable recommendation, No. XLV, from Dr. Edward Jarvis, who had recently written:

. . . the intelligent physician can see arrows of disease, invisible to any one else; watch their havoc, and know whence they come, and how they may be stayed; and there are many eminent medical men who have, as individuals, nobly used the means which their superior position and knowledge have placed within their control, in the *prevention* of *disease*, and in the promotion of public health. And we wish to increase the number of such professional men.[7]

One recommendation, No. XLI, might well have been written only yesterday, for it is as pressing an issue in the daily press of the middle of the twentieth century as it was in 1848. It reads, "We recommend *that measures be taken to prevent, as far as practicable, the smoke nuisance.*" One may reasonably assume that this subject will continue to be a matter of public discussion for generations still unborn.

Against these thirty-six recommendations whose soundness has been demonstrated by their full incorporation into the routine practices of public health, one finds only four of Shattuck's recommendations which experience has shown to be unimportant or, in some degree, unsound. One of these relates to a minor detail with regard to the format of printed annual reports. Another calls for control of inquests by the board of health; and still another for the management of cemeteries by the board of health. The fourth and last recommendation of dubious value urges that "whenever practicable, the refuse and sewage of cities and towns be collected, and applied to the purposes of agriculture." This was wholly in accord with the best thought of the time in England; but experience has shown that such a method of disposal is not generally "practicable" on economic grounds.

There remain ten recommendations of the report which are of particular interest to us. They are as sound as the thirty-six proposals which have been generally accepted; but their importance has not yet been fully realized.

Three of these recommendations (XVII, XXI, and XXXVIII) relate to the vital problems of housing and planning. We have accepted the necessity for health department control of the most obvious and glaring defects in housing; but this is merely curative and not preventive sanitation. Shattuck saw further into the future. He demanded that "in laying out new towns and villages, and in extending those already laid out, ample provision be made for a supply, in purity and abundance, of light, air and water; . . . that open spaces be reserved in cities and villages, for public walks; that

[7] Jarvis, Edward: *Communications*, Massachusetts Medical Society, Vol. VIII, p. 1, 1847.

wide streets be laid out; and that both be ornamented with trees."
He urged that "tenements for the better accommodation of the poor
be erected in cities and villages." It is true that he looked chiefly
to private philanthropy to attain the latter end; but we know today
that only public assistance, on the federal level, can possibly meet
our national needs.

A second challenge of the 1850 report is found in its suggestion
(XXX) that local boards of health should make "careful observation
of the sanitary evils of intemperance, and the local and personal
circumstances under which they occur." We have only begun to
realize that alcoholism is not primarily a moral or a social problem
but is a responsibility of preventive medicine as well.

Another of Shattuck's recommendations (XXXII) faces the challenge of mental and emotional disease, probably the greatest single
objective of the public health program of the future. His concrete
suggestion is a limited and perhaps, in its actual form, an unsound
one—that "the authority now vested in justices of the peace,
relating to insane and idiotic persons, not arrested or indicted for
crime, be transferred to the local Boards of Health." Yet his fundamental assumption is wholly valid; that the person of unsound
mind or emotional instability presents a problem for preventive
medicine rather than for legal medicine. All of our dealings with
such persons must be guided by expert psychiatric knowledge and
not, as is still too often true, by archaic and barbarous commitment
laws. The health officer faces a major opportunity in further
reform of these laws, and in providing preventive services which will
avoid the necessity for resorting to legal procedures.

Two of Shattuck's recommendations embody minor—but significant—suggestions as to the extension of our knowledge of disease
prevalence by more careful and detailed records to be kept by private
physicians (XLVI) and by systematic records to be kept in each
family "of the physical and sanitary conditions of its members"
(XLVIII).

Finally, three recommendations open up wide vistas in the area
of public health education. They suggest that "a sanitary association
be formed in every city and town in the State, for the purpose of
collecting and diffusing information relating to public and personal
health" (XXXVII); that "clergymen of all religious denominations
make public health the subject of one or more discourses annually,
before their congregations" (XLVII); and that "individuals make

frequent sanitary examinations of themselves, and endeavor to promote personal health, and prevent personal disease" (L).

In general, it will be seen that the 1850 report lays a sound basis for the development of health administration, vital statistics, sanitation, and control of foods and drugs. It opens the way for maternal and child health, school health, and the study of tuberculosis. Curiously enough, it ignores domestic (as opposed to maritime) isolation and quarantine, insofar as major recommendations are concerned. Obviously it could have no vision of the future developments of bacteriology or immunology (smallpox vaccination being the only specific procedure available). The causative agents of venereal diseases were unknown, and effective drugs for their treatment were not available. Public health nursing was not to come for a quarter of a century; and the cost of medical care was not recognized as a serious problem, although figures are quoted to indicate that the annual charges of physicians of the state averaged $800, with average collections of $600. On the whole, however, it is quite astounding that a report, written when public health practice was yet in its infancy and public health science yet unborn, should, out of fifty recommendations, include thirty-six which have been universally accepted and ten more which are now in process of attainment.

IV. Reasons for Approving the Plan Recommended

The fourth part of the report is devoted to cogent arguments as to why the fifty recommendations should be approved. Shattuck emphasizes that such a measure would be (1) practical, (2) useful, (3) economical, (4) charitable, and (5) of moral import, and, furthermore, (6) involved an important duty.

How well Shattuck knew the New England people and understood what would appeal to them! In this short outline he includes *all* those basic elements that are fundamental to Puritan doctrines, and that were then and are today the warp and woof of New England character and justly famed New England "conscience."

Shattuck prepared a bill for the legislature which he recommended for enactment. This bill contained the essential provisions for activating the recommendations of the report, and epitomized the principles of state and local health department organization, upon which all our modern concepts of public health practice are based. The bill was not passed, for its concepts were far ahead of the times.

The report was buried by the legislature and not disinterred for many years. It disappeared so completely that copies of the report are now one of the great rarities in medical literature.

Appendix

The appendix of the report contains thirty-two chapters upon widely varied subjects, all of which are related to the basic matters of the report. Some of them are actual sanitary surveys of small cities, such as Lawrence, Attleborough, and Lynn. The duties of a health officer are outlined, and the "Great Sanitary Act of June 22, 1797" is given in its entirety. Due emphasis is placed upon proper registration of vital data, and there is a chapter on nomenclature and classification of causes of death. Shattuck realized full well the importance of vital statistics as a sound public health measure and was leaving no stone unturned to promote this facility.

Perhaps the most interesting of all his recommendations is contained in his last chapter, "Books Recommended for Sanitary Libraries." This list is a comprehensive bibliography of the public health literature of this period. It gives us some idea of the breadth of Shattuck's knowledge and shows us clearly from whence he secured the wellsprings of his inspiration. For Shattuck, like so many other men of stature, did not create the fabric of great concepts from the gossamer found in the morning dew. His genius lay in the fact that he was able to take the ideas of others, the fragmentary threads of current knowledge and philosophy, and, utilizing his vision, his humanitarian instincts, and a clear and logical mind, weave a strong and serviceable pattern for public health practice on the framework of the political and social history of the nation. This pattern has endured for more than 100 years—a magnificent tapestry that will continue to be a guide and inspiration to students of preventive medicine for many years to come.

CHAPTER 28. *The National Quarantine and*

Sanitary Conventions

There is a tendency to consider evils suppressed as soon as a law against them is enacted.

D. F. LINCOLN, *1878*

The year 1857 was a memorable one. Dr. Wilson Jewell had been a member of the Philadelphia Board of Health for some eight years. A devastating epidemic of cholera had swept the nation during that period, invading his own city. During the same period, New Orleans had suffered from one of its worst periodic yellow fever invasions. The various large ports of the United States had attempted to follow the more advanced European countries in the matter of quarantine. These countries had utilized maritime quarantine in an attempt to prevent the invasion of the land by pestilence, but in America, all efforts along these lines had been signally unsuccessful. Dr. Jewell became deeply concerned with the antiquated and obsolete practice of maritime quarantine in Philadelphia and other American seaboard cities, and determined to attempt the establishment of a nationwide maritime quarantine code.

The success of the *Conference Sanitaire* in Paris in 1851 and 1852 suggested to him the value of a convention of delegates from the larger American seaports to consider this important matter.

Wilson Jewell was convinced that quarantine, as practiced, had serious defects. "They [the quarantine laws] advocated antiquated and obsolete doctrines; they embarrassed commerce, oppressed the merchant, imposed severe restrictions on the healthy, inflicted cruelties on the sick, and when rigidly enforced, became the ready means of disseminating and entailing disease and death."[1] He wished to

[1] See letter of Wilson Jewell to John H. Griscom in *Proceedings and Debates of the Third National Quarantine and Sanitary Convention*. Edward Jones & Co., Printers to Board of Education, New York, 1859, p. 3. This letter presented a brief history of the rise and progress of the Quarantine and Sanitary Conventions.

secure a uniform code of regulations operating alike in all the ports, and after much discouragement, and even opposition from various sources, he finally persuaded his board of health to permit him to correspond with the boards of health of Boston, New York, Baltimore, and New Orleans, "on the propriety of calling a convention of delegates from the various boards of health in the maritime cities of the United States for the purpose of a conference in relation to the establishment of a uniform system of revised quarantine laws."[2]

FIRST QUARANTINE CONVENTION

As a direct result of Dr. Jewell's initiative, the first Quarantine Convention met in Philadelphia, May 13, 1857. Twenty-six different authorities from nine states sent seventy-three delegates. Interest was apparently very keen. Boston sent her mayor and twelve delegates, among whom were Henry G. Clark, city physician of Boston, and Jacob Bigelow, a patriarch then in his seventieth year.

Edwin Snow, newly appointed health officer of Providence, came, and E. H. Barton, the yellow fever epidemiologist, was sent by New Orleans. René La Roche, D. G. Condie, and Henry Hartshorne ably represented the College of Physicians of Philadelphia.

This first meeting was harmonious, but quite ineffective. General principles of quarantine were discussed and specific propositions set forth as representing the sentiments of the convention. It was agreed that certain diseases might be introduced into a port by an infected ship—smallpox and, under suitable circumstances, typhus fever, cholera, and yellow fever.

These men recognized that smallpox was transmitted from person to person, but considered that the other diseases were introduced into a port largely because of foul conditions aboard ship, especially bilge water. General recommendations concerning vaccination of immigrants were suggested, and also certain methods for cleaning and airing a ship.

Wilson Jewell had drawn up a tentative quarantine code which he proposed. This code was discussed in great detail, with much quibbling over minor and wholly unimportant points. The delegates finally compromised on a few rather simple propositions relating to the quarantine of smallpox, cholera, typhus fever, and yellow fever.

These propositions provided for a full-time medical quarantine officer, appointed by the local board of health of each large port, who would be given power to inspect all vessels, quarantine those vessels

2 *Ibid.*, p. 5.

found infected, remove and care for the sick, unload the cargo in a safe place, and thoroughly cleanse and purify both the cargo and the empty vessel. Due provision was made for a subsequent convention. As an afterthought, it was suggested that all immigrants be vaccinated against smallpox.

The purposes of the convention were broadened by making the title "The Quarantine *and Sanitary* Convention." This apparently was a suggestion of Dr. Bigelow. Dr. Snow of Providence sneaked in a resolution at the last moment: "We recommend the adoption of a complete, accurate and uniform system of registration of births and deaths in all our cities as a necessary accompaniment of efficient sanitary measures."[3]

SECOND QUARANTINE AND SANITARY CONVENTION

The Second Quarantine and Sanitary Convention was called on April 28, 1858, in Baltimore. Twelve states were represented by eighty delegates. The following jurisdictions were represented: Boston, Providence, New York, Brooklyn, Newark, Philadelphia, Wilmington, Baltimore, Washington, D.C., Georgetown, Alexandria, Norfolk, Charleston, Savannah, and New Orleans. There were fifty-six delegates from outside Baltimore; Boston sent Dr. H. G. Clark, city physician, Dr. George C. Shattuck, and seven other physicians, as well as ten aldermen. Jacob Bigelow did not come.

Dr. Snow of Providence was present, as were René La Roche, Wilson Jewell, and Henry Hartshorne of Philadelphia. New York City was represented by three aldermen and three councilmen, *but no physician.*[4]

The chief accomplishment of the convention was the selection of two committees: one on "External Hygiene or Quarantine," and the other on "Internal Hygiene" or the "Sanitary Arrangement of Cities." We see the careful guiding hand of Wilson Jewell and his friends in this matter. He apparently felt that disease, even when it invaded a large city, would not spread if the city were thoroughly clean and wholesome.

The two committees were requested to bring in reports at the next convention. The title "Quarantine" included reports on (1) the history of quarantine, (2) reforms required to make quarantine more

[3] *Minutes of the Proceedings of the Quarantine Convention*, p. 46, held at Philadelphia by invitation of the Philadelphia Board of Health, May 13-15, 1857.

[4] *Proceedings of the Second Annual Meeting of the Quarantine and Sanitary Convention.* Baltimore, April 29, 1858.

efficient, and (3) proposals for uniform quarantine laws. The report on the "Sanitary Arrangement of Cities" included sewage disposal, water supply, disinfection, and birth and death registration. (Here again we see the hand of Dr. Snow.) Dr. Clark suggested the formulation of a "Sanitary Code for Cities," and he was forthwith asked to write it. If we may judge from the minutes, the delegates must have been thoroughly disappointed at the lack of results of this meeting.

THIRD NATIONAL QUARANTINE AND SANITARY CONVENTION

The Third National Quarantine and Sanitary Convention met in New York on April 27, 1859. If the second convention was a dismal failure, the third certainly was an overwhelming success. The *Proceedings and Debates*[5] fill over 700 closely printed pages. Delegates from outside New York numbered over 100. They came from as far as Canada and Alabama. Boston sent its mayor and apparently its entire board of aldermen, together with seven physicians. Dr. Jacob Bigelow, now seventy-two years old, came with the delegates, as did Dr. Henry Clark. Dr. E. M. Snow came from Providence with the mayor. René La Roche again represented Philadelphia, but for some reason Wilson Jewell was not able to come. Norfolk, Virginia, and Memphis were represented, but New Orleans sent no delegates—an ominous signal, for the Civil War was already in the making.

The New York Sanitary Association had twenty-one delegates. Among them appeared the names of Dr. Stephen Smith, Elisha Harris, and J. H. Griscom. The latter was elected president of the convention. The Academy of Medicine was represented by such outstanding personages as A. H. Stevens and J. W. Francis.

The report of Wilson Jewell's Committee on External Hygiene was read—paragraph by paragraph. It created a furor. The basic struggle soon began to revolve around yellow fever. Vainly did President Griscom point out that in fifty years New York had lost only 600 persons from yellow fever, whereas in twenty-five years, 12,300 had died of cholera. In the minds of the delegates, quarantine was intended primarily for the purpose of excluding yellow fever, and most of them believed that the whole matter of quarantine was a relic of superstition and ignorance.

Many of the delegates present had not been at the Philadelphia meeting, and were violently opposed to some of the clauses of

---

[5] *Proceedings and Debates of the Third National Quarantine and Sanitary Convention.* Edward Jones & Co., Printers to Board of Education, New York, 1859.

Jewell's report. Dr. Stevens, seventy years old, former president of
the American Medical Association, and the most prominent surgeon
of New York, was in a combative mood. The radical defect of the
report, in his mind, was that yellow fever was considered in the same
category with smallpox and cholera. He submitted the following
resolution:

. . . That in the absence of evidence establishing the conclusion that
Yellow Fever has ever been conveyed by one person to another, it is the
opinion of this convention that personal quarantine in cases of Yellow
Fever may be safely abolished.

The opponents of quarantine of the individual were well fortified
and entered into the discussion with great vigor.

Dr. John Francis, of the same age as Dr. Stevens, equally prominent and equally combative, rose to the fray. His praeceptor and
former partner had been the great Dr. Hosack, who had taught him
that "yellow fever was a specific disease, imported from the coast of
Africa, extending solely by germs derived from that original source."
He made a masterly plea for the contagious nature of the disease.
At the outset, however, he made the serious mistake of criticizing
the great patron saint of American medicine, Benjamin Rush, calling Rush's theory of the identity of fevers preposterous. Dr. Francis
showed that yellow fever was a specific disease, spread from person
to person, that the disease was always introduced into New York and
other Atlantic seaboard cities from some foreign port by ships, and
that climatic variations, hot summers, bad odors, and the like had
nothing to do with its propagation.

His argument was clear and unanswerable. He was willing to admit
that yellow fever might be produced from exposure to air emanating
from merchandise brought from an infected city, but he held to his
opinion and cited Chisholm as his authority that the person ill with
yellow fever is the true source of any epidemic and should not be
released, but quarantined until well.

Dr. Francis presented a truly remarkable and apparently spontaneous address, talking eloquently for more than two hours. He gave,
in masterly array, his reasons for believing that yellow fever is transmitted from person to person. He spoke from bitter personal experience. His father had died of that disease when Dr. Francis was a boy.
The child contracted the disease from his father, and his most vivid
memory, at seventy years of age, was the small coffin that had stood
in his little bedroom to receive him as soon as he should have died.

Dr. A. N. Bell, quarantine officer of Brooklyn, insisted upon the noncontagious nature of the disease, and he also spoke from personal experience. He had had the disease at Vera Cruz while he was a young naval surgeon on the frigate "Mississippi" during the Mexican War. His most impressive argument related to the French frigate "Gomer." This vessel in 1838 endured one of the most terrible ravages of yellow fever that had ever occurred on board a ship. "She discharged her patients at Pensacola, creating a panic among the population. To convince these people that their fears were groundless, a French surgeon wrapped himself at 10 o'clock at night in the bed clothes of a person who had died of the black vomit, immediately after the removal of the dead body, and slept the whole night through, without taking the Fever."

The debate became bitter and rather personal. Probably the tide of battle was turned by Dr. La Roche of Philadelphia, for he was generally recognized by his contemporaries as one of the great world authorities on yellow fever. He spoke for over an hour in opposition to quarantine. He was the author of a recent treatise on yellow fever in which he opposed the contagion or importation theory. "I believe," he said, "that a vessel, when it becomes dangerous to visit, owes the power of doing mischief not to the Yellow Fever cases that are or have been on board, but to a poison originating in her, or received and inclosed by her hold while in a sickly port. . . . I have yet to discover a satisfactory reason for quarantining the sick themselves, and still less, individuals in health, who arrive among us in sickly or healthy ships, or other-wise from infected places." Eventually, La Roche became quite abusive in his attack on Dr. Francis' point of view.[6]

Finally, on the third day, Dr. Stevens insisted upon a vote of the delegates, which he considered a vote of vindication and triumph. Elisha Harris saw the futility of this procedure and tried to obtain a compromise, with no actual vote to be taken. The general opinion of the delegates, however, was that a convention that fails to reach a conclusion is of no value.

Eighty-five delegates voted for the resolution, including Stephen Smith (one of the founders of the American Public Health Association in 1872). Elisha Harris voted in the affirmative, as did H. G. Clark of Boston, E. M. Snow, who was to be health officer of Provi-

[6] *Proceedings and Debates of the Third National Quarantine and Sanitary Convention, op. cit.*, pp. 179-80.

dence for almost thirty years, as well as many other men who were considered to be the leading physicians of their day. Only one other physician, together with three laymen, voted with Dr. Francis.

But scientific truth is not to be decided by popular ballot. We now know that Dr. Francis was correct in practically all of his arguments, and that the eighty-five who felt so triumphant over their victory were wrong. It was a hollow victory, which has been repeated time and again in scientific meetings throughout the world. How many times have we seen a courageous, clear-sighted man stand before his fellows and present the truth as it is revealed to him! How many times have we seen him lashed by the bitter scorn of his adversaries, beaten down and overwhelmed by the sheer weight of heavy-handed opposition of those who are regarded as the great authorities on the subject under discussion, finally avalanched into oblivion by the mass of popular opinion!

This controversy was so acrimonious that Dr. Henry Clark's "Sanitary Code for Cities" was almost forgotten. It was read and discussed perfunctorily. Old Dr. Stevens was contemptuous of the whole thing. He was a strong believer in personal and local community autonomy, and saw no reason why a plan of health organization that worked well in one city necessarily would be suitable for another. He saw absolutely no need for a state board of health. It represented too much interference with local affairs.

Dr. Clark's draft of "A Sanitary Code for Cities"[7] was really a most thoughtful composition which might be workable today, at least in its general outline.

Dr. Clark was city physician of Boston; other Massachusetts delegates who were registered at the convention were the mayor and eleven aldermen of Boston, none of whom took an active part in the discussions. Dr. Clark's consulting physicians who attended were Jacob Bigelow, John Jeffries, D. H. Storer, and James Ayer, all from distinguished Boston medical families. Dr. J. M. Moriarity, the port physician, was also registered. No other Massachusetts communities were represented at the convention.

Dr. Clark's "Sanitary Code" suggested a public health act which would provide for a state board of health together with a local board of health for each city and town. At least one-third of the members of the board of health should be doctors of medicine. A sanitary

[7] *Proceedings and Debates of the Third National Quarantine and Sanitary Convention: op. cit.* See Appendix E, p. 645.

survey should be made annually if ". . . the numbers of deaths shall exceed twenty-five to a thousand . . ."

The "Code" also provided for the supervision of sewage disposal, water supplies, interment of the dead, slaughterhouses, markets, lodginghouses, and dramshops, as well as control of epidemic disease and public vaccination. Other general provisions were included.

The "Sanitary Code" further provided for free public clinics for vaccination against smallpox and initiated the plan of certification of vaccination for children ". . . without which no child shall be admitted to public schools." Dr. Clark's list of town health officials and his report form for recording the sanitary conditions of premises are of special interest.

TOWN HEALTH OFFICIALS

1. A Registrar of births, deaths, and marriages, and regulator of funerals. He must be a physician.
2. Medical Health Officer.
3. Board of consulting physicians to function in epidemics.
4. Engineer or Surveyor.
5. Superintendent of cleaning of streets, of drains, and of burials.

APPENDIX A. REPORT FORM ON SANITARY CONDITIONS OF PREMISES BY HEALTH OFFICER OR INSPECTOR . . .

1. Prevalent sickness.
2. Overcrowding.
3. Ventilation.
4. Drainage.
5. Filth and rubbish.
6. Water supply.
7. Dead bodies in single living rooms.

Dr. Clark undoubtedly was familiar with Shattuck's famous document of 1850, for his recommendation in regard to a state board of health follows Shattuck's plan closely. Clark's "Code" was an excellent one, but the public health opinion of the nation had not yet developed to the point where it was ready to receive anything so revolutionary or altruistic. More than ten years were to pass before his own state of Massachusetts was ready to establish a state board of health.

The convention ended with a grand banquet to the delegates, at which no less than fourteen toasts were drunk. Even Dr. Snow, the austere Vermont Yankee, waxed eloquent when he gave a toast "to the ladies." (None were present.) The fourth toast was: "Medical Science—Instinct with Humanity, its Mission is Divine; it claims not the prerogative to give Life, but it may arrest the march of Death." Dr. A. H. Stevens was called on for the response.

FOURTH NATIONAL QUARANTINE AND SANITARY CONVENTION[8]

This convention was held in Boston, June 14-16, 1860. Jacob Bigelow, of Boston, was president. The largest representation of course, was from Massachusetts. Of the southern cities, only Baltimore, Savannah, and Memphis were represented—one delegate from each of the last two, and two from Baltimore.

The main topics taken up at this meeting were:

1. "Quarantine Regulations," including "A Code of Marine Hygiene." The committee report comprised "specific recommendations of principles and measures of quarantine, as severally applicable to yellow fever, cholera, typhus fever, and smallpox, having reference also to the variations which different localities require." Following the lead of the previous convention, the trend in this meeting seemed to be toward simpler and less stringent quarantine restrictions.

2. A "Report on Registration" by Dr. Edwin M. Snow of Providence. This report included a model "Ordinance in Relation to the Registration of Births, Marriages, and Deaths."

3. A "Report upon Legal Restrictions for the Control of the Sale of Poisons and Dangerous Drugs" by Dr. C. B. Guthrie of Memphis. This report evoked considerable discussion. One encounters an indication of things to come in the plaint (top of page 31, body of the *Proceedings*) that the "popular idea of an apothecary now-a-days, is that of a man who deals in a multitude of miscellaneous notions, and a few drugs."

4. "The Utility and Application of Heat as a Disinfectant" by Elisha Harris of New York.

5. A "Report on Civic Cleanliness and Economical Disposition of the Refuse of Cities" by E. L. Viele of New York.

Dr. Ordronaux stirred up a great deal of acrimonious debate because he requested a "Committee on State Medicine."

---

[8] See *Proceedings and Debates of the Fourth National Quarantine and Sanitary Convention.* George C. Rand & Avery, City Printers, Boston, 1860.

State medicine, in a word, is the application of the principles of medical science to the administration of justice and the preservation of the public health. It is a system of medical police, both *preventive* as well as *punitive* and *reformative*. In its origin it is not simply philanthropic, but also equitable and economic. . . . But inasmuch as many men from force of circumstance cannot obey the behests of the law of self-preservation, it devolves upon society in the aggregate to enforce such ordinances of physical government, as medical science has suggested for the hygienic well-being of its members.[9]

There was great opposition to the formation of this committee, as older members felt it would usurp the authority of other committees. *"The term 'State Medicine' seems to be not well understood."*[10] The only work published on the subject at that time was *State Medicine* by H. W. Rumsey of England, although, of course, Johann Frank's *Police Medicine* was compiled in the early part of the century.

Dr. Ordronaux was a fluent and brilliant speaker and apparently offended the other members of the convention because he talked too much and too well. After considerable debate, a committee was appointed "to report to the next convention such subjects of sanitary importance as in their judgment require investigation or legislation, for their permanent improvement."

We see several famous names among those present. Although neither took part in any discussion, both Edward Everett, the famous orator, and Dr. O. W. Holmes attended some of the meetings. The latter read a poem he had written in honor of the occasion; the final couplet is masterly:

> To guard is better than to heal,—
> The shield is nobler than the spear![11]

Other important public health men who were present at that meeting were:

Henry G. Clark, M.D., city physician of Boston, who drew up the "Sanitary Code for Cities" (see 1859 convention report).

John H. Griscom, M.D., of the New York Sanitary Association; one of the founders of the National Quarantine and Sanitary Conventions.

Alex H. Stevens, M.D., of New York, who had led debate at the 1859 meeting on the noncontagious nature of yellow fever.

[9] *Fourth National Quarantine and Sanitary Convention: op. cit.,* p. 67.

[10] It is some comfort to present-day health administrators to realize that our forefathers 100 years ago were as confused as we are in defining the term "state medicine."

[11] *Fourth National Quarantine and Sanitary Convention: op. cit.,* pp. 135-36.

Elisha Harris, M.D., of New York; later very active in the American Public Health Association.

A. N. Bell, M.D., of Brooklyn; one of the founders of that organization.

Wilson Jewell of Philadelphia; generally considered as primarily responsible for the formation of the first convention.

René La Roche, M.D., of Philadelphia.

C. P. La Roche, M.D., of Philadelphia.

S. B. Halliday, sanitary engineer of New York; called by Ordronaux "the American Chadwick, the American sanitary practitioner who explores night and day the purlieus of city life, and embodies in statistics the results of those observations."

Among the distinguished Boston physicians who were guests of the convention were James Jackson, J. Mason Warren, Charles E. Ware, George Bartlett, George H. Lyman, C. D. Homans, S. Cabot, Jr., Francis Minot, Henry I. Bowditch, and Oliver Wendell Holmes.

At the last session of the convention, plans were made to hold the next gathering in Cincinnati. I am unable to find even a foreshadowing of the death of the Quarantine and Sanitary Conventions. Yet the impending Civil War was foremost in the thoughts of all, and there was little inclination to give consideration to any other matter. Presumably, the outbreak of the war early in 1861 caused this fifth meeting to be postponed indefinitely. In fact, it was never held at all.

SECTION III. *The Period of Development*

THE CIVIL WAR TO WORLD WAR I

CHAPTER 29. *Military Sanitation*

WITH SPECIAL REFERENCE TO THE CIVIL WAR

Our grand business in life is not to see what lies dimly, at a distance, but what is clearly before us close at hand.

THOMAS CARLYLE

The Revolutionary War established a pattern of military sanitation that was maintained for more than 100 years. Benjamin Rush,[1] in his "Observations Made upon the Diseases which Occurred in the Military Hospitals of the United States during the Revolutionary War," noted that sick soldiers "recover health sooner and better in sheds, huts and barns than in the most superb hospitals. Hospitals are the sinks of human life in an army. They robbed the United States of more citizens than the sword." Rush pointed out that there was more sickness among men in tents than among those in the open air. Men under twenty were subject to the greatest number of camp diseases. "The southern troops were more sickly than the northern troops." (This has been true in all American wars including World Wars I and II.) "Native Americans were more sickly than the natives of Europe who served in the American army. . . . Typhus mitior [typhoid fever?] always prevailed most." Dysentery was the next most important disease. "A ship with a long-established crew may be very *healthy,* but if strangers are introduced among them, who are also *healthy,* sickness will be mutually produced." Thus we see that Rush was indeed a keen observer and a pioneer epidemiologist.

Mann (1759-1832)[2] has described the special medical problems of the War of 1812. He felt that a large proportion of the men in the

[1] Rush, Benjamin: "The Result of Observations Made upon the Diseases Which Occurred in the Military Hospitals of the United States during the Revolutionary War," *Medical Inquiries and Observations,* Fourth Edition, Vol. I, pp. 147-50, 1815.

[2] Mann, James: *Medical Sketches of the Campaigns of 1813-14.* H. Mann & Co., Dedham, Mass., 1816.

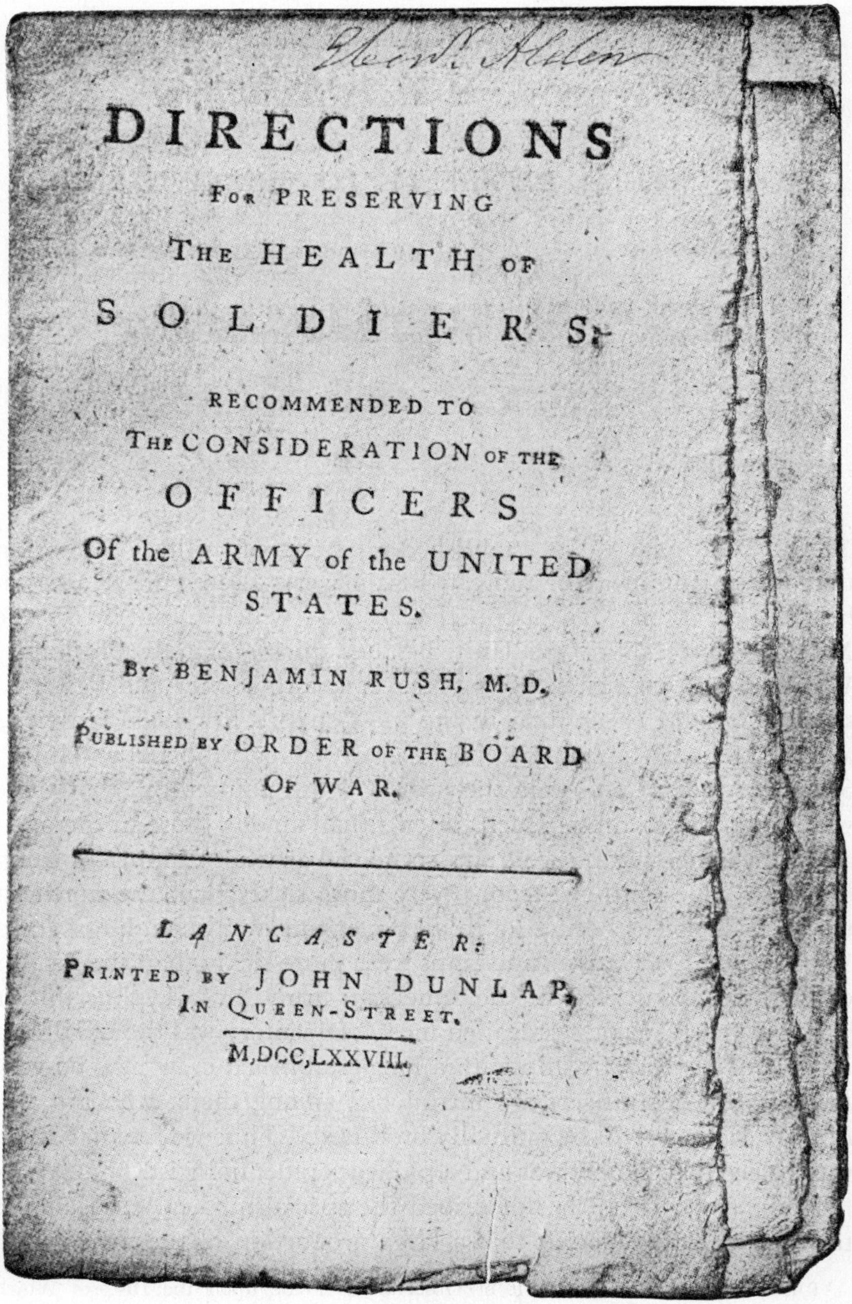

DIRECTIONS
FOR PRESERVING
THE HEALTH OF
SOLDIERS;
RECOMMENDED TO
THE CONSIDERATION OF THE
OFFICERS
Of the ARMY of the UNITED
STATES.

BY BENJAMIN RUSH, M. D.

PUBLISHED BY ORDER OF THE BOARD
OF WAR.

LANCASTER:
PRINTED BY JOHN DUNLAP,
IN QUEEN-STREET.
M,DCC,LXXVIII.

Fig. 24. Cover of pamphlet by Benjamin Rush on preserving the health of American soldiers in the Revolutionary War (1778).

army, when first enlisted, were not fit to be soldiers. Intemperance was an important factor in their inability to endure hardship and fatigue. A body of 5,000 men seldom furnished more than 3,000 who were capable of active field duty. Mann claimed that the officers were at fault. The quarters of the enlisted men were dirty and over-crowded. Sixteen to twenty men often occupied a room sixteen feet square. Their clothing was inadequate and their diet poor. Alcohol-ism was a major problem.

Adams[3] has recently made a record of American medicine during the course of the Civil War. He states that in the Mexican War ten American soldiers died from illness for every one who was killed by the enemy. In the Civil War, two-thirds of the 360,000 Union soldiers who perished were not killed in battle but died from infectious diseases.

Dr. J. J. Woodward[4] has given us an excellent picture of the im-portant "camp diseases" that were of chief importance during the Civil War. Malaria was so all-prevailing that it masked other condi-tions, and caused much confusion in differential diagnosis and in disease classification. Woodward believed in a combined symptom complex, which he called "typho-malaria," and this title became incorporated in disease nomenclature for many years. Indeed, it is quite possible that many of the soldiers suffered from a combination of the two diseases, malaria and typhoid fever. We do not know how much typhoid fever there was, but all the evidence points to a heavy incidence.

Woodward understood the epidemiology of malaria, and brought out many of its characteristic features. Its relationship to ponds and marshes was clear, as well as its seasonal incidence, but he was not sure that wet summers are sole factors in malaria production, for he noted that prolonged hot, dry weather may increase the intensity of malaria. We now know the reason why this is true, since those factors favor the development of anopheles mosquitoes. He noted the effect of prevailing winds on the intensity of malaria, as well as the relative safety of soldiers when they were exposed only during the day to malarious zones, with an opportunity to leave the area at night. This is also true since anopheles mosquitoes bite at night. He even noted that persons who inhabited the upper stories of a house were less likely to become infected than those on the ground floors.

[3] Adams, G. W.: *Doctors in Blue*. Henry Schuman, New York, 1952.
[4] Woodward, J. J.: *Chief Camp Diseases of the United States Armies*. J. B. Lippincott Co., Philadelphia, 1863.

Although Woodward did not think that a toxic gas from the decomposing vegetation of swamps could explain the origin of the disease, he accepted Mitchell's cryptogenic theory of its origin. We now know how near he came to a true explanation of the actual cause of malaria.

Woodward introduced an interesting classification of diseases due to "crowd poisoning." In this group he placed typhus fever, typhoid fever, and dysentery, as well as cholera and diarrhea. When his troops were confined within narrow limits, particularly in barracks, with poor toilet facilities and contamination of the area of the camp with feces and camp wastes, he found that dysentery and typhoid fever were sure to increase. Typhus fever, however, was not a serious problem during the Civil War. This is in great contrast to the history of armies in Europe. Why we escaped is not clear, for the disease had been quite prevalent in New York and in other port cities during the decade just preceding the Civil War.

Scurvy did not produce as many deaths as the army authorities had feared it would, but the "scorbutic taint" was always a great problem. The necessity for fresh vegetables and fruits in the soldiers' diet was understood, and great effort was made to provide them with potatoes, cabbage, and onions, but in the exigencies of campaigns this was not always possible. Woodward noted the influence of excessive fatigue, exposure, and nostalgia as the major factors in the production of scurvy, and pointed out that scurvy frequently was a complication of prolonged fevers, particularly typhoid fever. One of the important lessons learned and applied during the Civil War was the necessity for inclusion of fresh vegetables, such as onions, turnips, carrots, and potatoes, in the diet of the soldier.

Camp diarrhea was by far the most frequent of all camp diseases. Woodward stated that over 200,000 cases, with a mortality of about 0.5 per cent, were reported to the surgeon general in 1862. Woodward did not distinguish, however, between diarrhea and true dysentery. Chronic diarrhea, which in many cases may have been amoebic dysentery, was a frequent and debilitating disease that resulted in invalidism for many of the soldiers. There was no real information concerning the outcome of these cases, for most of them were sent home. The death rate was probably quite high.

"Camp measles" caused the army officers a great deal of distress. It was particularly prevalent among recruits. In some instances, nearly 50 per cent of the rural recruits developed the disease soon after entering camp. An epidemic in a regiment often lasted for two to three months, and persisted until all susceptibles were attacked. Many of the young soldiers died, usually with a complicating pneumonia. Woodward believed that measles was more severe in its total manifestation in the army barracks than in civil life.

Acute respiratory disease, which Woodward called "catarrh," was, of course, highly prevalent, but caused no serious disturbance of military plans. No true epidemic of influenza appeared during the entire war. Lobar pneumonia was a frequent complication of catarrh, and it was highly fatal. Of 11,001 cases reported prior to July, 1862, 2,134 died, a case fatality rate of nearly 20 per cent.

Rheumatism caused a good deal of concern to army authorities. They made no distinction between rheumatic fever and rheumatoid arthritis. More confusion occurred because malingering was most often encountered among the soldiers who complained of bone and joint diseases. Furthermore, because cases of scurvy sometimes developed bone and joint symptoms, the diagnosis in these patients was often confused with rheumatism. Venereal disease did not give the army authorities great concern. Woodward developed a classification of "Enthetic Diseases," i.e., *implanted diseases*. In reality, they were the venereal diseases plus a few cases of rabies, glanders, and snake bite. During the year July 1, 1861, to June 30, 1862, some 9,000 cases of syphilis and 15,000 cases of gonorrhea were reported, a ratio of 1 case of syphilis infection to each 30 soldiers; in gonorrhea the ratio was 1 to 19. These figures compared most favorably with the British data for the Crimean campaign of 1855, where the over-all ratio for venereal disease was 1 to 2.5 men per year, as compared with the American ratio of 1 to 11.8 soldiers. Woodward felt that one of the chief influences in the low American venereal disease rate was the distance of the large camping grounds from the cities, but he also admitted the possibility of better recording by the British.

Epidemic jaundice was frequent and troublesome, with some 11,000 cases reported during the first year of the war. The disease was not due to malaria, as many believed, since it was most prevalent in the winter months. The death rate was low, but disability in some cases was severe.

As in all wars, the Civil War resulted in a great national improvement in medical care and sanitary science. The army served as an excellent course in postgraduate training for physicians in the newer surgical techniques and in the utilization of anesthesia. Out of the war grew social betterment, particularly improvement of nursing techniques. We now realize that the training of nurses in the United States was initiated as a direct result of the experiences of the Civil War. The actual establishment of courses for the training of nurses in hospitals took place in 1866, the year after the war ceased.

The chief public health lessons that were learned during the war were:

1. Better understanding of the principles of "crowd diseases."
2. Increased knowledge of the epidemiology of malaria.
3. Realization of the importance of proper disposal of human feces, and other wastes, in the prevention of typhoid fever and dysentery.
4. Increasing realization of the great importance of fresh vegetables in the prevention of scurvy, with implementation of this knowledge.
5. An understanding that prolonged fever, such as typhoid fever, or such factors as exhaustion and monotonous food, might bring out the "scorbutic taint" in soldiers who otherwise might not develop this condition.
6. The great advantage of trained female nurses in proper care of the sick.
7. The great value of ether and choloroform anesthesia in surgery.

In the following chapter we shall discuss the United States Sanitary Commission, which was a voluntary organization, formed at the outset of the war to care for the soldiers. At least two important developments came from that organization, namely:

1. The value of a nationwide co-ordinated voluntary organization in promotion of community health.
2. The utilization of the *health education pamphlet,* which considers a specific subject and which is written by an expert for a definite audience and a special purpose.

CHAPTER 30. *The United States Sanitary*

Commission and the Civil War[1]

Social influences exert their power, either good or bad, upon all who come within their reach.

E. H. JANES, *1876*

The United States Sanitary Commission was our first nationwide voluntary health organization. It was initiated by war conditions.

War, with its resultant profound disturbance of social life, always initiates or activates special problems in medical care and in public health. Each war is a different situation, producing quite different combinations of circumstances. Therefore, each war has its own peculiar sanitary problems. It is also an axiom that every major American war has resulted in a great upsurge in scientific knowledge, particularly in medical science. Community administration of public health affairs has improved after each war. Physicians who have served in the wars have received a postgraduate course of medical education, and have learned the value of co-ordination of community-wide health services, to the great subsequent benefit of the communities to which they return. Each war has also brought us new and important epidemiological knowledge.

The Revolutionary War was characterized by the severe epidemics of smallpox and the acute respiratory diseases, particularly influenza, pneumonia, and measles. There was great privation, with nutritional disturbances of various sorts. The medical lessons learned in this war were of paramount medical value to the new nation. The War of 1812 and the Mexican War were of too short duration to present outstanding medical problems.

As Adams[2] has emphasized, the Civil War had many more casual-

[1] See *United States Sanitary Commission, A Sketch of its Purposes and Work.* Little, Brown & Co., Boston, 1863.
[2] Adams, G. W.: *Doctors in Blue.* Henry Schuman, New York, 1952.

ties from disease than from guns and cannon. Dysentery led all the
rest. Typhoid fever was devastating. Pneumonia was not outstanding
as a cause of death, probably because the army lived in the open in
small tents, or camped in barns and small buildings rather than in
large barracks. Malaria loomed large, and surgical infections, particularly those following amputation, were most troublesome. The
major nutritional disturbance was scurvy. Yellow fever and cholera
were completely under control, for the simple reason that the ports
were blockaded.

When the Civil War broke out, the War Department had no conception of what the medical and sanitary problems would be and
was not equipped in any way to meet the coming emergency. The
medical officers had little understanding of camp sanitation, and no
sound knowledge of preventive medicine or military hygiene.

The very recent experience of the British in the Crimean War
and the development of a nursing service for soldiers by Florence
Nightingale in 1855 were just beginning to attract general attention.

Dr. S. G. Howe of Boston, husband of the famous Julia Ward
Howe, was a personal friend of Miss Nightingale, and Dorothea
Dix, founder of the mental hygiene program in America, was a lifelong friend of the Howes. Dr. Elizabeth Blackwell, America's famous
woman physician, was also familiar with Miss Nightingale's work,
as were many others.

Acting on the inspiration of the work of Miss Nightingale, a small
group attempted to secure official recognition from the federal government for a voluntary war relief association. Leaders in the group
were Mr. Bellows, a minister from New York; Dr. Valentine Mott,
a prominent New York doctor; Dr. A. A. Bache, a grandson of
Benjamin Franklin; Dr. S. G. Howe of Boston; Dr. Elisha Harris,
who later took an active part in founding the American Public
Health Association; Mr. F. L. Olmstead, the great landscape architect; and other prominent citizens. Mr. Olmstead was executive
secretary, and the organization was called the United States Sanitary
Commission.

The government authorities told the initiators of the commission
of their doubts and misgivings concerning the feasibility of its plans.
President Lincoln feared it might be "a fifth wheel to the coach,"
not only needless but also embarrassing to the proper prosecution
of the war. The War Cabinet supposed that some clergymen, sensitive
women, and a few physicians had concocted a sentimental scheme,
which had little solid foundation in common sense and efficiency.

Strong opposition to the whole idea developed in the surgeon general's office and throughout the army medical staff.

Soon, however, the Secretary of War was faced with reality. The first Battle of Bull Run completely demoralized the army medical service, and as the battle casualties accumulated, the people began bitterly to criticize the neglect of the sick and wounded as well as the lack of hospital facilities and medical supplies.

On June 9, 1861, President Lincoln approved the formation of the United States Sanitary Commission, and gave it limited powers to oversee the promotion of the health and welfare of the volunteer army. Dorothea Dix, although she was approaching her sixtieth birthday, was appointed superintendent of army nurses. She was ill suited for this job and did not do it well.

Funds for the organization were obtained from voluntary sources; local chapters were established in all the states and local communities. The nucleus of each of the local chapters was the Ladies' Aid Society. The primary purpose of these societies was to provide medical supplies and nursing care to sick and wounded soldiers.

The activities of the United States Sanitary Commission were divided into three major parts:

    I. Camp Inspection Service.
    II. Division of Supplies.
    III. Service Division of General Relief.

I. Camp Inspection Service

The Camp Inspection Service was most unpopular with the regular medical officers of the army. Undoubtedly there was much to criticize, and it is also true that the sanitary inspectors, who had little authority, were often officious and dogmatic. One colonel stated: "One of your Inspectors came about my camp, and put me through the closest set of questions I ever had to answer. I do believe there were hundreds of them. Well, I did not like it and told him so. In fact, I told him that I hoped I might never see him in my camp again." But the day came, after a great battle, when the same colonel welcomed the same inspector with grateful thanks, for the inspector now was active in the Service Division of General Relief and brought nursing care and supplies to the wounded.

The list of inspectors, all, of course, volunteers, contains the names of the foremost physicians of the day: men who were destined, in years to come, to shape the medical and educational as well as the public health policies of the nation.

Inspector-in-chief was Henry G. Clark of Boston, who had written the "Sanitary Code" for the Third National Quarantine and Sanitary Convention. Boston was represented by such great names as Dr. S. L. Abbott, Dr. James Ayer, Dr. Henry I. Bowditch, Dr. S. Cabot, Dr. J. Homans, Dr. J. B. S. Jackson, Dr. Edward Jarvis, Dr. Francis Minot, and Dr. George C. Shattuck. Dr. Edwin Snow, health officer of Providence for almost thirty years, was an inspector. From New York there came Dr. Gordon Buck, Dr. John W. Draper, Dr. A. Jacobi, Dr. Alfred C. Post, and Dr. Stephen Smith. The latter was to be instrumental in founding the American Public Health Association in 1872. Philadelphia furnished Dr. John Bell, Dr. S. Mitchell, and Dr. G. R. Morhouse. Cincinnati sent Dr. G. Mendenhall. The list is a most distinguished one.

The distribution of educational material, usually in the form of pamphlets that were issued by the commission, was one of its most valuable activities. The subjects were varied, and included:

1. "Advice as to Camping," which had first been issued by the British Government Sanitary Commission.
2. "Crimean War Directions to Army Surgeons in the Battle-field."
3. The value of vaccination.
4. Quinine as a prophylactic in malaria.
5. Reports on amputations.
6. Treatment of fractures.
7. Venereal disease control.
8. Scurvy.
9. Dysentery.
10. Pneumonia.
11. Malaria.

There was also a pamphlet of rules for preservation of the health of the soldier.

These pamphlets are a historical landmark, for they initiated a special technique of health education which, in later years, developed into enormous proportions and became one of the standard procedures of health education in America.

II. Division of Supplies

The most active division of the whole commission was that of supplies. It was very effective in distributing food, clothing, and gifts from families to the soldiers at the front. It was the only agency in the country for this purpose. Miss Louisa Schuyler reported in a letter of January 13, 1863, that, despite confusion and criticism, over 25,000 boxes had been distributed to the soldiers by the commission without loss.

The local ladies' aid societies supplied three types of materials classified as:

1. Hospital "furniture," such as blankets, sheets, pillows, quilts, towels, and the like.
2. Personal clothing: socks, shirts, drawers.
3. Hospital delicacies: tea, spirits, jelly, beef stock, and so on.

For example, in two summer months, the hospitals of the Army of the Potomac received, among other things, 43,000 sheets, 88,000 shirts, and 7,000 jars of jelly.

Mary Livermore,[3] a volunteer nurse, was most effective in organizing a nutrition program for the soldiers. In the Vicksburg campaign, the soldiers' diet consisted of meat, hardtack, and coffee, with no fruit or vegetables. Scurvy developed, which she controlled by giving the soldiers raw onions and raw potatoes dipped in molasses. Miss Livermore developed a general slogan for all local communities: "Don't send your soldier a letter, send him an onion." The onions and potatoes were collected by the local ladies' aid societies, which visited every home, secured the contributions, and utilized the local schoolhouse as a collecting point and storehouse. From these central points, the vegetables were collected and distributed to the whole army.

When spring came, Miss Livermore arranged for "victory gardens"[4] for convalescent soldiers. The Sanitary Commission furnished seeds, plants, and expert advice, and when July 4 arrived, the children pledged their firecracker money to buy vegetables for the soldiers.

All these activities were later to be consolidated under the Red Cross. Clara Barton, who was later to found the Red Cross in America in 1882, was apparently never connected directly with the Sanitary Commission. She was attached to the Ninth Army Corps as a volunteer nurse, and was active in bringing food and supplies to the wounded.

[3] Greenbie, M. L. B.: *Lincoln's Daughters of Mercy.* G. P. Putnam's Sons, New York, 1944.
[4] This term "victory gardens," so widely utilized in World War II, was apparently coined by Miss Livermore.

Another distinguished social worker, Louisa Schuyler, who organized the New York State Charities Aid in 1872, and thus became the creator of modern social work in America, was a volunteer nurse for the New York Division of the United States Sanitary Commission and was active in its organization.

III. *Service Division of General Relief*

Mr. Olmstead, as executive secretary, soon demonstrated the great value of the Sanitary Commission to the army. He provided for nursing care in the field by volunteers. Those courageous women often carried on their work directly behind the battle lines. During the Peninsular campaign, he devised a system of ambulances for rapid removal of the wounded from the field of battle. This system later became incorporated in the medical care service of all our modern community hospitals.

As the war progressed, the Service Section of General Relief of the Sanitary Commission became more and more efficient. At the great battle of Gettysburg, more than 20,000 wounded were left on the field, with little or no official medical or hospital units for their care. This entire number, which included the men in gray uniforms as well as those in blue, were cared for on the field by volunteer nurses and were evacuated to dressing stations and temporary hospitals by the volunteers of the United States Sanitary Commission.[5]

In summary, the United States Sanitary Commission was loosely organized and, in some instances, poorly administered. It had considerable difficulty with its finances, and had no clear-cut and definitely assigned administrative responsibilities. It did cut across well-established lines of military authority and often was, as Lincoln had anticipated, "a fifth wheel to the coach." Some of its personnel were officious, tactless, and bungling. A great deal of sentimentality and impracticality was wrapped up in the whole bundle of philanthropic and well-intentioned activity.

Although it was a sanitary commission, its achievements in the field of sanitation were negligible. But, despite its faults, the United States Sanitary Commission met a great need and fulfilled its responsibilities to a remarkably successful degree, due largely to the heroic self-sacrifice and sincere devotion of its volunteers.

[5] See *United States Sanitary Commission Document 71* on operations during and after the Battle of Gettysburg.

A very important contribution of the United States Sanitary Commission to the social life of America was the introduction of the concept of the volunteer, unofficial, *health and welfare association*. The Sanitary Commission demonstrated not only that a citizens' group could affect governmental action, but also showed the value and power of organization in promotion of public welfare. Small, isolated groups, working independently, accomplish nothing, but a well-planned and well-organized co-ordination of effort by small groups in each community, *with the support of a central organization*, can influence public opinion, educate great masses of people, and bring about profound reforms in social structure.

Furthermore, the Sanitary Commission influenced the entrance of nursing into the social and political life of the nation. In fact, immediately after the close of the war, the first school of hospital training for nurses was established in Boston.

As we have already noted, Miss Louisa Schuyler, who was active in the United States Sanitary Commission, continued her welfare work after the war, and in 1872 organized the New York State Charities Aid. This association was to play an important part in the promotion of the health and welfare of New York State and, indirectly, the whole country. We shall meet many of these volunteers again in subsequent chapters.

CHAPTER 31. *City Health Departments: Their*

Early History

WITH SPECIAL REFERENCE TO NEW YORK CITY

Away, then, with crowded cities, the 30 feet lots and alleys, the artificial reservoirs of filth, the hotbeds of atmospheric poison. Such are our cities. They are great prisons built with immense labor to breed infection and hurry men prematurely to the grave.   NOAH WEBSTER, *1799*

The early development of public health administration in the United States was centered in the local communities. In fact, practically all the important developments in public health during the first seventy-five years of the nineteenth century were carried out in cities and towns.

RAPID GROWTH OF THE URBAN POPULATION

One of the social factors that has had a very important effect upon the public health has been the rapid growth of the urban population of the United States during the past century. There has occurred a continuous migration from the farm and village to the city. Furthermore, the foreign immigrants who came to America in enormous and ever-increasing numbers at the beginning of the twentieth century settled in our cities, even though most of them originated in the country. During the last half of the nineteenth century the city population increased three times as fast as the rural, and during the present century the urban increase has been four times as fast as that of the country areas. In 1880 less than 3 per cent of the people lived in cities of over 1,000,000 population. In 1950 this rate had increased to over 20 per cent.

Figure 25 illustrates the relative growth of the urban and rural

populations of the United States for the years 1850 to 1950. The
two trend lines cross about 1915, and it is quite apparent that
the present trends will continue for years to come.

The history of the growth and development of public health in
America from 1850 to the present time would have been very different indeed if the two lines on the graph had remained as parallel
from 1880 to 1950 as they were from 1850 to 1880. This would have
resulted in 60,000,000 rural dwellers in 1950, which is about the

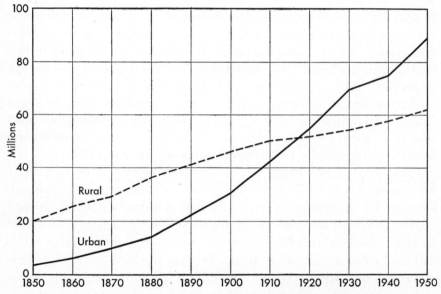

Fig. 25. Growth of urban and rural populations of the United States, 1850-1950.
(Rural people are those who live in communities of less than 2,500 population.)
(From *Statistical Bull.*, Metropolitan Life Insurance Co., Vol. 32, Sept., 1951, as
based upon various reports of the Bureau of the Census.)

actual 1950 number, and 40,000,000 city people instead of 90,-
000,000. There would have been few cities of over 1,000,000 population and no large industries. The people would have been
conservative, staid, independent, resistant to change, and slow to
accept modification in their mode of life. Local self-government
would have maintained its prominence in the social and political
philosophy. Full-time local health services would have been few in
number. Mass methods for prevention of communicable disease
as well as sanitary measures for purification of water supplies, for
sewage disposal plants, food sanitation, milk pasteurization, and

many other advances that have been made in public health protection would not have been consummated. It must be remembered that the rapid growth of cities has resulted first in appalling sanitary conditions, for the simple reason that the rural people who moved to the cities brought with them the family and village customs. Hygienic measures that were quite adequate in sparsely settled areas were completely unsuited to the city dweller. Thus, sickness and death rates increased to such a degree that the specific sanitary problems were first recognized, then faced, and finally a solution was obtained. But in every instance it was the people of the cities who initiated the improved procedures, whether they related to environmental sanitation, communicable disease control, health education, or public health administration. As we develop our discussion of the history of public health and preventive medicine during the second part of the nineteenth century, it will become quite clear that the rapid change of population from a rural to an urban economy, with all that this migration entails, has been a major factor in molding the pattern of the public health procedures of our nation.

Local boards of health were organized before 1800, but their development was slow, and their activities were extremely limited. Chapin[1] has informed us that only five principal cities established boards of health between the years 1800 to 1830. Chicago initiated its health service in 1867. Even as late as 1875, many large cities had no health departments at all. Perhaps the best record was that of Providence, Rhode Island. Dr. Edwin M. Snow began his duties as superintendent of health of Providence in 1856, and served continuously until he was succeeded by Dr. Charles Chapin in 1884. Chapin continued in this office for forty-eight years—to 1931.

Dr. Snow dealt almost exclusively with the abatement of nuisances. His principal responsibilities were to clean the streets, maintain clean yards, prevent overcrowding, and remove dead animals and decaying materials. As the years passed, he assumed the supervision of the cleaning of yard privies. After many years he became concerned with the purity of the water supplies of the city. Quarantine was not an important part of his duties.

Chapin[2] has emphasized the fact that health services in the cities of the United States, during the first half of the nineteenth century, were based on three major errors. It was believed that:

[1] Chapin, Charles: "History of State and Municipal Control of Disease," *A Half Century of Public Health*. American Public Health Association, New York, 1921, p. 137.
[2] *Ibid.*

1. Disease bred in filth. Thus the etiology of all infections was an essential element of the putrefactive process.
2. All kinds of filth were dangerous.
3. Infectious diseases were always air-borne. Decomposition and fermentation gave rise to poisonous gases. These noxious gases were carried for a long distance through the air, resulting in widespread epidemics. It was not realized until after the middle of the century that water might be a vehicle of infection.

Since these errors were accepted generally, it becomes obvious that public health procedures which were based on error were, for the most part, quite ineffective.

In a previous chapter (see page 122) we have described the general attitude toward quarantine for prevention of household infections. Since it was believed that disease was not transmitted directly from person to person (with the exception of smallpox), it was felt that there was no community advantage in isolating a person who was sick with a fever, nor was it considered of any great value to quarantine an infected family. Thus household quarantine languished. In most cities and towns, health services were applied sporadically and intermittently. There would be a recrudescence when epidemics threatened, but as the contagion disappeared the health department quietly expired.

The concept that each community should maintain a continuous, effective, local health service grew slowly; so slowly, in fact, that it did not penetrate to all parts of the nation for nearly 100 years. The development of this concept can be traced through the records of New York City,[3] and for this reason we shall use this city as an illustration of municipal health department growth.

NEW YORK CITY: DEVELOPMENT OF ITS HEALTH SERVICES

In 1799 the New York state legislature granted New York City the authority to pass and enforce local health laws. John Pintard was appointed city inspector of health in 1804. From 1810 to 1838, the city health inspectors were a branch of the local police department. They were concerned chiefly with the control of epidemics— particularly outbreaks of yellow fever and smallpox. At the outset there was one inspector and one assistant inspector, but more were

[3] New York City is used as an illustration because (1) its development is quite representative of other American cities and (2) the records are more readily available. Other municipalities would have a very similar story to tell.

added during epidemic periods. Cornelius B. Archer, who was city inspector in 1845, secured, for the first time, the enactment of a local regulation for registration of vital statistics. In 1852 T. K. Downing, then city inspector, established two bureaus: (1) Registry and Statistics; (2) Sanitary Inspection.

For the most part, the activities of the city health inspectors were comparable to those of our present-day local sanitary inspectors. They were not responsible to the board of health, however, but usually were political appointees assigned to the police department.

The board of health was an advisory body which functioned only in epidemic periods. Maritime quarantine was organized under this board, and during epidemic periods of smallpox, yellow fever, and cholera, quarantine laws were enforced by it. The board of health consisted of the mayor, the city recorder, the commissioner of state quarantine, and five other members. This board appointed the quarantine officer, who was always a physician, and whose duty it was to inspect all ships arriving from foreign lands.

At the beginning of the century, New York City had a population of about 60,000. At first its growth was very slow, but in the fourth decade there began a period of rapid growth, so that by the middle of the century the city had a population of 500,000.

By 1857 New York City had the highest death rate of any of the large cities of the world. Sanitary science had been making great advances in western Europe for more than twenty years, but the New World had not kept abreast of the times. The death rates of London and Berlin had been reduced to 25 per 1,000 population; and Paris boasted a death rate of only 28, whereas in New York the death rate, instead of declining, had risen from 25.1 per 1,000 population in 1840 to 36.8 in 1857.

The reasons for this were manifold. As we have noted, the city had increased very rapidly in population and its character had changed. In the previous fifteen years a horde of immigrants had poured into and through the port of New York—nearly 2,500,000 of them. Many of these poor people were the destitute, starving Irish, who were fleeing from their potato famine. They arrived without resources, in a terrible state of malnutrition, and crowded into the basement tenements under desperately filthy and foul conditions, where they died in appalling numbers. Deaths from diarrheal diseases of infancy increased 250 per cent. Smallpox, typhus fever, and cholera, as well as erysipelas and cerebrospinal meningitis, swept through these wretched hovels, slaying the helpless victims by the thousands. In the first six months alone of the year 1858, 425 persons died in New York City of smallpox—and yet vaccination had been known for over fifty years.

In 1858 the city had no sanitary protection whatever. D. B. Eaton described the situation vividly:

Men elected by party caucuses were treated as competent to administer the science of health and solve the problems of sanitary precaution. It is no wonder that the exercise of sanitary authority soon became a greater peril than miasma and contagion; that political doctors became the agents of partizan and unnecessary city officers; that mayors of New York, by no means scrupulous or timid, did not dare for a whole term to even call a meeting of the N. Y. Board of Health; that of 48 health wardens and assistants, more than half were keepers of corner groggeries (the other half were partizan repeaters and bullies); and that nearly the whole sanitary force of the city was in reality a scandal and a peril to a civilized community.[4]

The New York Sanitary Association[5]

In 1856 the Academy of Medicine of New York pointed out these evil conditions to the state legislature, without result. Two years later the Academy of Medicine renewed its efforts. In order to secure action and promote proper legislation, the New York Sanitary Association was formed (1859). It was composed of laymen and Academy members. Frederick E. Mather, a layman, was president, and Peter Cooper was on the council; but a physician, Dr. J. H. Griscom, the first vice-president, and Dr. Elisha Harris, the secretary, had the burden of drafting the legislation and of guiding the public health reform bill through the state legislature. The medical members of the council were Dr. Isaac Wood of New York Hospital; Dr. A. C. Post, one of the great surgeons of the country; Dr. E. R. Peaslee, who had succeeded Oliver Wendell Holmes at Dartmouth as professor of anatomy; and three others who were later to take an active part in public health affairs in New York City: Dr. Joseph Smith, Dr. C. R. Agnew, the young aristocrat who had recently returned from his studies in Europe, and young Dr. Stephen Smith, who had yet to win his spurs in public affairs.

[4] Eaton, D. B.: *Sanitary Regulations in England and New York.* J. W. Amerman, New York, 1872, p. 31.
[5] From the *Reports of the New York City Sanitary Association.* Academy of Medicine, New York, 1859.

Dr. Griscom drew up the bill which proposed a board of health for New York City. In the light of our present experience, we know that he proposed a completely unworkable organization. The board of health was to be made up of a heterogeneous group of eleven men, including the mayor, the chairman of the board of aldermen and the city council, the chief of police, a representative from each of the three medical colleges, the president of the Croton Aqueduct Board, and others. The bill would have taken away the jobs of the incompetent sanitary wardens, and would at least have brought some honesty and sanitary knowledge into play in amelioration of the tragic sanitary situation. The sponsors of this bill made a good fight, and marshaled their facts well, but were naive and inexperienced in legislative matters and were completely outmaneuvered by their opponents in the state legislature. They got little support from those who should have helped them most. Thus they lost the battle.

Though the New York Sanitary Association had such a short and inglorious existence, the experience gained in this skirmish served only to test the mettle of two men who were to become great leaders in the development of the public health in the city and the nation. Elisha Harris and Stephen Smith gained valuable knowledge and experience from this initial bitter defeat. It was their first encounter with the stupidities and machinations of political chicanery. They were destined to fight many a battle together, and eventually to mold the foundations of city, state, and national health services for all America.

The Third National Quarantine and Sanitary Convention, 1859 (Held in New York City)[6]

In a previous chapter we have presented a summary of the deliberations of the Third National Quarantine and Sanitary Convention, with special emphasis on its major interest, namely, maritime quarantine. Another very interesting development of this convention was the initiation of a discussion on sanitary measures. Dr. John Bell of Philadelphia read an extensive report on "The Importance and Economy of Sanitary Measures to Cities."[7] This report was concerned chiefly with the cleaning of streets, the control of sewage and sewer gases, the city water supply, and to some degree housing. It discussed also public parks and recreation and the sanitation of

[6] *Proceedings and Debates of the Third National Quarantine and Sanitary Convention.* Edward Jones & Co., Printers to Board of Education, New York, 1859.

[7] *Third National Quarantine and Sanitary Convention: op. cit.*, pp. 523-24.

schoolrooms and public buildings. The control of slaughterhouses and other nuisances was also presented. Public workhouses were advocated and intemperance was deplored. Another important topic dealt with the great danger of interment of the dead within the city. Attention was drawn by Dr. Bell to the report of Dr. Griscom[8] upon "Improving the Conditions of the Laboring Classes in the City of New York," in which he stated:

Crazy old buildings, crowded rear tenements in filthy yards, dark, damp basements, leaky garrets, shops, out-houses, and stables converted into dwellings, though scarcely fit to shelter brutes, are the habitations of thousands of our fellow-beings dwelling in this wealthy, Christian city.

The chief causes of mortality in New York City were attributed to bad food, bad clothing, damp and impure air, and overcrowding in filthy, unventilated, miserable cellars:

The fearful aggregate of infant mortality in New York . . . is at once the fruit and the proof of the contaminated air they breathe, in the wretched habitations of the poor, where confined and ill-ventilated apartments render healthy respiration impossible.[9]

We have quoted at some length from this report in order to emphasize the fact that the authorities believed in the theory that odors and miasma which arose from filthy human living were the most important source of illness. They also believed that the chief functions of the sanitarian were to promote community cleanliness and provide for suitable disposal of community wastes.

Although the Civil War (1861-1865) interrupted all progress in sanitary affairs throughout the nation, it taught a great many lessons in public health and medical care that were soon to be applied to civil life. In 1865, at the end of the Civil War, there was no board of health in New York City. The aldermen were summoned to meet as a board of health only in the face of an emergency. There was a health commissioner, but he had no prescribed duties. The "health wardens" were placed in the Street Cleaning Department, which had an appropriation of nearly $1,000,000 a year. Theoretically the health wardens were also quarantine officers, although their major duty was the abatement of nuisances. There were scores of these officers, generally saloonkeepers and political henchmen of Tammany Hall. The city government was completely dominated by

[8] *Third National Quarantine and Sanitary Convention: op. cit.,* pp. 441-639.
[9] *Third National Quarantine and Sanitary Convention: op. cit.,* p. 526.

Tammany and the citizens had found it impossible to break the hold of this political machine on civic affairs.

Dorman B. Eaton, a lawyer, who in 1859 had already manifested interest in the public health, drew up a new public health bill for the New York state legislature in 1864. This bill was based on the English sanitary system. It was framed to form a *metropolitan board of health* which would include various outlying districts adjoining Manhattan Island, such as Brooklyn, the Bronx, and so on (these are now a part of the City of New York). The bill was intended to remove the control of city health services from politics, but Tammany was able to defeat the bill in the state legislature with ease.

Stephen Smith enters the picture at this stage. He began his career as a young surgeon in New York, at the middle of the century. He was placed in charge of the typhus fever wards on Welfare Island, where he noted that a large number of the victims came from the same city address. He visited this dwelling, which was located in the slums, and found the most shocking conditions of poverty, filth, overcrowding, and destitution. He interested William Cullen Bryant, the poet, who at that time was editor of the *Evening Post*, in a crusade for sanitary improvement of the city. This occurred in 1855. This episode gave Stephen Smith a crusading public health spirit that was to grow with the years.

The Citizens' Association

In the early sixties a Citizens' Association was formed which consisted of 100 leading New York citizens, with Peter Cooper as its president. The purpose of this association was to break the stranglehold which Boss Tweed of Tammany had on the government of the city.

The Citizens' Association selected a Committee on Public Health which was composed of New York's most distinguished doctors. They were largely instrumental, as we shall see, in promoting Eaton's health bill which was mentioned above.

The Sanitary Survey of 1864

The Public Health Committee of the Citizens' Association, on the defeat of Eaton's bill in 1864, decided to make a sanitary survey of New York City in order to demonstrate and document the actual intolerable conditions. A sum of $22,000 was appropriated for this purpose. Stephen Smith organized this study with great energy. He divided the city into twenty-nine districts, and selected twenty-nine of his young medical associates to make the survey. He gave to each a detailed outline of his duties and in July, 1864, the work began. These young men combed their territories thoroughly. Detailed colored maps were drawn and sketches of bad situations were made. Every tenement, every brothel, every dark and dismal corner, was penetrated. The conditions that were uncovered far exceeded the expectations of the survey committee. Dr. Elisha Harris edited the report and it was published in full in 1865.[10]

The report received the attention which it so well deserved. Eaton again drew up a bill for the New York state legislature which provided for a metropolitan board of health. The area to be covered included Brooklyn, the Bronx, Queens, Westchester County, and other localities contiguous to Manhattan.

Again its purpose was to wrest the control of sanitary affairs from the political gang. Dr. Smith framed the sanitary features of the bill and defended it eloquently before the hearings of the state legislature in Albany in 1865. Despite its eminent backing, the health bill was defeated for a second time. The city inspector denied vehemently that unsanitary conditions existed in the City of New York. This inspector was, as Dr. Smith tells us in *The City That Was*,[11] a grossly ignorant ward politician but, as he had upwards of $1,000,-000 annually at his disposal, he had a prevailing influence on the legislature when any bill affected his interests.

The matter assumed so much public interest that the following year the measure became an important political issue. Seventeen candidates who had voted in opposition to the measure in 1865 were defeated. Most opportunely, a cholera epidemic appeared in New York at this time. Finally, in 1866, the bill, which established the Metropolitan Board of Health, was passed.

We have discussed these events at some length because the report of the sanitary survey is one of the important keystones in the establishment of the sound principles of local municipal health organization in our nation. The young men who organized this study were soon to become the public health leaders of America. They were responsible for the establishment of the American Public Health Association, and were key members of the indomitable group that

---

[10] Smith, Stephen, and associates: *Report of the Sanitary Conditions of the City of New York*. D. Appleton & Co., New York, 1865.

[11] Smith, Stephen: *The City That Was*. Frank Allaben, New York, 1911, pp. 166-67.

carried it through its difficult neonatal period. They organized the National Board of Health and took a very important part in the establishment of state and local health services throughout the nation. Stephen Smith was to survive until his one-hundredth year, and thus he lived long enough to see the full fruition of his courageous pioneer work.

The *First Annual Report of the Metropolitan Board of Health* in 1866 was a wonderful document with detailed epidemiological charts, vital statistical tables, and current data. It was the work of Elisha Harris, who was corresponding secretary and registrar of vital statistics. Edward B. Dalton[12] was made sanitary superintendent and D. B. Eaton was counsel. Stephen Smith was not appointed to the first board as a sanitary commissioner; in fact, his name does not appear until 1869. The Metropolitan Board of Health lasted four years—until 1870.

The politicians of New York City did not like the Metropolitan Board of Health. It set a bad precedent for them since the city voted for an expenditure of funds over which the politicians had no control. In 1869 Elisha Harris succeeded Dalton as sanitary superintendent, with Moreau Morris as his assistant. We are not clear about all the details of political intrigue, but apparently Dr. Harris was not a good politician and Morris, who was most ambitious, saw a way to realize his ambition by undermining his chief. In any case, in 1870, New York City was excluded from the Metropolitan Health District by the state legislature and the New York City Board of Health was formed. Dr. Harris was out of office and Dr. Moreau Morris was made sanitary superintendent. Dr. Stephen Smith was demoted to membership in the Committee on Vital Statistics.

But a precedent had been set and a solid, local health service had been established. Thus, from that day on, New York was to have a health department. It has been a department which has survived all vicissitudes, has innovated important procedures, and has produced such great public health personalities as Stephen Smith, Elisha Harris, Charles F. Chandler, Ernest J. Lederle, Hermann M. Biggs, William H. Park, Josephine Baker, Charles F. Bolduan, Shirley W. Wynne, and Haven Emerson—to mention only a few.[13]

[12] Dr. Dalton had been a colonel in the Civil War and was highly regarded as the man who organized the ambulance system for care of the wounded.

[13] Further details of New York City Health Department history may be secured from the following articles:

Rosen, George: "Public Health Problems of New York City," *New York State J. Med.*, p. 73, January, 1, 1950; Weinstein, Israel: "Eighty Years of Public Health in New York City," *Bull. New York Acad. Med.*, 23:221-31, 1947.

Philadelphia, Baltimore, Boston, Chicago, New Orleans, and other great cities were to have their health department vicissitudes and achievements, each more or less paralleling those that we have just described. The pattern was set and the basic principles of organization were established.

The formation of the American Public Health Association in 1872 proved to be the cohesive force that served to cement the foundation stones of the public health structure. The association was formed by municipal health officers and from its very outset had a profound influence in the advancement of health services, first in the large cities, then in the smaller municipalities. Finally, after more than fifty years, its influence permeated to the most remote sections of the nation through organization of adequate health services for rural areas.

CHAPTER 32. *The American Public Health*

Association

We shall have next year, I doubt not, the American Sanitary Association, which will live until her work shall be performed and her need shall be no longer.

JOHN H. GRISCOM, *1860*

Dr. Stephen Smith of New York, in his "Historical Sketch of the American Public Health Association,"[1] gives us the chain of events that led up to the organization of the association. In 1856 Dr. Wilson Jewell, a member of the Philadelphia Board of Health, secured a resolution from his board which entailed the calling of a Quarantine Convention of the boards of health of the cities of Boston, Baltimore, New York, and New Orleans to consider the establishment of a uniform system of revised quarantine regulations. Dr. Jewell was stimulated to undertake this matter because of the success of the Sanitary Conferences held in Paris in 1851 and 1852.

Sanitary conventions were held, as we have already noted, in 1857, 1858, 1859, and 1860. The fifth was to have met in Cincinnati in 1861, but the organization as such was destroyed by the Civil War. At the Fourth National Quarantine and Sanitary Convention in Boston in 1860, Dr. John Griscom indicated the sentiment of the meeting when he said:

We shall have next year, I doubt not, the American Sanitary Association, which will live until her work shall be performed and her need shall be no longer [great cheering].[2]

But over twelve years were to pass before this hope could be realized.

At the end of the Civil War, the pioneers in sanitary reform were

---

[1] Smith, Stephen: *Reports and Papers of the American Public Health Association,* 1879, Vol. V, pp. VII-LIV. Houghton Mifflin Co., Boston, 1880.

[2] *Proceedings and Debates of the Fourth National Quarantine and Sanitary Convention.* George C. Rand & Avery, City Printers, Boston, 1860, p. 146.

stimulated to renewed zeal. As Smith notes, "Though the Civil War proved so disastrous to the Convention, as an organization, the seed planted was not destroyed."[3]

The passage of the Metropolitan Health Law of New York in 1866, ". . . which has been declared officially and judicially to be the most complete piece of health legislation ever placed on the statute books,"[4] resulted in the organization of many new municipal boards of health. State boards of health began to be organized in 1869. Obviously the time had come to form a health officers' association for mutual benefit and stimulus.

THE ASSOCIATION IS FORMED

On April 18, 1872, Dr. Stephen Smith called a meeting of a few of his friends at the City Health Department office at 301 Mott Street, New York City, to consider the formation of a nationwide association of those persons who were interested in public health. It was an opportune time to plan for such an organization, and Dr. Smith was the logical person to initiate the movement.

He had been interested in public health matters for years. He was one of the founders of the short-lived New York Sanitary Association in 1859. He sat in on that famous debate on the contagious nature of yellow fever in the National Quarantine and Sanitary Convention, which met in New York that same year. He took little active part in this meeting, but gained a great deal of experience. He was the active, driving force that had secured the support of the Citizens' Association of New York in making the survey of the sanitary conditions of New York City, which was reported in 1865. He was appointed to the Metropolitan Board of Health when it was founded in 1866, and to the New York City Board of Health, which succeeded the Metropolitan Board in 1870. He was undoubtedly the most active and influential person in the public health field in the whole nation.

Dr. Smith was in constant correspondence with other leading health officers throughout the country. In April, 1872, he had written to some of his friends, inviting them to come to New York to consider the feasibility of organizing a stable, nationwide public health association. Seven men met in his office that first afternoon. Dr. E. M. Snow, health officer of Providence, was asked to take the chair. He was only fifty-three years old, but was dean of the group insofar as health work was concerned, for he had been health officer of his city

[3] Smith, Stephen: *op. cit.*, p. x.
[4] Smith, Stephen: *The City That Was.* Frank Allaben, New York, 1911, p. 158.

since 1856, and had been in attendance at the National Quarantine and Sanitary Conventions of 1858, 1859, and 1860. Dr. J. H. Rauch came to the meeting from Chicago. He had already shown his aggressiveness in promoting health work in the West. He had been sanitary superintendent of Chicago for the past five years and had just won nationwide renown because of his sanitary work during and following the great Chicago fire of 1871. Dr. J. Ordronaux was the only other person present who had attended any of the National Sanitary Conventions. He was a lawyer as well as a doctor, and primarily interested in medical jurisprudence. He had gone to the Boston meeting in 1860, and though a very young man (twenty-nine years old) had quite overwhelmed the conference with his erudition and oratorical talent; but he lived a life of frustration, and time was to show that he was not greatly interested in the broad new concepts of public health.

Dr. C. C. Cox, health officer of Washington, D. C., came to the meeting. He was not destined to take an important part in the future affairs of the association. He was to present an excellent paper on the "Necessity of a National Health Organization" at the Cincinnati meeting in May, 1873. He attended the Philadelphia meeting in 1874, where he read a paper on "Sewage and Drainage," but apparently his connection with the association ceased. He was no longer on the membership roll in 1879, the fifth anniversary, and dropped out of sight. E. H. Janes was apparently a satellite of Dr. Smith. He was a New York City sanitary inspector at the time, April, 1872, and he continued with this health department either as assistant sanitary superintendent, or in one capacity or another for many years. He had ahead of him a good deal of hard work for this new public health association, but he received little recognition. He seems to have been one of those men who are always "assistant" to someone else. Whenever his name is mentioned in the minutes, it seems to be as an afterthought: "Such and such men were present at the meeting—and E. H. Janes." His life work was more closely linked with Elisha Harris than with anyone else, and he named one of his children for Harris. He did excellent spadework, presented some good papers at the association meetings, and never missed a session. Like one of the Disciples, he was simply an undistinguished "Simon Peter's brother."

The last member of the group was Carl Pfeiffer, an architect. Dr. Smith invited him because they were both interested in housing for the poor. Dr. Smith understood the necessity for inclusion of those persons who were interested in the public health but who were not physicians. This preliminary invitation to Carl Pfeiffer established the precedent of nonmedical membership in the American Public Health Association and established also its broad policy of inclusion in the membership of all those groups that are professionally interested in this field. Mr. Pfeiffer proved a loyal and valuable contributor to the association. We find a number of good papers from his pen in the *Reports and Papers of the Association,* relating chiefly to tenements and housing. At the fifth anniversary we find that he was still an active member.

This first afternoon's meeting was devoted to a preliminary discussion of the purpose and value of an association of public health men. Dr. Snow had to return to Providence that afternoon because of illness in his family. The others of the group reconvened that evening at the New York Hotel and were joined by three recruits: Dr. Moreau Morris, Dr. Heber Smith, and Dr. Elisha Harris.

Dr. Moreau Morris was obviously a politician. He had been health commissioner of New York before the Metropolitan Board was founded in 1866, and was absorbed into the Metropolitan Board of Health as sanitary inspector. He then became New York State cattle inspector for two years, 1869-1870. At the time of this meeting he was superintendent of the New York Board of Health (1870-1872). He took little part in the discussions, but was made a member of the executive committee of the association, and attended the meetings of 1873, 1874, and 1875. He did not come to the fifth anniversary meeting, but was registered as an active member with residence in Binghamton, New York. He then dropped out of sight until 1889, when we find his appointment as sanitary inspector in charge of the New York City public schools. He read one or two papers before the annual association meetings, but they are not outstanding, and he contributed little to the association:

Dr. Heber Smith, who was in charge of the United States Marine Hospital Service at Stapleton, Staten Island, came over for the evening meeting. He was not much interested in public health, and although he continued as an active member of the association for several years, he took no active part in it and contributed little to its development.

The third man of the evening group was Dr. Elisha Harris. He had been in public health work since 1855, the year he was made chief of the Quarantine Hospital at Staten Island. He had taken part in the National Quarantine and Sanitary Convention in 1860 and had aided in the Sanitary Survey of the Citizens' Committee of New York City in 1865. He was well versed in vital statistics; he was interested in housing and understood the principles of communicable disease control. He was destined to take an active part in every important public health advance of his generation. In fact, it can truly be said that Stephen Smith and Elisha Harris, with the able assistance of John Rauch, bore the heaviest part of the burden of the early years of trial and difficulty of the American Public Health Association.

The evening group got down to serious business. They elected a Committee of Permanent Organization and made Stephen Smith chairman. They then selected representatives of state health departments, such as Dr. George Derby of Massachusetts, C. B. White of Louisiana, and Jerome Cochran of Alabama. To this list were added a few university professors, such as William Clendenin of Ohio and Henry Hartshorne of Pennsylvania. They also asked the surgeon general of the army and the navy to designate members to sit on the permanent committee. They specifically invited the surgeon general of the Marine Hospital Service, Dr. John Woodworth, to serve on the committee. (They forgot to name Dr. Snow on the committee; Dr. Janes came in at the tail end as usual. He was honored by selection on the organization committee in the customary way, but as an afterthought . . . "and Dr. Janes.")

THE EARLY YEARS OF THE ASSOCIATION

An organization meeting was called for September 12, 1872, at Long Branch, New Jersey. There was an excellent and very encouraging attendance at this meeting. Dr. Snow did not come down from Providence, but it was the only meeting he was to miss during his long period of health activity. Heber Smith of the Marine Hospital Service did not get there, but all the others who had met in New York in April were at this meeting. They were joined by J. M. Woodworth of Washington (of the United States Marine Hospital Service). Professor C. F. Chandler, who was a chemist at Columbia University and who later became health commissioner of New York City, was there as well as Henry Hartshorne, who taught hygiene at the University of Pennsylvania, and who was a voluminous writer. Dr. William Clendenin of Cincinnati, who was a professor of surgery at

Miami Medical College and who had been health physician of Cincinnati since 1865, came to this meeting. C. B. White, sanitary director of New Orleans, came and was made second vice-president. The other officers elected at this meeting were:

Stephen Smith	President
Edwin Snow	Vice-President
Elisha Harris	Secretary
John Rauch	Treasurer

These four were the stalwarts who served as a cohesive nucleus and kept the organization from disintegration during the perilous years that were ahead. They borrowed money from their own families to print the transactions, rotated the important offices among themselves, and gave boundless energy and abundance of their own time and thought to make the association a success.

At the September meeting they elected a few new members, who were to play a very important part in national health affairs. One of these new members was J. S. Billings, who established the Surgeon General's Library and became the greatest American physician of his day. He was to take a very important part in determining the policies of the new association. J. M. Toner of Washington, who proved a tower of strength to the association, was elected at this time, and also J. L. Cabell, of Charlottesville, Virginia, who was later to be president of the National Board of Health during its entire existence.

Edward Jarvis of Boston, philosopher and pioneer in mental hygiene, was chosen for membership. Ezra Hunt of New Jersey, who was to play such a fine part in rural health promotion, was elected to membership also, as was A. N. Bell of Brooklyn, an authority on maritime quarantine. He was to establish *The Sanitarian* the very next year and to edit it through the rest of his life. He was the only other one of the group who had taken part in the early National Quarantine and Sanitary Conventions. (He attended the 1859 and 1860 meetings.)

The association was well launched at the Long Branch meeting. Almost all the charter members selected at that meeting took a real interest in the infant organization and gave it strong support. The first regular session was held the following spring in Cincinnati, at the same time and place as the American Medical Association meeting. They had an excellent program. It is probably the only meeting

Elisha Harris ever missed, but Dr. Smith, Dr. Snow, and Dr. Rauch came, together with most of the other charter members. Billings attended, and Jarvis and Toner were made members of the executive committee.

The following resolution was adopted:

. . . That a committee . . . be appointed to consider . . . the best plan for the appointment and organization of national, State, and local boards of health . . .[5]

Dorman B. Eaton, the famous attorney who had drafted the New York Metropolitan Board of Health laws and who was to draft the National Board of Health law, was placed on this committee.

A New York meeting was held on November 11 of this same year, 1873. This was the second actual session, with fine attendance and a good program. H. B. Baker, who was the health officer of the new state Health Department of Michigan, was there. The attorney, D. B. Eaton, came and also S. O. Van der Poel, quarantine officer of the Port of New York. Gen. F. H. Walker came down from New Haven. He was superintendent of the United States Census and read a fine paper on this topic. The meeting was so small that practically everyone gave a paper; some of the contributions were poor, but most of them were very good indeed.

The next meeting at Philadelphia in November, 1874, was poorly attended, for enthusiasm had begun to wane. The four pillars of the association were there, of course, "and E. H. Janes," who had never missed a meeting. J. S. Billings, Ezra Hunt, A. N. Bell, J. M. Toner, and a handful of new members made up the assembly. There were few state health departments as yet, and those that had been established had taken little part in the association's affairs. Baker of Michigan came, and Cox of Washington, D. C., attended for the last time; but Derby of Massachusetts was not there, nor Cochran of Alabama, nor Hewitt of Minnesota. The association was due for a long, hard struggle for survival. Dr. Samuel Gross submitted a resolution relating to sponsorship by the association of a *National Board of Health* that was to be of great import to the association, but nothing was done about it at this meeting.

The Baltimore meeting of November 9, 1875, was quite well attended. Dr. J. M. Toner was president of this meeting, succeeding Dr. Smith. He had been president of the American Medical Association in 1873, and was at the height of his career. He added great

[5] *Reports and Papers of the American Public Association,* 5:16, 1879.

prestige to the young association and took real interest in its meetings. John Rauch was elected first vice-president at this meeting,
Edwin Snow was made president-elect, and Elisha Harris continued
as secretary.

Health education techniques were discussed for the first time, and
the functions and duties of a state board of health received serious
consideration.

The association began to get into its stride, and the next meeting
at Boston seems to have been a critical one. The Boston meeting of
1876 had an excellent program. Dr. Edwin Snow was president this
year. New names began to appear on the program. Professor Wm.
Ripley Nichols of Massachusetts Institute of Technology gave a
paper, and J. P. Kirkwood, the sanitary engineer who had pioneered
in water purification, was there. Henry I. Bowditch, who had
founded the first board of health in Massachusetts in 1869, was present; and Charles F. Folsom, who had succeeded George Derby as
secretary, represented the Massachusetts State Board of Health. A. L.
Gihon, of the United States Navy, who was a pioneer in syphilis
control, was elected to the executive board. Six of the group of ten
who first met in New York in 1872 were present, "including E. H.
Janes." Edward Everett Hale made an inspiring address, and the
great clinician, Austin Flint, read a paper on nutrition, "Food and
Its Relation to Personal and Public Health."

Henry G. Clark, pioneer in municipal health administration, who
wrote the "Municipal Sanitary Code" for the National Quarantine
and Sanitary Convention of 1859 and was city physician of Boston
in 1856, was present at the Boston meeting, but took no part. He
was an old man and his active public work was done.

The fifth meeting was held in Chicago, on September 25, 1877, in
honor of Dr. J. H. Rauch, who was president that year. He had done
a great deal for Chicago, and was one of Chicago's most important
citizens. He had made a careful study of the climate and geological
features of the area. He had planned its park system, for he believed
that public parks had a beneficial effect upon the "moral, physical,
and sanitary conditions of a large city." Over a million trees had
been planted in Chicago's parks on the treeless prairie soil during
the previous ten years, and they have remained, to this day, as a living
monument to the great citizen of his beloved city.

Dr. Rauch's presidential address was upon "The Sanitary Problems of Chicago, Past and Present." The breezy, optimistic spirit of

the rapidly expanding West is well illustrated in this address. He was introducing a new land to many of the members of the association who had never before been beyond the Allegheny Mountains.

College health promotion service was first described at this meeting. Professor Edward Hitchcock gave an excellent description of the experience of the Department of Physical Education and Hygiene at Amherst College during the previous sixteen years. Dr. Charles Hewitt, state health officer of Minnesota, discussed health education in the common schools, and Elisha Harris began to hammer away at more complete and authentic records of deaths and causes of death. Professor Edmund Andrews of Chicago introduced a new topic, "Treatment of the Needy Poor"; and Dr. Harris pointed out that there are "links in the chain of family misfortune and pauperism that should be broken by sanitary and medical means."

One event of the session in Chicago delights us. Dr. E. H. Janes finally was given the recognition he deserved and was elected secretary. He was one of the original group that met with Dr. Smith in April, 1872. He had attended every meeting, had borne more than his share of the burden of organization, and had received no consideration. As we have noted, his name had always been mentioned as an afterthought. Now he was no longer "and E. H. Janes," but national secretary of the association. Apparently Stephen Smith did not get to the Chicago meeting, but Snow was there, with Ezra Hunt, J. S. Billings, A. N. Bell, and Henry Hartshorne of the University of Pennsylvania. C. N. Hewitt, state health officer of Minnesota, and Henry B. Baker of Michigan were active at the meeting. The state health departments were beginning to make themselves a real force in public health affairs.

Richmond, Virginia, was chosen for the meeting of 1878. This meeting was an important one. During the summer a devastating epidemic of yellow fever had occupied everyone's mind. It was perfectly obvious that something must be done, on a nationwide scale, to curb the spread of epidemic disease. Each state had its own sanitary regulations. Many of the states and not a few of the large cities had no health departments to enforce the sanitary laws. The long-felt need for a national health service was in the mind of every thoughtful man. The association decided to do everything it could to forward the necessary legislation, and a large committee was appointed as advisory to the executive committee to formulate the national legislation. The association had before it a task which was to give it strength and perseverance, but which was to divide its leaders and nearly bring about its downfall. Out of this committee and its activities was to grow the National Board of Health.

It is interesting to note that the greatest enemy the association ever had, Dr. John B. Hamilton of the United States Marine Hospital Service, was elected to membership at this meeting in Richmond. He was the man who was eventually to destroy the National Board of Health in 1883. Dr. John Woodworth, surgeon general of the Marine Hospital Service, also was at the meeting in November. He died the following March, and Dr. Hamilton succeeded him. Dr. J. L. Cabell of the University of Virginia, who was soon to be president of the National Board of Health, was elected president of the American Public Health Association at this meeting. Hamilton was to attack other members of the association and cast suspicion on their motives, but he never attacked Dr. Cabell, and he did not need to attack Stephen Smith, for he won him over to his point of view.

State health departments were at last obtaining a voice in the association. Five of the six members[6] elected to the executive committee were executive officers of state health departments.

Stephen Smith gave an historical sketch of the American Public Health Association at the seventh annual meeting in Nashville in 1879. The small group of men who met in his office in April, 1872, had grown by now to an organization which consisted of almost 600 members. About 90 per cent were physicians; the remainder were civil engineers, educators, architects, and a few laymen who were vitally interested in public health affairs.

There were two women members of the association in 1879. Dr. Emily Blackwell of New York, the first woman member, was elected in 1873. She took no active part in the association and attended few of the meetings. Mrs. Elizabeth Thompson, who was elected in 1878, was a philanthropist who gave the funds for investigations of the Yellow Fever Commission during the terrible epidemic of 1878.

This was the seventh anniversary of the association, and all its general policies, which have been carried through down to the present day, were well established. It had admitted nonmedical members from the very start; its interests were varied, and included health administration, communicable disease control, sanitary engineering, health education, industrial hygiene, housing, food sanitation, and

[6] J. Rauch, Illinois; C. B. White, Louisiana (ex-president of state board of health); C. W. Chancellor, Maryland; J. T. Reeve, Wisconsin; and C. N. Hewitt, Minnesota.

school health promotion. The subject of vital statistics was of serious concern to the association. Nutrition and its relation to disease processes had been discussed, and the influence of environmental factors on health and welfare of the community had all been given due consideration. Three modern public health objectives are conspicuous by their absence: laboratory service, public health nursing, and maternal and infant hygiene. Mental health promotion had been considered very briefly, and the problems of remedial care of the sick poor had been mentioned.

During the first seven years of the association's existence, emphasis on health administration had shifted from municipal health activity to state health organization, and the association was just beginning to interest itself in a national health program.

The real leaders in the promotion of preventive medicine and public health of the nation had emerged. There were still on the membership roll the names of some forty men who had been charter members of the association in 1872,[7] but only a handful of these men had taken an important part in the establishment of the association. The most devoted of them had been:

Stephen Smith of New York, Edwin M. Snow of Providence, Elisha Harris of New York, J. H. Rauch of Chicago, Ezra Hunt of New Jersey, E. H. Janes of New York, A. N. Bell of Brooklyn, J. S. Billings of Washington, Dorman B. Eaton, the attorney of New York, C. B. White of New Orleans, J. L. Cabell of Virginia, J. M. Toner of Washington, and C. N. Hewitt of Minnesota.[8]

Around this group of thirteen men the association had revolved. They were to give it the permanence and strength that it needed to weather the difficult and strenuous years that were before it. Each year they were to depend upon the strength of the young members that were being added to the roll. None was to give greater strength than George M. Sternberg, who first participated in the association's affairs in this year, 1879. This small group of men were the true public health pioneers of America and to them the whole nation owes a deep debt of gratitude.

[7] Dr. S. O. Van der Poel, of Albany, once health officer of the Port of New York, was rather characteristically listed as a member since 1871—a year before the association was founded.

[8] Dr. Woodworth, of the Marine Hospital Service, a devoted member, had just died.

CHAPTER 33. *The American Medical Association:*

Section on State Medicine and Public Hygiene

> *What will become of the physician and his practice if the public takes care of its own health, more than at present? Will the medical profession be useless? No. It will be the prophet of the future and direct men to govern their bodies in order to get the full amount of work and joy that is possible.*
>
> HENRY I. BOWDITCH, *1874*

Almost at the same time that the American Public Health Association was founded, the American Medical Association established a section on *state medicine*. This was not a mere coincidence but is an illustration of the fact that new social concepts gradually increase in importance to the point where they become so impelling that they demand general recognition and consideration.

The *Transactions of the American Medical Association* report the authorization of a section on state medicine in 1872, but the *Sanitarian*[1] states that a section on state medicine and public hygiene was authorized in 1873. Under the title of "Section on State Medicine and Hygiene," it held its initial sessions at the meeting in Detroit in 1874. At that time, as at present, there was some misunderstanding and much debate as to the meaning of the term "state medicine." The general definition of the Medical Council of Great Britain was selected, and adopted by the section: "State Medicine consists of the application of medical knowledge and skill to the benefit of the community." It encompassed the following titles:

Forensic medicine
Toxicology
Morbid anatomy

[1] *Sanitation*, Vols. I, II, III, 1873, 1874, 1875.

Psychological medicine
Law of evidence
Preventive medicine
Vital and sanitary statistics
Medical topography
Sanitary engineering

This was a most comprehensive appreciation of the function of the community in the promotion of public health. It was a new concept of medicine and quite in contrast with the application of medical knowledge to the benefit of the *individual,* which for many years had been the province of curative medicine. The obvious sentiment of the association in authorizing this section was that organized medicine should take an active interest in the promotion of the public health.

Dr. A. N. Bell was the chairman of the first session at the meeting in Detroit in 1874, and A. B. Stuart of Minnesota was the secretary. The first subject for discussion was "state medicine." Dr. Henry I. Bowditch of Boston, already in his sixty-fifth year and long a student of public health, submitted a paper describing the Massachusetts State Board of Health, which had been functioning for five years under his direct supervision. The following unanticipated resolution was submitted to the section: "That it is expedient at this time to petition Congress for the establishment of a National Sanitary Bureau."

A bill had been introduced into the United States Senate three years previously which provided for a federal health service, but it had not received much consideration. The resolution was apparently somewhat of a surprise to the section. We find from the minutes that the question was discussed at length. Dr. Bell, the chairman, opposed the resolution, for he believed that work should first be directed toward organizing state boards of health, of which there were only six. Dr. Bowditch agreed with Dr. Bell. Jerome Cochran of Alabama, in discussing Dr. Bowditch's paper, opposed "the present establishment of a National Board of Health," and criticized the details of organization of the Massachusetts State Board of Health, but for some reason he voted for the resolution, as did Kedzie and Baker of Michigan. The resolution finally passed.

The second session in 1874 was devoted to a consideration of "defective drainage." All discussion emphasized the fact that permanent drainage decreased malaria in a community by at least 50 per cent. In Michigan alone, 20,000 miles of ditches had been dug during the previous ten years (Kedzie), with direct and striking effect, producing a decrease in malaria.

The third session was devoted to a discussion of the "effects of alcohol," a subject in which Dr. Bowditch was much interested. Attendance had been poor at the first session of the state medicine section, but quite a few were attracted from other sections for the later discussions. J. L. Cabell was at this final session, as was Ezra M. Hunt of New Jersey. J. M. Toner was president of the American Medical Association, but did not attend these sessions, despite his great interest in public health.

Dr. Toner was one of the few men who was ever elected president of both the American Medical Association and the American Public Health Association. He wrote extensively in the fields of public health and on the medical history of America. At this meeting of the American Medical Association in 1874, his presidential address was entitled, "Syphilis in Relation to National Health." This address was the initiation in America of the concept that the control of venereal disease is a direct responsibility of the public health service. He was a farsighted and courageous man.

From the very beginning, the Section on State Medicine and Hygiene interested itself in a campaign to establish state health departments in every state. In 1873 there were only three state health departments; Massachusetts, California, and Michigan. The association sent a letter each year to each of the state governors urging the necessity for a state department of health. At the meeting of 1879, the Section on State Medicine and Hygiene could report nineteen state boards of health.

Dr. Henry I. Bowditch was chairman of the section in 1875 and again discussed the National Council of Health. He believed it unwise to precipitate the measure or to agitate the matter in Congress, when there were so few state boards of health, so few state medical societies, and so little national sentiment for a public health department. "Physicians must be educated to this end, and the public must gradually be inducted into the merits and advantages of such a measure."

He was right, as time was to prove. He served on the National Board of Health when it was founded four years later, and saw it disintegrate and go down to defeat only four years after its organization, because of the very weaknesses that he pointed out in 1875. Dr. R. C. Kedzie of Michigan was made chairman of the section that year, 1875, and Ezra Hunt, a man born to be an association secretary and to serve in that capacity with one organization or another most of his life, was made secretary of the section.

The name "Section on State Medicine and Hygiene" was changed in 1900 to "Section on Hygiene and Sanitary Science" and in 1909 to "Section on Preventive Medicine and Public Health." Finally, in 1922 the name "Section on Preventive and Industrial Medicine and Public Health" was adopted.

At first the section had considerable weight and influence in the public health affairs of the nation, but its influence waned with the growth of the American Public Health Association. Its membership was limited to physicians, whereas the American Public Health Association had a representative membership of all types of public health workers. The section has always been one of the smaller special sections of the American Medical Association, but it has had good programs and a representative medical membership. The American Public Health Association was composed at the outset almost entirely of physicians, but as it grew in membership it fell into the hands of the numerous nonmedical groups that were not interested primarily in the medical aspects of disease prevention. Many physicians who were working in the public health field resented the fact that the policies of the A.P.H.A. were determined by public health nurses, health educators, statisticians, and sanitary engineers. They turned to the Section on Preventive Medicine of the American Medical Association for leadership. They received little encouragement, however, for the great mass of the American medical profession was interested in clinical rather than preventive medicine, and the policies of the American Medical Association were determined by a highly conservative House of Delegates. From 1920 on, the Section on Preventive Medicine and Public Health of the American Medical Association steadily lost its influence, and for years the leadership and stimulus to public health advancement in the United States came largely from the American Public Health Association together with the various voluntary public health agencies which were, for the most part, interested in some special field of health protection or promotion. (See chapter on "Voluntary Health Agencies.") This is still true down to the present day.

The term "state medicine," which was cordially accepted by the American Medical Association in 1873, later became an anathema to the whole of organized medicine, and as time passed it developed quite a different meaning and connotation from the adopted definition of those early days.

CHAPTER 34. *State Health Departments:*

Early Organization

The first and largest interest of the State lies in this great agency of human power—the health of the people. Herein is all its strength. This creates and manages all its wealth, and the chief responsibility of government is to protect it, and if possible, to enlarge it and make it more productive.

EDWARD JARVIS, *1874*

During the Colonial period, the public health acts, as well as other laws, were enforced on a colony-wide, and not on a local community, basis. Local self-government by the cities and towns did not emerge until late in the eighteenth century.

With the establishment of the United States, each state assumed sovereign power, but the state gave permission to the separate local communities to establish local laws. In 1797, for example, Massachusetts granted state-wide authority to towns and cities to establish local health services; but the state itself assumed no responsibility in public health affairs. Even such matters as maritime quarantine were carried out by the local community.

It is true that certain states assumed an active role in maritime quarantine. The reason was that these states had but one main port —as New Orleans for Louisiana, and Charleston for South Carolina —and thus, in effect, the state did give aid, and sometimes a subsidy, to maritime ship quarantine. At first the states assumed no responsibility for medical care. During the Colonial period, the various colonies passed numerous acts which regulated the practitioners of medicine, but the newly organized states were loath to pass any laws which infringed on personal liberty and private enterprise.

However, during the early part of the nineteenth century, conditions became so notoriously bad in the field of medical care and medical education that drastic action had to be taken. Inferior medical schools sprang up at every crossroad, quacks abounded, and

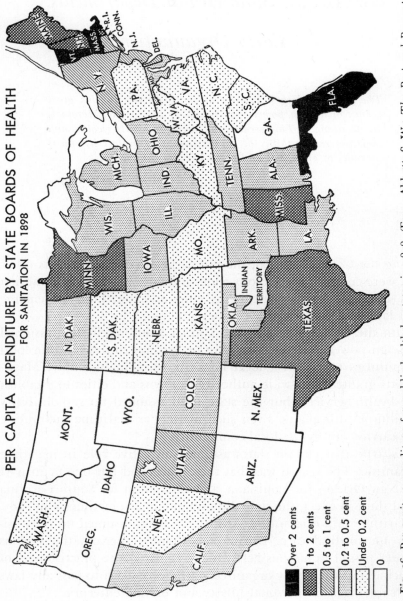

PER CAPITA EXPENDITURE BY STATE BOARDS OF HEALTH
FOR SANITATION IN 1898

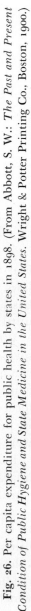

Over 2 cents
1 to 2 cents
0.5 to 1 cent
0.2 to 0.5 cent
Under 0.2 cent
0

Fig. 26. Per capita expenditure for public health by states in 1898. (From Abbott, S. W.: *The Past and Present Condition of Public Hygiene and State Medicine in the United States*. Wright & Potter Printing Co., Boston, 1900.)

medical practice was chaotic. To meet this situation the various states adopted measures which tended to restrict the practice of medicine to those who had at least some formal preparation.

As we have noted previously (see Chapter 20), Samuel Thomson, the highly successful botanical practitioner of the early part of the century, was one of the most influential factors in forcing state legislation for control of medical practice. Thomson's influence had spread far afield. Alabama's Medical-Practice Act, which restricted incompetent practitioners, was passed in 1823. But in 1832 the act was amended to exclude from the operation of this restrictive law any person "practicing medicine on the botanical system of Dr. Samuel Thomson, provided if he shall bleed, blister, give calomel, opium or laudanum, he shall be liable to the penalties of the act."

The first activities of the state in relation to medical affairs of the people were developed as welfare functions, rather than as public health measures. These initial acts related to state responsibility for custodial care of the insane, and were initiated through the activity of Dorothea Dix and her friends (see page 209).

The necessity for proper recording of vital data on a uniform, statewide basis was recognized early in the nineteenth century, and one of the initial activities of the American Medical Association in public health was the effort expended by this association to secure statewide recordings of deaths, births, and marriages.

In 1844 Massachusetts passed a law which required the recording and analysis of vital data by the state, and which designated the secretary of state as the collector of vital statistics. This law remained on the books of the state for over 100 years. Even though a State Board of Health and Vital Statistics was established in 1869, the vital data of the state continued to be collected by the secretary of state. Lemuel Shattuck was influential in securing this early legislation.

THE LOUISIANA STATE BOARD OF HEALTH[1]

The first state board of health was established in Louisiana. It was founded to prevent the further inroads of yellow fever.

Dr. Joseph Jones, the great Confederate patriot and competent public health officer, states:

[1] The data on the formation of the Louisiana State Board of Health are taken from the original *Reports of the Louisiana State Board of Health*, 1856, 1860, 1866, and 1867-1871. They may be found in the archives of the Surgeon General's Library, Washington, D. C.

Louisiana had been deprived in 1853 of thousands of her citizens in the most frightful epidemic she had ever witnessed. It had not confined its ravages to New Orleans, but had spread to the distant parishes of the country.[2]

To meet this situation, Act 336 of the Louisiana state legislature, "An Act to Establish Quarantine for the Protection of the State," was passed in 1855. Section 2 provided that "there shall be a *Board of Health,* composed of nine competent citizens of the State to be elected as follows: Three by the Council of New Orleans on joint ballot, and six to be appointed by the Governor, by and with the advice and consent of the Senate; the said members shall be selected in reference to their known zeal in favor of a quarantine system." The first report of this board was issued in January, 1857. It contained the results of the board's activities for 1855 and a portion of 1856. Dr. A. Forest Axon[3] was president of the board, H. D. Baldwin, secretary.

A second report was issued in 1860. At this time Dr. Deléry was president of the board, Dr. George Dermeyer was secretary.

During the Civil War there were no reports by the board. In 1866 the board issued a very short and incomplete report. A summary of five years' activity was reported in one volume for 1867-1871. From that date on, the annual reports were completed regularly. The board in 1867 was made up of nine members—six appointed by the governor and three by the city council. At this time Dr. S. A. Smith was president of the board and Dr. Dermeyer was secretary. Dr. P. B. McKelvey was director of the Mississippi River Quarantine Station.

Dr. Baldwin, in the 1855-1856 report, gives a good analysis of mortality. The data selected were from April 1, 1855, to May, 1856. The table on page 315 (No. 13) summarizes the number of deaths that occurred from the most prevalent diseases. These data were for New Orleans and did not include the whole state. The total number of deaths from zymotic disease was 4,671 out of a total of 9,085 deaths from all causes. Only 25 deaths were attributed to cancer. The following year from May 1, 1856, to December 31, 1856, there were only 3,806 deaths. During that summer there was no cholera and little yellow fever.

[2] Jones, Joseph: "President's Report to the Louisiana State Board of Health, 1882," *Medical and Surgical Memoirs,* Vol. 111, Part 1, p. CLI; see also Friedman, Ben: "The Louisiana State Board of Health, Established 1855," *Am. J. Pub. Health,* 41:1279, 1951.

[3] Friedman states that Samuel Choppin was the first president of the board: *Am. J. Pub. Health,* 41:1281, 1951.

Table 13

Important Causes of Death in New Orleans*
1855-1856

CAUSE OF DEATH	DEATHS	CAUSE OF DEATH	DEATHS
Yellow fever	2,670	Diarrhea	262
Cholera	885	Teething	223
Consumption	652	Tris nacentium	200
Infantile convulsions	383	Enteritis	195
Stillbirth	307	Typhoid fever	187

* SOURCE: Reports of Louisiana State Board of Health.

The 1860 report gives a total of 7,341 deaths—of which 826 were due to consumption and 132 to "lock jaw." Total deaths in 1867 were 10,096. The reports do not give the population of the area from which these mortality data were secured, so that one can only guess at the specific death rates.

Jones gives the following data (Table 14) for this period:

Table 14

Yellow Fever Deaths in New Orleans*
1855-1867

YEAR	POPULATION	TOTAL DEATHS	DEATH RATE PER 1,000	YELLOW FEVER DEATHS	DEATH RATE PER 1,000
1855	158,980	10,096	63.50	2,670	16.80
1856	161,404	5,689	35.24	81	0.50
1860	168,670	7,341	43.52	15	0.09
1866	178,042	7,754	43.55	185	1.00
1867	181,269	10,096	55.57	3,107	17.10

* SOURCE: Jones, Joseph: *Medical and Surgical Memoirs,* Vol. III, Part I, p. CCXCVI, New Orleans, 1890.

The Louisiana Board of Health certainly was not very effective. Dr. Stanford Chaillé,[4] in the annual address to the Louisiana State Medical Society in 1879, was emphatic on this point:

Louisiana has legislated on *paper* a State Board of Health and Vital Statistics; but in reality we have no state, merely a city, board of health, organized under laws which nobody except politicians (and a designing or an ignorant class of these) can possibly approve.

Dr. Chaillé says further in this address:

[4] Chaillé, Stanford E. (orator of the Louisiana State Medical Society for 1879): "Address on State Medicine and Medical Organization." Democrat Publishing Company, New Orleans, 1879.

In regard to State Boards of Health, the following facts deserve to be better known; after thirty years of effort by the medical profession, Massachusetts, in 1869, legislated into existence the first State Board of Health and Vital Statistics organized in the United States.

THE MASSACHUSETTS STATE BOARD OF HEALTH[5]

As we have noted previously (see Chapter 27), Lemuel Shattuck of Boston, in his sanitary report of 1850,[6] had strongly urged the formation of a state board of health in Massachusetts and had outlined a suitable type of organization to secure this desired end. This report received scant consideration by the Massachusetts legislature and was disregarded by the medical men of the state. Shattuck died in 1859, without any indication that this very important effort of his would bear any fruit.

But Shattuck had a friend, Dr. Edward Jarvis, who practiced medicine in Concord. Here Shattuck had lived before he moved to Boston and here he had awakened in Jarvis an interest in vital statistics and in the public health.

Edward Jarvis was born in Concord in 1803, and was graduated from Harvard Medical School in 1830. He became interested early in sociological matters. He aided Dorothea Dix in establishing suitable state hospitals for the insane and took an active part in that campaign. He was also chairman of the committee of the Massachusetts Medical Society which aided Shattuck in preparing his report of 1850.

The analysis of mortality data of the seventh national census of 1850[7] was greatly improved through Dr. Jarvis' aid, for he submitted a plan for proper classification of disease nomenclature. In 1860 the United States government delegated Dr. Jarvis to work out the statistics of the eighth national census.

During the Civil War we find Dr. Jarvis' name listed as one of the active members of the United States Sanitary Commission, and in 1869, in the *Atlantic Monthly*, we find a series of very interesting popular articles on "The Increase of Human Life" by Dr. Jarvis.[8]

[5] Many of the data from this section were secured from Eleanor J. MacDonald: "A History of the Massachusetts Department of Public Health," *Common Health*, Vol. 23, 1936.

[6] *Report of the Sanitary Commission of Massachusetts—1849*. Dutton & Wentworth, Boston, 1850.

[7] De Bow, J. D. B.: *Mortality Statistics of the Census of 1850*. The Seventh Census, Washington, D. C., 1855. See appendix, p. 45.

[8] Jarvis, Edward: "The Increase of Human Life," *Atlantic Monthly*, 24:495, 581, 711, 1869.

Apparently it was through the continued interest of Jarvis, after the death of Shattuck, that the concept of a Massachusetts state board of health was kept alive. Finally, in 1869, ten years after Shattuck's death, and twenty years after his report was compiled, the Massachusetts state legislature passed an act, on June 21, creating a State Board of Health. The men most directly concerned in actually securing this legislation were Dr. Henry I. Bowditch and Dr. George Derby.

The act authorized the appointment of seven persons who should constitute the Board of Health. Four important areas of activity of the Health Department were included in this act: (1) vital statistics, (2) communicable disease control, (3) epidemiology, and (4) environmental sanitation. Dr. Bowditch was chosen as chairman of the first Massachusetts State Board of Health and Dr. Derby as secretary. Bowditch served for ten years, but Derby died in 1874, and was followed by Dr. C. F. Folsom, who served until 1879.

The great motivating force of the Massachusetts State Board of Health was Henry I. Bowditch. He was one of the greatest American physicians of his generation, perhaps one of the greatest of the nineteenth century. His major interest was the control of tuberculosis, and in 1862 he published his famous epidemiological study on "Consumption in New England."[9] As a result of this study, he felt that the states should take an active part in the investigation of all contagion. It now seems probable that it was largely through his influence in the state legislature that the state board of health bill was passed.

He was a man of great vision, far ahead of his day. This is clearly brought out in his article on "Preventive Medicine and the Physician of the Future," which was published in the *Fifth Annual Report of the State Board of Health of Massachusetts,* 1874.[10]

One of Bowditch's greatest contributions to public health was his address before the International Medical Congress in Philadelphia in 1875[11] on the subject, "State Medicine and Public Hygiene in America." It is in this address that he pays tribute to Shattuck for the part he played in promoting public health in America.

Dr. C. F. Folsom was an assistant of Bowditch during the early part of his career and, through Dr. Bowditch, was appointed secretary to

[9] Bowditch, Henry I.: "Consumption in New England," *Transactions of the Massachusetts Medical Society,* 1862.

[10] Bowditch, Henry I.: "Preventive Medicine and the Physician of the Future," *Fifth Annual Report, Massachusetts State Board of Health,* p. 31, 1874.

[11] Bowditch, Henry I.: "State Medicine and Public Hygiene in America," *Tr. Internat. M. Cong.,* Philadelphia, 1875.

the state Board of Health in 1874. Later, Dr. Folsom followed Dr. Bowditch as a member of the National Board of Health (see Chapter 36).

The friends of Dr. Folsom established a professorship at Harvard Medical School in his honor, called the Charles Follen Folsom Teaching Fellowship in Hygiene. This fellowship eventually led to the establishment of the first full-time department of preventive medicine in a medical college. Thus the chain remains unbroken, for an original idea of teaching preventive medicine to medical students was carried through Shattuck, to Jarvis, to Bowditch, to Folsom, to Rosenau, and finally reached full fruition in the disciples of that great teacher. All this occurred in less than 100 years. The initial goal was reached when Dr. Milton J. Rosenau was selected as first full-time professor of preventive medicine in America in 1912. The nucleus of his department was the Folsom Fellowship.

The Massachusetts State Board of Health terminated after ten years of activity and great usefulness. It was merged into the Massachusetts Board of Health, Lunacy and Charity (in 1879). Drs. Bowditch and Folsom then both withdrew from state service. The state Board of Health was not reorganized until 1886, with Henry P. Wolcott as chairman.

Other state health departments were established in rapid succession following the organization of the Massachusetts Board of Health in 1869.

OTHER STATE BOARDS OF HEALTH

The state Board of Health of California was organized in 1870, that of the District of Columbia in 1871, and those of Virginia and Minnesota in 1872. Michigan organized its health department in 1873, Maryland in 1874, and Alabama in 1875. Other states followed in rapid succession. By the end of the century all the states, with eight exceptions, had organized state health departments. The last state to form a board of health was New Mexico in 1919. It began late, but within a short time it had one of the best state health departments in the nation.

The state Board of Health of California deserves special mention, for it was formed in a pioneer country during a period of robust, but primitive, social organization.[12] Its existence was due in great part to Dr. Thomas Logan.

Dr. Logan went to Sacramento during the early "gold-rush" days.

[12] See Jones, Guy P.: "Early Public Health in California" (a series of articles), *California Health,* 1944.

He brought with him from South Carolina instruments for measuring precipitation, temperature, and humidity. He kept meteorological records, did epidemiological investigations, and organized the state Medical Society. He became one of California's most distinguished citizens, and in 1870 drafted the bill which provided for the state Board of Health. The legislature passed his bill and he was made the first chairman of the board.

In 1871 the American Medical Association met in San Francisco. Dr. Logan urged its members to aid in the organization of a national health council. His plan was to promote a national sanitary bureau, which was to be organized in the Department of the Interior. This bill was introduced in 1871 through the influence of Dr. Logan, but it did not pass the national Congress. However, as a result of the consideration of these matters and again through the influence of Dr. Logan, a Section on State Medicine of the American Medical Association was formed in Detroit in 1873.

Logan was a worthy representative of the best in this pioneer field of public health.

The first ten states to organize state health departments were as follows:[13]

STATE	DATE	OFFICERS
1. Louisiana	1855	A. Forest Axon, Pres.
		H. D. Baldwin, Sec'y.
2. Massachusetts	1869	Henry I. Bowditch, Chairman
		George Derby, Sec'y.
3. California	1870	Henry Gibbons, Pres.
		T. M. Logan, Sec'y.
4. Minnesota	1872[14]	Charles N. Hewitt, Sec'y.
5. Virginia	1872	L. S. Foynes, Sec'y.
6. Michigan	1873	H. B. Baker, Sec'y.
7. Maryland	1874	E. L. Howard, Sec'y.
8. Alabama	1875	Jerome Cochran (1879)

(Governed by a Committee of the State Medical Society (1875-1879)

9. Wisconsin	1876	J. T. Reeve, Sec'y.
10. Illinois	1877[15]	John H. Rauch, Pres.
		E. W. Gray, Sec'y.

[13] The Kingdom of Hawaii, now the Territory of Hawaii, organized a health department in 1850, with Dr. T. C. Booke as its chairman. Thus, when Hawaii becomes a state, it will head the list as the earliest of the state health department organizations. See "The 100th Anniversary Report of the Hawaii Board of Health, 1950."

[14] According to Patterson the Health Department of the District of Columbia was organized in 1878, but in *Bulletin 184* of the U.S.P.H.S., 1932, the date is listed as 1871. There has been an annual report since 1872.

[15] Mississippi, New Jersey, North Carolina, and Tennessee also organized their state health departments in 1877.

The foregoing data are from the *Historical Directory of State Health Departments in the United States of America* by R. G. Paterson, Ph.D., published by the Ohio Public Health Association, April, 1939.

CHAPTER 35. *The Conference of State and*

Provincial Health Authorities

of North America

To secure true progress in hygiene those already skilled must acquire more skill; and those who are leaders, more knowledge.

J. S. BILLINGS, *1789*

This august and venerable organization has been one of the most potent forces for the promotion of the health of the American people. For many years, this association of state and provincial health officers has held an important annual meeting to discuss matters of common interest. The policies that have been formulated at these meetings have been of nationwide importance. The conference originated as the Sanitary Council of the Mississippi Valley.

THE SANITARY COUNCIL OF THE MISSISSIPPI VALLEY

In 1878 a severe epidemic of yellow fever occurred in Louisiana. The control of the disease was in the hands of the Louisiana State Board of Health, which was "in effect the local Board of Health of New Orleans."

The Mississippi Valley states were much alarmed by the apparent inefficiency of the Louisiana State Board of Health in handling this outbreak and so, for their own protection, organized a protective council. The first meeting was held in Memphis on April 30, 1879. It was called by J. D. Plunket, president of the Tennessee State Board of Health. The following delegates attended: R. C. Kedzie, president of the Michigan State Board of Health; J. H. Rauch, secretary of the Illinois State Board of Health; R. W. Mitchell of Memphis, representing the National Board of Health; J. D. Plunket, president of the Tennessee State Board of Health; J. M. Taylor of the Mississippi State Board of Health; S. M. Bemiss of New Orleans, representing the National Board of Health; Samuel Choppin, president of the Louisiana State Board of Health; and D. C. Holliday of the Auxiliary Sanitary Association of New Orleans.

J. D. Plunket was made president, and J. H. Rauch secretary. The recommendation was made that towns and states report immediately the presence of yellow fever. The council adopted a policy of friendship with the National Board of Health, which at that time was engaged in a bitter struggle with the New Orleans health authorities concerning the nature and the control of the existing epidemic of yellow fever (see page 335).

The council met again at the time of the annual meeting of the American Medical Association in Atlanta, Georgia, on May 6. This group was joined by the officers of the National Board of Health— James L. Cabell, president; T. J. Turner, secretary; and J. S. Billings and Stephen Smith.

The council discussed inland quarantine, including such matters as ship and railroad quarantine and sanitation, disinfection of mail, cleaning of freight cars, and notification of disease incidence. The next day the council had a joint meeting with the National Board of Health.

At the Atlanta meeting, Rauch was selected to represent the National Board of Health in the Mississippi Valley. He then went to Washington for a conference with the National Board of Health, and on June 1 he was sent to New Orleans under confidential instructions from the executive committee of that board. He made an inspection of sanitary conditions there and attempted to prepare a general quarantine code.

An epidemic of yellow fever broke out in Memphis shortly thereafter. Dr. Rauch busied himself inspecting interstate commerce, causing a great deal of concern to railroads and ships, particularly to river boats. He made rules for isolation of the yellow fever patients and for disinfection of the sickroom. He recognized that yellow fever was due to "germs" and believed that this germ flourished in decaying organic matter and filth.

Dr. Rauch, as representative of the National Board of Health, worked up and down all of the Mississippi Valley during the summer of 1879; he felt sure that in the end he should be congratulated on the outcome of a successful demonstration in railroad and river sanitation. Dr. Jones of New Orleans did not think so.

Dr. Rauch, who was secretary of the Sanitary Council of the Mississippi Valley, was also secretary of the Illinois State Board of Health. For this reason, the minutes of the Sanitary Council of the Mississippi Valley were published in the annual report of the Illinois State Board of Health in 1880.

A meeting of the council was held in Nashville on November 21, 1879, after the yellow fever season ended. Dr. Jerome Cochran, who was to play such an important part in all the state health department activities throughout the country in the years to come, represented Alabama at this meeting. A spring meeting was held in St. Louis on April 21, 1880. The report of this meeting does not say who attended. We know Dr. Plunket was there, also Dr. Rauch. Apparently there were delegates also from all the member states. A resolution was made to support the bill before Congress to increase the efficiency of the National Board of Health. They believed this bill to be "wise and judicious." A fall meeting was held in New Orleans in December of the same year. Up to this time New Orleans had not taken an active part in the council meetings. Now for the first time since the organization meeting in April, 1879, New Orleans was represented by Dr. C. B. White of the New Orleans Sanitary Association and Dr. D. C. Holliday of the New Orleans Medical Association. No representative of the Louisiana State Board of Health, nor of the New Orleans City Health Service, was present. Dr. E. F. McCormack of Kentucky made his initial appearance in public health affairs at this meeting. The discussion of this meeting centered around the question: "Shall the National Board of Health be entrusted with the executive control of the quarantine of the Mississippi Valley?" Dr. Kedzie of Michigan, president of the council, made a strong plea for the unification of this service.

Dr. Kedzie made an important address at the April meeting of the Sanitary Council of the Mississippi Valley, which was held in Evansville, Indiana, in 1881. Since he initiated certain very important concepts concerning the necessity for interstate cooperation in public health affairs, we have selected excerpts from his paper.[1]

When the representatives of the health organizations of the Valley met at Memphis to organize the SANITARY COUNCIL OF THE MISSISSIPPI VALLEY, there was in every heart a stern determination that such scenes should never again occur in this Valley if human wisdom and energy could prevent them—that never again should a steamer like the

[1] Kedzie, R. C.: Address published in the *Annual Reports of the Illinois State Board of Health,* pp. 151ff., 1881.

"Emily B. Souder" or "John D. Porter" carry lamentation, mourning and woe from one end of the Valley to the other—that the safety of our people should be secured at whatever cost—that in any possible conflict between public health and commerce, the benefit of any doubt should always be given to the public health, while commerce must bide its time; but that, when the people of the Valley were made secure against the pestilence in every form, the rights of business and trade should be fully recognized and protected.

The deliberations and consultations at Memphis developed the conviction, entertained with singular tenacity by every one present, that a health organization, to successfully solve these questions of public health as related to commerce, *must not be limited by State lines,* but must have jurisdiction commensurate with the area of danger, and must embrace the whole field, which may be either the starting point of yellow fever (and any pestilence) or the wide region into which it may spread. If the action of State authority, limited by State lines, were adequate for this work, then a plural-State organization was uncalled for, and the SANITARY COUNCIL OF THE MISSISSIPPI VALLEY had no claim to be, but was an impertinence and intrusion into the affairs of men from the outset. But the sanitary history of the Valley in years gone by—the lessons of 1878, in the broken business and shattered health of her people—nay, the thousands upon thousands of fresh-heaped graves, uttered a solemn warning not to lean upon the broken reed of State control. When each State acts for itself in sanitary matters, concert of action with other States becomes impossible. But as in the movements of a great army in an engagement, so in the battle for public safety, concerted and harmonious action is essential to victory. In disconcerted action upon any common subject by neighboring States, bickerings and suspicions will arise; each State will surmise that the authorities of the other State will consider the certain advantage of the business prosperity of its own citizens rather than any possible dangers which may threaten the health of a distant community beyond its borders. In all such contests, so far as the public confidence is concerned, the fear is as fatal as the fact. Recriminations ending in reprisals, is the brief history of every such inter-State contest. To avert this, some authority which, by overleaping State lines, shall harmonize State action, becomes the demand alike of public safety and of commercial enterprise. . . .

Soon after, Congress passed a bill giving the National Board of Health enlarged powers for dealing with pestilential epidemics, and a reasonable sum of money to defray the necessary expense. The States of the Valley welcomed this assistance from the General Government, and felt that in a matter of National importance, and affecting so many States, the friendly intervention of the General Government was fitting and right, and that the Government was only discharging a duty in so doing. . . .

By 1880 the public confidence has been so restored by the wise action of the National Board and the harmonious action of the State and municipal boards of health, that though there was a dreaded outbreak of yellow fever, there was no panic, and the interruption of travel and trade was very small. Sanitarians congratulated themselves that they had found a solution of the vexed problems relating to the public health of the Valley. But, by an inscrutable Providence, Dr. Choppin (of New Orleans) was removed by death; and by an equally inscrutable Providence, his successor in office, Dr. Joseph Jones, instead of working cordially with the National Board of Health to secure the highest well-being of the whole valley, has expended his energies in thwarting the efforts of the National Board, and obstructing every sanitary movement which he did not originate or govern. Soon charges were made against the health authorities of Louisiana, and at last the State Board of Health of that State came to an open rupture with the National Board of Health.

Then came a demand from the necessary number of States for a special meeting of the SANITARY COUNCIL which met in New Orleans, in December 1880, and after discussion and careful consideration of the whole subject, it passed unanimously the following preamble and resolution:

WHEREAS, Experience has shown that measures of quarantine under the sole direction of local and State boards of health have not succeeded in protecting this Valley from invasions of yellow fever; and

WHEREAS, Our people habitually view with distrust all announcements of local boards where those acts and announcements are of a character to affect the commercial interests of the locality directly concerned; Therefore,

Resolved, That in our opinion the General Government alone, acting through its sanitary agents, should have the direction and control of national and maritime quarantine.

Dr. Jones continued his combat with the National Board of Health and the Sanitary Council of the Mississippi Valley as actively and vehemently as only an unreconstructed states' rights Confederate veteran could, and eventually his side was to win the battle.

The Sanitary Council of the Mississippi Valley continued its activities through 1884; it supported the National Board of Health as effectively as it could in its struggle with the Louisiana State Board of Health. Despite all of its efforts, however, the National Board of Health was destroyed largely through the efforts of John Hamilton in 1883 (see page 337).

The feeling of the Sanitary Council of the Mississippi Valley on that matter is well shown in a resolution that was passed at its annual meeting in Memphis on March 24, 1884.[2]

WHEREAS, The Supervising Surgeon-General of the United States Marine Hospital Service has opposed, and in a manner defeated, important measures for the promotion of public health interests in the United States, which have been advocated by our leading sanitarians and by this and other sanitary organizations in this country; and whereas, the representatives of the Marine Hospital Service in the National Board of Health have not contributed to the success of the important work of that board; therefore

Resolved, That in any associated action which we may contemplate, either as executive sanitary officers or as voluntary associations, it behooves us to consider the Marine Hospital Bureau as inimical to the public health interests, which it is our duty to protect, and as a danger which we should not disregard. For, although neither the chief of the service nor his subordinate officers are known in sanitary organizations like this, they are able to so place themselves before Congress as to secure the ends they have in view.

Resolved, That as delegates representing the health organizations in the several States and municipalities hereinafter mentioned, and collectively, as the Sanitary Council of the Mississippi Valley, we earnestly memorialize Congress to so amend the act establishing the National Board of Health as to dispense with the representative in that board from the Marine Hospital Service.

The council served a very useful purpose in that it succeeded in getting the Mississippi Valley states to act in unison on health matters of mutual interest, but it embraced only a small part of the total area of the nation. Obviously, an organization of all the states should be formed to consider and to regulate public health affairs of interstate import. An annual conference of state boards of health was a necessity, and in 1884 it finally came into being.

THE CONFERENCE OF STATE HEALTH OFFICERS

This conference was a direct outgrowth of the Sanitary Council of the Mississippi Valley. Dr. C. N. Hewitt, health officer of Minnesota, conceived the idea of a conference of representatives of *all the state boards of health* in 1879. He brought the matter up at the Sanitary Council of the Mississippi Valley, which was held in Nashville in

[2] Minutes of the Sanitary Council of the Mississippi Valley held on March 24, 1884. Published in the *Sanitarian,* May, 1884.

1879. At this meeting a small committee was appointed to "arrange a plan for cooperation between all the State Boards of Health of the Union." Dr. Hewitt was chairman; other members were Pinckney Thompson of Kentucky, E. L. Griffin of Wisconsin, Samuel Choppin of New Orleans (who died shortly afterward), and two others—T. A. Atchinson and C. A. Rice.

In 1880 Dr. Hewitt made a report to the Sanitary Council of the Mississippi Valley in St. Louis in which he recommended the organization of a council of state health officers. No action was taken. Dr. Hewitt explained the reasons for this lack of action in the *Tenth Annual Report of the State Board of Health of Minnesota,* 1884, as follows:

There has been apparent all the time, a fear on the part of some of the Friends of the National Board of Health that the council now proposed would be in some sense antagonistic, and that it would weaken also the American Public Health Association, by withdrawing the representatives of state boards of health therefrom. Both objections have appeared to me to be of little weight as compared with the necessity, *which is constantly increasing,* for a union of state boards of health for cooperation, as specified in the attached plan. At a meeting held in Washington this summer, for the purpose, after discussion of various elaborate plans proposed by a committee, a temporary organization was effected upon the suggestion of this board through its delegate (namely, Hewitt).

The following plan for the completion of that organization will be submitted at the adjourned meeting to be held next October, 1884, in St. Louis. It is to be hoped that it will, in essentials, be adopted there.

This board is firm in the conviction that this is a practicable way to meet a self-evident want, i.e., hearty, intelligent and constant cooperation between the sanitary authorities of states, in inter-state sanitary work, and this irrespective of any national board of health, whose organization does not recognize and seek the cooperation of such state boards of health, as necessarily independent, and whose functions cannot be delegated to, or supplanted by, any other organization.

This organization shall be known as the Council of State Boards of Health of the United States. The objects of this Council shall be:
1. Closer acquaintance and more intimate professional relations between the executive officers and members of said boards.
2. Better opportunity and facility for the consideration and discussion of subjects belonging to their peculiar department of sanitary study and work by members and officers of said boards.
3. Better facilities for comparing and discussing methods, and for con-

sidering mutual relations, and devising plans for mutual cooperation in the following directions:

(a) The collection and collation of the history and statistics of disease prevalence.

(b) Mutual notification of disease prevalence, particularly epidemic diseases.

(c) The interstate control of epidemics.

(d) State legislation for sanitary purpose, and the comparison of the sanitary legislation of the different States, and of legislation necessary to be had by the States.

(e) The common study, by committees, of the history of epidemics as affording a knowledge of their origin, the laws of their propagation and the best means of their control, particularly of any existing epidemics, and the collection and preservation of data and documents which are not to be obtained after their cessation.

(f) The establishment of such relations with similar organizations in other countries as will make available for said boards the latest information as to the existence or spread of epidemics liable to be imported into this country.

(g) To enable any board to ask and receive the advice and experience of practical sanitary work in relation to local boards of health; the enforcing of sanitary laws; means of popular enlightenment; how to reach and influence all classes of the people; and make the rules of hygiene operative in trades, and in family and personal life. These and similar questions constantly arising can in this way receive satisfactory attention and discussion from the practical standpoint of active and working State Boards of Health.

Dr. Hewitt finally was able to complete the organization, and the first meeting of the council was held on Tuesday, October 14, 1884. It was concomitant with the meeting of the American Public Health Association in St. Louis. Dr. Hewitt was elected president of the Council of State Health Officers and Dr. McCormack of Kentucky was elected secretary. Thirteen state health departments were represented at that first meeting.

Dr. A. J. Chesley, secretary and executive officer of the Minnesota State Department of Health has furnished the author with the following details of the organization of the council.[3] There was an informal conference of representatives of various state boards of health at the November, 1883, meeting in Detroit of the American Public Health Association to decide whether they should create a

[3] Personal letter, dated January 26, 1954, from Dr. Chesley.

separate organization of state health officers. The outcome of this meeting was a delegation to the American Medical Association meeting in May, 1884, in Washington to consider the expediency and methods of forming the desired organization. Dr. A. L. Gihon, president of the American Public Health Association, proposed that the organization be formed as a section of the A.P.H.A. A committee was appointed consisting of Drs. J. E. Reeves, West Virginia; C. W. Chamberlain, Connecticut; Stephen Smith, New York; H. B. Baker, Michigan; and C. C. Fite, Tennessee. This committee presented a resolution that "there shall be a National Conference of executive officers and other representatives of State boards of health, during the meetings of the American Public Health Association, and at other times and places if so desired. All questions shall be determined by votes by States, each State being entitled to one vote. The officers shall be a chairman and secretary." This resolution was adopted. "After a general and rather informal discussion of some of the important questions connected with the work of State boards of health, the Hon. Erastus Brooks of New York was elected Chairman, and Dr. J. N. McCormack of Kentucky, Secretary for the ensuing year." The conference adjourned to meet on October 13, 1884, in St. Louis.

Dr. Brooks was chairman at this meeting, and the Dominion of Canada was represented by Dr. Charles W. Covernton of Ontario and by Dr. Peter H. Bryce of the Provincial Board. The Canadians took an active part in the discussions. The general outline for the conference was called the "Minnesota plan," because Dr. Charles N. Hewitt had repeatedly advocated the establishment of a council of the state boards of health of the United States.

The Canadian provinces had membership in the National Conference of State Boards of Health from the very outset, as is shown by the roster from time to time, and the various subjects discussed seemed always to include the provinces.

The change of title of the organization is shown in the *Proceedings of the Twelfth Annual Meeting* in 1897 at Nashville, Tennessee. Here it is called the Conference of State and Provincial Health Authorities of North America.

This conference, which has remained in continuous existence since its formation, has always been an unobtrusive and simple organization; nevertheless it became *the most effective* single cohesive force in promotion of public health throughout the nation. Its effectiveness through the years has been due in no small part to the continuity of its traditions and leadership.

The principles adopted at its early meetings and the program laid down by Hewitt have been its *constitution* and *by-laws* down through the years. It has maintained the integrity of state health services and has emphasized the primary responsibility of the state for the promotion of the health of its people. It has always been a strong supporter of a national health service, but has maintained from the outset that the sovereign powers of government rest and abide in the state.

The wheel of human destiny revolves slowly, and sometimes requires many years to traverse its whole circumference. The Sanitary Council of the Mississippi Valley was organized to protect the Valley states from the doctrine of inviolability of the principle of the right of the state of Louisiana to determine its own destiny irrespective of the rights of other states. The council did its utmost to promote a national board of health which would assume responsibility for public health matters of interstate import. It failed in this effort.

Yet by the middle of the twentieth century, federal health organization had advanced much further than the Sanitary Council of the Mississippi Valley had anticipated. In addition, through development of national sources of revenue, the federal government determined and controlled state as well as nationwide policies in regard to all matters relating to the public health. The very stone which the builders rejected, i.e., a national health service, and which was so scorned and spurned by Joseph Jones, has become the keystone of the structure.

Through all these years, the Conference of State and Provincial Health Authorities of North America has retained its independence and its influence, although it has always worked closely with the federal health services. No small part of its prestige has been due to the devoted efforts of Dr. A. J. Chesley, who has been for a great many years the executive officer of the Department of Health of Minnesota. Dr. Hewitt was founder of the organization. Dr. Chesley carried on the purposes and traditions of the conference and gave it stability and purpose. He served continuously as secretary of the conference for a period of over thirty years.

CHAPTER 36. *The National Board of Health*[1] 1879-1883

> *State Medicine is the application by the state of medical knowledge to the commonweal, and embraces every subject for the comprehension of which medical knowledge, and for the execution of which the legislative and executive authority of the government is indispensable.*
>
> STANFORD E. CHAILLÉ, *1879*

Very few people in the United States, even among that group most actively engaged in national public health affairs, realize that the United States once had a National Board of Health.

It is a dramatic story, and, like all dramas, has its heroes, struggling against overwhelming odds; its villain, who possesses the intelligence and aptitudes that all villains are supposed to exhibit; its comedy; its periods of calm which usually precede stormy outbursts; its climax, anticlimax, and finale.

The idea of unified, correlated national health services had been germinating slowly since the epidemic of yellow fever in 1793. Four National Sanitary Conventions had been held from 1857 to 1860, and the question of a nationwide quarantine service was discussed at these meetings. At the first meeting of the American Public Health Association in 1872, Dr. C. C. Cox, health officer of Washington, D. C., gave an excellent discourse on the necessity for a national health organization and outlined its functions and a suitable organization.

A meeting attended by representatives of many state and city health departments was held in Washington in 1875 to discuss plans

[1] Smillie, W. G.: *Am. J. Pub. Health,* Vol. 33, No. 8, August, 1943. Reproduced by permission.

for a federal health organization, but this convention met with little success. The three existing national government departments that already possessed medical officers—namely, the Army, the Navy, and the Marine Hospital Service—flew into a jealous dispute as to which should be most prominent in the new organization; and the meeting closed in dissention. Dorman B. Eaton, the distinguished lawyer who had drafted the pioneer Metropolitan Board of Health Act of New York in 1867, and also had drawn the act for the New York State Board of Health, was asked to prepare a draft of a bill which would create a National Board of Health. He did so, placing the medical departments of the Army, Navy, and Marine Hospital Service on the same footing. This proved fatal. Both the Army and the Marine Hospital Service rejected the bill and each at once endeavored to secure legislation from Congress which would make its service more prominent in national sanitary work.

The yellow fever epidemic of 1878 precipitated the issue. This devastating outbreak swept up the Mississippi Valley from New Orleans, causing great loss of life and paralyzing industry. The Valley states realized that the invasion came to them from the river, and blamed the Louisiana authorities for lax sanitary administration. They felt that their only hope against future disaster lay in a co-ordinated health service under national auspices.

In April, 1878, Dr. J. M. Woodworth of the Marine Hospital Service succeeded in getting a bill through Congress which conferred quarantining powers on his department, but he was given no appropriation to carry out the objects of his bill.

When Congress convened in 1879, the sentiment of the public was unmistakable. There must be no repetition of the disaster of 1878. The Army and the Marine Hospital Service both sponsored bills relating to a National Health Department. Dr. Stephen Smith thought that Dr. Woodworth's bill was the only one that could pass, and thus he sponsored it. But the act that Congress finally accepted in March, 1879, was sponsored by the American Public Health Association and drawn by Mr. Eaton. It transferred from the Marine Hospital Service all the health duties and powers hitherto conferred upon it, including all maritime quarantine. Surgeon General Woodworth, a fine, sincere, talented man, had worked very hard for his bill and sincerely believed it was the best that had been proposed on national health legislation. Upon its failure, he collapsed, and within a few days he was dead.

The new act created a National Board of Health, consisting of seven physicians, no two from any one state, and a representative from the Army, the Navy, the Marine Hospital Service, and the Department of Justice. The members were appointed by the President and had the following duties:

1. To obtain information on all matters affecting the public health.
2. To advise governmental departments, the commissioners of the District of Columbia, and the executives of the several states on all questions submitted by them—or whenever in the opinion of the board such advice might tend to the preservation and improvement of the public health.
3. Report to Congress a plan for a national health organization, special attention being given to quarantine and especially regulations to be established between the states, as well as a national quarantine system.

The following men were appointed to membership on the board, and $50,000 was appropriated for this work: J. L. Cabell, J. S. Billings, T. J. Turner, P. H. Bailhache, S. M. Bemiss, H. I. Bowditch, R. W. Mitchell, Stephen Smith, S. F. Phillips, and T. S. Verdi.

The board was an excellent one. Dr. Cabell, professor at the University of Virginia, was one of the most distinguished physicians of his day; Stephen Smith had done more to advance the public health than any man in the nation. Henry I. Bowditch, the Boston representative, was the pioneer in state health work in New England; J. S. Billings was to become the foremost physician of the land.

On June 2, 1879, Congress passed a second act, giving the new board wide quarantine powers, and appropriated $500,000 for its quarantine work. This act had one clause which proved to be a fatal weakness: It gave these quarantine powers for a period of four years only, and a re-enactment bill was necessary for a continuation of the work.

The National Board of Health started its work most auspiciously. Eight quarantine inspectors were employed, covering the coast from Maine to the Rio Grande. Familiar names appear: Elisha Harris was assigned the coast from Portland to New York; A. N. Bell was given Norfolk to Brunswick, Ga.; and Jerome Cochran, from Key West to Pensacola. In theory, the National Board of Health aided states in enforcing their quarantine regulations, but in practice, since the board had the funds, it dictated the quarantine policies. From

January 12 to June 3, 1880, the board spent $284,000, and during the next fiscal year, $202,000 was expended for hospital construction and quarantine purposes. It sent a yellow fever commission to study conditions in Cuba, with Dr. Chaillé of New Orleans as chairman and Dr. Sternberg as secretary. The board members themselves were very active on a variety of sanitary matters and published some excellent reports.

But serious trouble was not far off. Dr. Joseph Jones was secretary of the Louisiana State Board of Health. He was a man of tremendous energy and strong opinions. He had been an officer in the Confederate Army, and was an indomitable foe to anyone who did not agree with his ideas. Although he had lost the Civil War, he had not lost his belief in states' rights. He wrote Dr. Cabell in the summer of 1880:

The Board of Health of the State of Louisiana cannot delegate its quarantine powers to any other organization, whether created by a National Congress or by other individual States.[2]

Shortly thereafter an epidemic broke out in the delta below New Orleans. Sternberg visited the zone and made the diagnosis of yellow fever. Samuel Bemiss, the member of the National Board of Health who lived in New Orleans, wrote Dr. Jones the facts in a rather superior manner, stating that the board could be drawn upon for necessary funds for disinfectants, sanitary inspections, and necessary equipment in order to control the epidemic. He stated just how funds were to be allotted and indicated that approval of all expenditures must, of course, be in his hands. This statement has a familiar sound to present-day health departments that receive federal grants-in-aid, but most modern state health officers are not so conscious of the principle of state sovereignty as was Dr. Jones. Dr. Jones responded that the Louisiana State Board of Health had investigated the "malaria fever" of the rice lands and that necessary health measures had been taken, thus putting young Sternberg in his place. Sternberg made a second visit and again made a diagnosis of yellow fever. A neutral commission was then selected to study the matter. Dr. Mitchell, the board member from Memphis, and Sternberg went along. The commission decided that the epidemic was malaria,[3] and Dr. Jones won the first round.

[2] *Reports of National Board of Health*, p. 605, 1880.
[3] From the description of the cases, Sternberg may have been wrong. It is more probable that there were cases of both yellow fever and malaria at the same time. Diagnosis was purely symptomatic and very difficult.

On July 15, 1880, a vessel called the "Excelsior" came to New Orleans with a cargo of coffee. Five days later one of her crew developed yellow fever. She had been held in quarantine a few days in the lower delta, and it is possible that her crew was infected from the cases diagnosed as yellow fever by Sternberg. Meanwhile, the coffee had been sent to a number of interior cities. Dr. Bemiss, National Board member in New Orleans, telegraphed the facts to the health officials of these various cities. This was an unprecedented thing to do and was an interference with commerce. Dr. Bemiss writes:

A great deal of excited discussion arose in consequence of this action of the National Board in relation to the cargo of the "Excelsior."

The upper Mississippi Valley states had no confidence in the Louisiana quarantine service and stood by the National Board of Health in this controversy. But apparently Dr. Jones was more than a match for Bemiss. He stung like a hornet, for he was never satisfied with one encounter, but always returned to the attack.

In 1881 the National Board appointed as its inspector a worthy opponent for Dr. Jones in Dr. S. E. Chaillé. He had been a famous Confederate war officer, was a professor in the medical college, and perhaps the most beloved physician of Louisiana. His appointment appealed to local sentiment and was a very wise move on the part of the National Board of Health. But trouble began for Dr. Chaillé almost at once. To forestall any outbreak and to be prepared for emergencies before the yellow fever season began, he asked the Louisiana State Board of Health for the right to station his inspector down the river at the state quarantine station, and also asked to have access to the New Orleans death reports. The Louisiana State Board of Health were indignant, and felt that they had been grossly insulted. They would have no federal "spies" in their midst. But the New Orleans Auxiliary Sanitary Association—a group of businessmen— supported Dr. Chaillé. One suspects they did so because of the threat of embargo from the Sanitary Council of the Mississippi Valley, which had insisted upon federal supervision of the Louisiana quarantine officers. Dr. Cabell wrote from Washington directly to the governor of Louisiana requesting his co-operation. The governor supported the National Board of Health, and Dr. Jones lost the second round.

His own letters testify that he did everything in his power to make life miserable for Dr. Patton, the federal inspector who was stationed at quarantine.[4]

The year 1882 was the most active and productive of the National Board of Health. The report of the year is a book nearly 6 inches thick devoted to various sanitary investigations that were carried out by members of the board, or that were authorized by the board. Many of these studies are basic, well planned, and efficiently executed. But the gadfly at New Orleans was more tormenting than ever before. All states, says the report rather plaintively, are willing to co-operate with the National Board of Health except Louisiana.

On May 1, before the yellow fever season began, Dr. Chaillé wrote the new governor of Louisiana asking if the National Board inspector could again be stationed at state quarantine. The governor replied in the affirmative, stating:

The inspector is expected, in accordance with the original authorization of Congress, to aid and assist our state quarantine officer. It must be understood that he shall not supervise, control or direct the actions of the state quarantine officer.

Dr. Patton was again assigned to quarantine by Dr. Chaillé, but Dr. Jones kept up a continual battle against what he considered the effrontery of the federal government in invading his state and attempting to supervise his work. Dr. Chaillé wrote at the end of the summer:

I shall hope never again to occupy such unpleasant and detrimental circumstances as my office has brought me during the past two years.

When Congress was considering the appropriation for the National Board of Health that summer, the New Orleans press accused the board of "manufacturing yellow fever in the Mississippi Valley" to frighten the national legislative body to give it more funds and continue its work. A telegram from the National Board secretary, Dr. Turner, was misquoted by one of the New Orleans papers to say that if the National Board were not supported, it would be necessary for the upper Valley states to resort to the "trusty shotgun" for the purpose of enforcing quarantine against yellow fever. The Louisiana State Board of Health flew into a rage and passed the following resolution:

[4] See Dr. Chaillé's defense of Dr. Patton in letter to Dr. Jones, September 5, 1881, p. 339, of *Reports of National Board of Health.* See also Vol. III, compiled works of Dr. Jones.

WHEREAS: the National Board of Health by the emission of such innuendos and incendiary publications violates the conventionalities of official intercourse in a gross and unwarrantable manner, showing what it would do if it once had the power, and reflecting most aristocratically upon the self governing power of the American people

Be it *resolved,* that the telegram of Secretary Turner be copied and forwarded to President Cabell, with the request that in the future their communications be couched in more decorous language when alluding to this Board.

Few of the friends of the National Board of Health seem to have realized that while the controversy in New Orleans was raging, a much more dangerous foe within the shadow of the National Capital was quietly plotting its destruction. When Surgeon General Woodworth died, a young Marine Hospital Service officer, John Hamilton, was appointed to the position. His rise in the service had been phenomenal. He had taken no part in the advancement of public health in the nation and was not even a member of the American Public Health Association. He had no knowledge or experience in the field of quarantine, nor, in fact, had he any knowledge or experience in the fields of sanitation and public health. He was forceful and intelligent, and must have been an expert in political intrigue. He knew that if Congress did not re-enact the quarantine law by June 2, 1883, the National Board of Health must terminate. Since the bill of April, 1878, had granted quarantine powers to the Marine Hospital Service, these functions would revert to him and to the Marine Hospital Service if the National Board of Health were discontinued.

Quietly and effectively he did his utmost to bring discredit upon the National Board of Health and its activities. He accused the members of the board of misuse of funds, of extravagance, and incompetence. He insinuated that leading sanitarians, such as Rauch, Kedzie, Elisha Harris, and Wirt had used funds of the board to corrupt local health officers, and claimed that they had packed the Indianapolis meeting of the American Medical Association in securing endorsement of the National Board of Health.

Congress gave consideration to extension of the activities of the National Board of Health in 1884. Colonel George Waring, secretary of the board in 1884, in his remarks before the Committee of Public Health of the House of Representatives, stated:

In Dr. Hamilton I knew was centered the only effective opposition to the National Board of Health. I accused him of misrepresentation to lash him into appearance before this Committee rather than, as has been his practice hitherto, "at the button hole."

Waring pointed out that Hamilton's quarantine work (in the Brownsville epidemic) "has been injudicious and unskilled," and insisted that the Marine Hospital Service had no facilities at all except curative ones, and was engaged in one specific duty: the cure of sick sailors.

The defenders of the National Board of Health were good sanitarians but poor politicians. It was true that the members of the board had been overzealous; they had tried to move too rapidly, and in this sense they had been extravagant. They had made the fatal mistake of encroaching on the prerogatives of the individual states, and the representatives of these states in the Congress did not relish this taste of federal centralization of power. There had been no more widespread epidemics, and memory of past disaster is notoriously short. The real statesman profits by past experience and plans for the long future, but not the politician.

Despite the support of the American Public Health Association, the Sanitary Council of the Mississippi Valley, the state departments of health of Massachusetts, New York, Illinois, Michigan, and many others, the re-enactment bill of June 2, 1883, failed to pass. A small grant of $10,000 was given the National Board of Health to continue its investigations and advisory functions, but all its quarantine powers reverted to the Marine Hospital Service.

Stephen Smith, of all the national sanitarians, saw the importance of a *National Public Health Service*. He had favored Woodworth's bill in 1879. He was cited by Hamilton in 1883 as favoring transfer of the National Board's powers to the Marine Hospital Service; but Smith, in his address before the Public Health Committee of the House of Representatives in 1883, made his stand clear. He wished to confer all public health duties and powers on the National Board of Health, but to incorporate in the National Board the officers, the staff, and the activities of the Marine Hospital Service. He foresaw that Congress would lose interest in the National Board of Health, but would continue to support a service agency that had full-time career officers and was incorporated as an integral part of national government machinery.

In retrospect we realize that Stephen Smith was right. The unwieldy board of experts, each living in a different community and attempting to carry out administrative duties, with no cohesion, no real unity of opinion, and no central authority, was an impossible administrative machine. A centrally guided service, such as actually developed, had unity and purpose, but unfortunately lacked intelligent leadership. The public health policies for a great nation for many years were determined solely by the opinions—sometimes the whims and personal prejudices—of a single individual. It would have been a much better plan if Dr. Stephen Smith's half-formulated plan of 1883 could have been carried out, thus salvaging the really important features of the National Board of Health and incorporating in it a service agency with full-time personnel, an *esprit de corps,* and a strong central administrative machine. The members of the National Board of Health, selected by the President of the United States because they were public health experts, should have been continued as a board of health and should have served as a permanent policy-forming body, advising and aiding their administrative officer. The Marine Hospital Service was the most logical existing national agency with which to vest this national public health function. The surgeon general should have been made the executive officer of the board, and all actual administrative responsibility should have been centered in him. It was a great opportunity to have organized a close-knit, effective National Health Service, but there was no single man who had the vision or the power to solve this simple problem.

CHAPTER 37. *Environmental Sanitation*

ITS DEVELOPMENT DURING THE NINETEENTH CENTURY

The prevention of disease requires a definite knowledge of causes and contributing circumstances of the inception, progress, and injurious results of maladies by which lives are jeopardized or destroyed.

ELISHA HARRIS, *1877*

In previous chapters we have discussed different phases of environmental sanitation in connection with the development of various types of health services and have presented the prevailing theories in regard to the influence of the environment upon health, as well as its baleful influence in the production of specific diseases. In this chapter we shall present the developing concepts and the gradual advances that have been made concerning the importance of safe water supplies, adequate systems for sewage disposal, waste and refuse disposal, and the removal of "sanitary nuisances." Disinfection, insofar as it relates to disease-preventive procedures, will be considered. Food sanitation and particularly the development of a safe, adequate milk supply will be included, as well as a discussion of housing, with its good or bad influence upon the health of city dwellers.

COMMUNITY WATER SUPPLIES

At the beginning of the nineteenth century, as we have already noted, household water supplies consisted of (1) individual shallow wells and (2) running streams or other surface waters. For purposes of convenience and economy, communities began to bring water by a conduit from a distance of several miles to a group of houses; these first conduits were made of wood. The water supply was furnished by a private corporation. These community water supplies were not

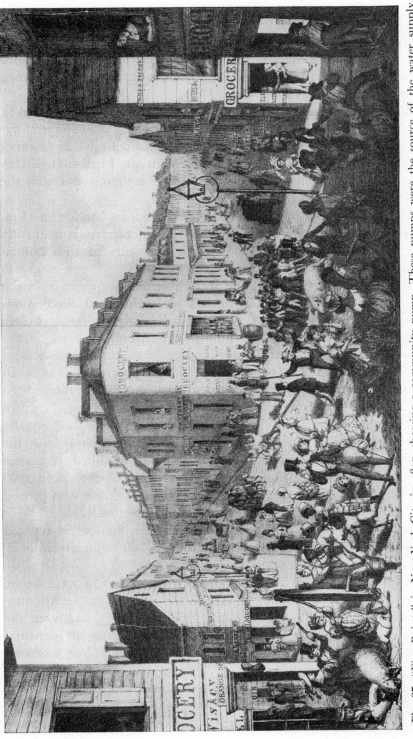

Fig. 27. "Five Points" in New York City in 1827, showing a community pump. These pumps were the source of the water supply for the great majority of the people throughout America during the nineteenth century. (Courtesy of Harry S. Mustard.)

considered to be a public health achievement. In fact, it was generally believed that any clear water which was free from perceptible odor and color was healthful. Running brooks or springs were supposed to be the best source of supply.

Slow sand filtration of community water supplies was initiated in England in 1829 by the Chelsea Water Company. James Simpson was the engineer. In 1856 Berlin, Germany, instituted sand filtration of its water supplies. This filter was constructed by English engineers. The primary purpose of these sand filters was merely to clarify the water, and not to prevent illness.

The Broad Street pump epidemic of cholera in London in 1849, which was studied so brilliantly by Snow,[1] demonstrated conclusively that a community water supply which was polluted with human wastes could be very dangerous.

In retrospect, we find it almost incredible that sanitary authorities did not profit immediately by Snow's epidemiological observations which were begun in 1849. John Snow's analysis of the cholera epidemic of London was first published in pamphlet form in the summer of 1849. The second edition was based on more extensive observations and more complete data. It was published in 1854. In this report he demonstrated conclusively that cholera was transmitted by "fecalized" water supplies. Simon did not accept this theory in full. Simon believed that "fecalized water and fecalized air equally may breed and convey this poison." Farr immediately saw the significance of Snow's observations but gave only qualified acceptance to Snow's theory. Not until the repeat epidemic of cholera in 1866 was he convinced. In this outbreak, Farr was the one who proved that polluted water was the chief source of infection.

Budd,[2] who began his classical studies of water-borne typhoid fever in 1857, was the only outstanding English authority who accepted Snow's theories completely.

Despite this lack of full acceptance of the theory of water-borne cholera, the London Board of Health did make vigorous attempts to prevent fecal pollution of water supplies, and gradually, as the years passed, the concept of water-borne epidemics of intestinal infection began to penetrate America. Thirty years later, when all

[1] Snow, John: *On the Mode of Communication of Cholera*, Second Edition. John Churchill, London, 1854. (Reprinted in *Snow on Cholera*. The Commonwealth Fund, New York, 1936.)

[2] Budd, William: *Typhoid Fever—Its Nature, Mode of Spreading, and Prevention.* London, 1874. Republished by American Public Health Association, New York, 1931.

controversy had subsided, Sir John Simon, who had stood aloof from Snow during his lifetime, stated that Snow's theory of the transmission of cholera by polluted water was "the most important truth yet acquired by medical science for the prevention of epidemics of cholera."[3]

Sir John Simon's theories[4] on sanitation were presented to America in 1876 by the Massachusetts State Board of Health. His major thesis was that "of removable causes of disease, the chief is uncleanliness." He distinguished between bad odors and microscopic agents in disease production.

Infecting powers should never be regarded as a mere question of stink. The agents which destroy the stink of filth may leave all its powers of disease production undiminished.

This was a new and revolutionary idea. Since the days of Benjamin Rush, the medical profession as well as the laity had believed firmly that disease arose from emanations of decay; the worse the smell, the greater the danger of infection. Water which was clear and sparkling and free from odor was considered quite safe and pure. It was believed that running water purified itself "every seven miles" as it dashed over the rocks and foamed down steep valleys. Simon pointed out clearly the dangers of stream pollution and the necessity of securing a community water supply which was free from exposure to human wastes. He emphasized the danger of filth in the transmission of disease for some distance "through appropriate channels of conveyance."

C. F. Chandler, who was analytical chemist for the Metropolitan Board of Health in New York in 1869,[5] reported that many cases of lead poisoning which were "hitherto unaccountable" could be attributed to the use of lead-lined water cisterns and lead pipes of the household water supplies.

In 1866 James P. Kirkwood, an engineer, was sent to Europe by the city of St. Louis to study the clarification of river water. He published a report in 1869 on "Filtration of River Water," and in 1871 Poughkeepsie installed the first water filtration plant in America. Kirkwood was the designer. Hudson, New York, followed suit

[3] Simon, John: *English Sanitary Institutions.* Cassell & Co., London, 1890.
[4] Simon, John: *Filth Diseases and Their Prevention.* First American Edition reprinted by the Massachusetts State Department of Health, Boston, 1876.
[5] *Fourth Report of the Metropolitan Board of Health of the State of New York.* D. Appleton & Co., New York, 1870.

in 1874, and Columbus, Ohio, and Toledo, Ohio, built water filtration plants in 1874 and 1875. The primary purpose of these plants was clarification of the water, in order to remove suspended matter and color. It was not a program of disease prevention.

At the very first meeting of the American Public Health Association in 1872, Austin Flint of New York read a paper on "The Relations of Water to the Propagation of Fever."[6] He described an outbreak of typhoid fever that occurred in North Boston, Erie County, in 1843. Twenty-eight of the forty-three villagers developed typhoid fever within a few weeks. One of the neighbors was accused of poisoning the community well and Dr. Flint was called in as a medical examiner. He proved that the deaths were due to typhoid fever and not to poison. Years later Flint read Budd's[7] reports on the water-borne character of typhoid fever (1857 and subsequently). Suddenly he realized that the North Boston outbreak was water-borne. After a lapse of twenty years, he worked out in detail the epidemiology of this little epidemic and demonstrated the first known outbreak of water-borne typhoid fever in this country. Flint reported this episode at the first meeting of the American Public Health Association.

William Ripley Nichols, a professor of engineering at the Massachusetts Institute of Technology, wrote, in 1879, a chapter entitled "Water: Drinking and Public Water Supplies" for Buck's *Hygiene and Public Health*.[8]

He stated that there are two views concerning polluted water:

The belief is universal that there is some connection between filth and disease. Filth is decaying organic matter of animal or vegetable origin. The dispute is upon the points:
a) Filth can originate specific disorders.
b) Filth simply forms a medium for something by which disease is carried.

He concluded that most nonmedical sanitarians and many medical authorities believed that air and water serve as disease-agent transmitters. He continued:

Others assert that water which is not polluted to an extent to inspire disgust by taste and smell is fit to drink. . . . It is important to consider the source of the polluting filth. I do not know that there is any proof

[6] Flint, Austin: "The Relations of Water to the Propagation of Fever," *Reports and Papers of the American Public Health Association*, 1:164-72, 1873.
[7] Budd, William: *op. cit.*
[8] Buck, A. H.: *Hygiene and Public Health,* Vol. I, p. 210. William Wood & Co., Philadelphia, 1879.

that public sewage when largely diluted is injurious to drink. There is strong evidence that dejecta from persons who are sick with certain particular diseases may communicate the disease to others if taken into the stomach.

Nichols suggested a dual system of water suply. A poorer type of water might be supplied to street hydrants and be used for fire protection, street cleaning, and for industrial purposes. Household supplies should be of a pure quality and should be supplied to the amount of 15 to 20 gallons per person per day. In discussing sources of community water supplies, he noted that rain water was insufficient. He already saw the danger of pollution of river water by heavy manufacturing. His chief objection to ponds and lakes as a source of supply was the growth of algae which gave objectionable tastes to the water. He realized that ground water might be polluted by privies or cesspools, and cited the *Fifth Annual Report of the Massachusetts State Board of Health* concerning two family epidemics of typhoid fever that were spread by privy-polluted wells.

We learn from the same author that the initial sand filters of Poughkeepsie, Hudson, Columbus, and Toledo had been "more or less" successful. He presented an illustration in Buck's text of a cross section of a slow sand filter—2 feet of sand—and stated that it is "simply a mechanical operation." He also mentioned alum as a suitable agent for clearing turbid waters. Drinking water on board ship can be rendered safe by adding permanganate of potash until the water is faintly pink. "The most simple method of treatment of impure water is boiling."

Coagulation Filters[9]

Adolphus Hyath in 1884 patented *aluminum sulfate* as a coagulant for muddy waters. (Whipple states that Prof. A. R. Leeds was the real inventor of this process.) A mechanical filter, utilizing alum, was installed in Somerville, New Jersey, in 1884. Rapid sand filtration, using aluminum sulfate as a coagulant, was first designed and installed in Providence, Rhode Island, by the great sanitary engineer, E. B. Weston, in 1893.

Chlorination

Chlorination of public water supplies is a comparatively recent innovation. Cruickshank recommended bleaching powder as a dis-

[9] Whipple, George: "Fifty Years of Water Purification," *A Half Century of Public Health*. American Public Health Association, New York, 1921, p. 163.

infectant for sewage as early as 1800. A Committee on Disinfectants of the American Public Health Association in 1885 designated chloride of lime as the best disinfectant. In 1897 in Maidstone, England, chloride of lime was used to disinfect the water distribution mains following an epidemic. In 1896 George W. Fuller of the Louisville Experiment Station first used chloride of lime as a method of rendering polluted water safe for consumption. The method was put into commercial application by engineer George H. Johnston in 1908 in the Chicago stockyards.

The Lawrence Experiment Station

The great training ground for sanitary engineers in the United States was the Lawrence Experiment Station. It was established in 1886 by the Massachusetts State Board of Health under the guidance of its president, Dr. Henry P. Walcott. This station studied the principles of the purification of water and of sewage. The young engineers who contributed to these studies became our great sanitary engineers. Hiram F. Mills was an important factor in the establishment of the station. Allen Hazen was in charge of the station from 1888 to 1893. At the outset William T. Sedgwick was director of bacteriological research. He was aided by E. O. Jordan. Thomas M. Drown was the sanitary chemist. Ellen H. Richards, W. F. Miller, and Frederick B. Stearns were other initial members of the research group. Each of them was to make his own significant contribution to American sanitary science during the coming years.

The studies at the station resulted in the establishment of the Lawrence city filter in 1893. This was the first scientifically controlled demonstration of water purification.

In 1892 George E. Fuller, while working at the station, differentiated the characteristics of the typhoid bacillus:[10]

1. Noncoagulation of milk.
2. No acid formation in milk.
3. Production of turbidity without gas in the Theobald Smith tube of glucose broth.

The most notable man in the whole group was William T. Sedgwick. In 1892 he published, in the annual report of the Massachusetts State Board of Health, his fine epidemiological studies of the waterborne typhoid epidemic in Lawrence and Lowell. As Winslow has

[10] Fuller, George E.: *Boston M. & S. J.,* September 1, 1892.

said, "Sedgwick was indeed the first scientific American epidemiologist."

Sedgwick was a brilliant teacher. Singlehanded he developed America's first informal school of public health at the Massachusetts Institute of Technology. He was the school.

Another great name in the municipal water purification field was George C. Whipple, who wrote the chapter on "Fifty Years of Water Purification" in *A Half Century of Public Health*, 1921. The reader who has an interest in the development of water purification in the United States is referred to this comprehensive report.[11]

SEWAGE DISPOSAL

Shattuck in the 1850 *Report of the Sanitary Commission of Massachusetts* recommended that cities install sewerage systems as a sanitary measure; but Shattuck was far ahead of his time. In 1860 there were only ten municipal sewerage systems in the whole United States; by 1880 this number had grown to over 200. These sewers were all discharged into lakes or streams without any previous purification.

In the cities, individual households gradually installed water closets which were drained into "cesspools." This device was a large, closed, bricklined tank which was buried in the back yard, and was emptied at night at appropriate intervals and with attempts at secrecy.

This system of sewage disposal met with general community disapproval because of the bad odor which was created. In 1851, when President Millard Fillmore first installed a permanent bath and water closet in the White House, these innovations met with great popular disapproval. Not only were they unsanitary but undemocratic as well.

The great objection to the installation of sewers was the danger of *sewer gas*. Pettenkofer's prestige influenced all thinking in sanitary matters during the middle of the century. He believed that disease emanates from the soil, and that poisons are elaborated there. Thus the rise and fall of ground water had a profound influence on the health of a community. Gases formed in sewage were identical with the poisons found in the soil. During the last half of the century the English sanitarians insisted that fecal pollution of water was an essential source of infection and that sewer gas was not dangerous.

[11] See also "Historic Review of the Development of Sanitary Engineering in the United States during the Past 150 Years," *Tr. Am. Soc. Civil Eng.*, Vol. 92, 1928; "Century of Progress through Sanitation," Symposium, Part 2, *Am. J. Pub. Health*, 43:15, 1953.

They used the strong argument that the workers in the London sewers were not affected in health by their occupation. Their opponents, however, pointed out instance after instance that could be cited where cholera, typhoid fever, pneumonia, erysipelas, arthritis, and particularly diphtheria were "undoubtedly produced by sewer gas when all other possible causes examined had been eliminated." In fact, Ford[12] stated that "all diseases are more or less affected by these effluvia." He described the investigation of an epidemic of diphtheria in New York in 1872 in which defective drainage of the subsoil was the undoubted cause of the outbreak. "There is good reason," Ford stated, "for supposing that morbific agents which produce enteric fever, cholera, diarrhea, and dysentery may exist in sewer air." In this chapter of the text he described, in great detail, the construction of water closets, with emphasis on the importance of traps for prevention of escape of sewer gas into a dwelling.

In 1877, when the Prince of Wales had a severe case of typhoid fever, it was discovered that there was an *unused* cesspool under the house in which he lived. His disease was attributed to the gas from this source. As late as 1892, George Wilson wrote an article on "Sewer Gas and Its Dangers,"[13] in which he emphasized the fact that cases of diphtheria, ulcerated throat, membranous croup, puerperal fever, septicemia, and hospital gangrene "all have been found associated with drainage defects, but why sewer gas should be the apparent cause of so many dissimilar diseases has not been fully explained."

The Massachusetts State Board of Health, which was organized in 1869, began very early to assume leadership in the study of stream pollution and sewage disposal. Professor William Ripley Nichols of the Massachusetts Institute of Technology made a study in 1874 on "The Present Condition of Certain Rivers of Massachusetts."[14] In this report he pointed out the great danger of sewage from human sources, no matter how dilute, which may find its way into a riversource of community water supply. This was a revolutionary idea in America and was not widely accepted. In the *Report of the Massachusetts State Board of Health* of 1877, one finds an extensive report by Nichols on the dangers of stream pollution. In that same volume

[12] Ford, William H.: "Soil and Water," chapter from Buck's *Hygiene and Public Health*, 1879.

[13] Wilson, George: *Handbook of Hygiene and Public Health*, Seventh Edition, 1892.

[14] Nichols, William R., in the *Fifth Annual Report of the Massachusetts State Board of Health*, pp. 63-152, Boston, 1874.

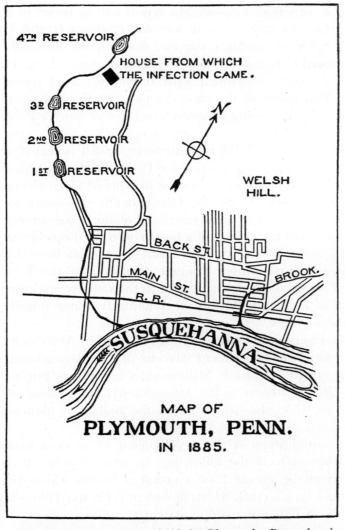

Fig. 28. Water-borne typhoid in Plymouth, Pennsylvania. (From Sedgwick, W. T.: *Principles of Sanitary Science and Public Health.* The Macmillan Co., New York, 1902.)

we find an article by the engineer, E. S. Cheesborough of Chicago, on "Sewerage—Its Advantages and Disadvantages."

Europe and particularly England, with her good sanitary engineers, were far ahead of America in matters of community sewage disposal. Thus it was most logical that Rudolph Hering should be sent to Europe in 1881 by the National Board of Health to study the practice of sewage disposal. His report will be found in that rare volume, the 1881 *Report of the National Board of Health*.[15] Hering made an extensive summary, together with a series of beautifully detailed colored charts, of the sewer systems of eleven large European cities. The article concluded with twenty-two solid pages of references! This is one of the most extensive bibliographies in public health literature. Hering's tremendous piece of work was buried in the report of 1881.

In 1885 an epidemic of typhoid fever, which occurred at Plymouth, Pennsylvania, was studied by L. H. Taylor.[16] This town of about 8,000 suffered from 1,104 cases of typhoid fever within a short space of time, with 114 deaths. The epidemic was shown to be due to the pollution of the small reservoirs of the water supply system of the town with the dejecta of a farmer who lived on the watershed. He had a severe case of typhoid fever; his excreta were thrown on the frozen ground, which drained directly into the town water supply. This epidemic demonstrated to the sanitary engineers of the nation that human pollution of community water supplies is an ever-present danger.

The first important study of sewage disposal in America was made at the Lawrence Experiment Station of the Massachusetts State Board of Health. Hiram F. Mills made a report on "Purification of Sewage" in the *Report of the Massachusetts State Board of Health* of 1890, in which he demonstrated the biological nature of sand filtration.

Other initial steps in the development of modern concepts of sewage disposal were the following: In 1893 *chloride of lime* was used to treat the sewage from a group of houses which discharged their wastes into a creek which flowed into Croton Lake—a part of the New York City water supply system.

This same year *trickling filters* for sewage disposal were devised by Corbett in England. In 1908 George H. Johnson of Chicago used *bleaching powder* in purification of highly polluted Bubbly Creek. In 1910 *liquid chlorine* was introduced as a measure for purification of water supply and of sewage.

William T. Sedgwick's text on *Principles of Sanitary Science and the Public Health,* which was published first in 1902, became a classic, and went through many editions. Sedgwick was the great

[15] Hering, Rudolph, in the *Report of the National Board of Health,* Appendix 4, p. 99, 1881.
[16] Taylor, L. H., in the *First Annual Report of the Board of Health and Vital Statistics of Pennsylvania, 1886.*

leader of his generation in the field of environmental sanitation, and his students from the Massachusetts Institute of Technology constituted a dynamic strength and power that was to prove an important factor in public health advancement in America during the next fifty years.

REFUSE AND WASTE DISPOSAL

This section might well be called the rise and decline of garbage disposal as a health department function. For over a century, the disposal of refuse and wastes that accumulate from community living was one of the major activities of the municipal health department. The reasons for this great concern for potentially putrid material are quite clear. We have already noted in a previous chapter that Benjamin Rush, in his *Inquiries*,[17] considered that accumulations of filth were a very important factor in production of disease. He believed that the great yellow fever epidemic of Philadelphia in 1793 was initiated by a pile of rotting coffee at Ball's wharf, and he was quite specific about the dangers of various accumulations of community wastes, such as rotten cabbage, rotten hemp, bilge water, musty books, old paper money, dead fish, privies, pigsties, tanneries, and the like. Rush's ideas were quite representative of those of the educated people of his time.

Whenever an epidemic of illness occurred, the city health authorities made haste to institute an extensive clean-up campaign. The cholera epidemic that invaded America through New York in 1832 was checked in Boston by the intensive activity of every citizen in such a cleansing of the city as had never been known. These measures undoubtedly did some good in the prevention of cholera, since privies were cleansed, manure piles were eliminated, and flies were brought under some degree of control.

Disposal of refuse also reduces the rat population and thus reduces the spread of rat-borne infections such as plague. But North America luckily did not suffer from an invasion of bubonic plague in the nineteenth century. Though rats were very prevalent in the cities and rural areas as well, no serious epidemic of rat-borne disease occurred in North America during the entire century.

The general concept throughout the world was that a clean city is a healthy city. On the other hand, if a city allowed filth to accumulate then disease would be the inevitable result. The Sanitary Survey of

17 Rush, Benjamin: *Medical Inquiries and Observations*, Fourth Edition, Vol. IV, 1815.

New York City in 1865 by Stephen Smith and his associates[18] was concerned primarily with the neglect by the city authorities of ordinary cleanliness. In fact, Clark's "Sanitary Code for Cities," which was published in the 1859 report of the Third National Quarantine and Sanitary Convention, related chiefly to disposal of refuse and waste and to their importance as producers of disease.

Since municipal filth "produced disease," it became the function of the board of health to abate nuisances, and to clean or to supervise the cleaning of the streets, alleys, and back yards. A large part of the local health department budget was allocated to sanitation, and a great proportion of the personnel was employed as street cleaners and nuisance abators. The inevitable happened. The health department fell into the hands of politicians. It was generally recognized that a political retainer who was too stupid to be appointed as a policeman and too awkward to be a good fireman, could at least be utilized in the sanitary department as a street cleaner, and thus add to the voting strength of the party in power. For this reason, garbage and waste disposal became more and more a center of political intrigue, with the result that the health department was subjected to strong political pressure which forced it to employ incompetents and laggards.

Meanwhile, sanitary engineers were devising various methods for disposal of garbage. The early reports of the American Public Health Association,[19] contain extensive discussions of these matters. A special committee on garbage and refuse disposal was formed, which reported each year. Rudolph Hering, the sanitary engineer who was sent to Europe in 1881 by the National Board of Health to study municipal sewage disposal, became chairman of the American Public Health Association's Committee on Garbage and Waste Disposal, and made extensive remarks on this subject in the reports of 1891, 1894, 1895, 1896, and subsequently. In the annals of the meeting of 1902, we find that Rudolph Hering made a voluminous report on methods of disposal of garbage and refuse. Various procedures which municipalities may employ were suggested, such as:

1. Feeding to swine.
2. Dumping on land.
3. Dumping into large volume of flowing water.

[18] Smith, Stephen, and associates: *Report of the Sanitary Conditions of the City of New York.* D. Appleton & Co., New York, 1865.
[19] *Reports and Papers of the American Public Health Association,* 29:129-33, 1903.

4. Ploughing into soil.
5. Extracting grease.
6. Cremating the organic matter.

In this same issue C.-E. A. Winslow published,[20] with P. Hansen, his first scientific article on the public health subject, "Some Statistics of Garbage Disposal for the Larger American Cities in 1902." Dr. Winslow had joined the association that year. He was destined to take an active part in its organization for more than fifty years, and was to be its president and editor of its journal. His first paper was a carefully tabulated report of the type of garbage disposal that was employed in 155 American cities. Truly, garbage disposal was big public health department business in 1902.

Chapin in his textbook on *Municipal Sanitation in the United States*[21] in 1901 devoted over 100 pages of description to "Refuse Disposal" and over 100 pages more to "Nuisances and Nuisance Abatement." Nearly one-fifth of the book is concerned with these matters.

However, Chapin was a realist and a very clear thinker. He was health officer of Providence, Rhode Island, for over forty years, and he became the greatest city health officer that this country has ever produced. Furthermore, he was his own severest critic. His logical mind told him that all the municipal activities in city "housekeeping" were excellent in themselves, but were not the business of the health department. The esthetic side of city cleanliness was important, but did not have much effect upon the mortality or morbidity of the community. Thus, in 1912 we find this very clear statement in Chapin's *Sources and Modes of Infection:*

Except for a few diseases, or except for very indirect effects, the cleansing of streets, alleys, and back yards, of dwellings and stables, the regulation of offensive trades, and the prevention of nuisances generally, have, so far as we can see, no effect on the general health, nor any value in the prevention of specific diseases.[22]

Flies

The housefly was an important sanitary menace during the last half of the nineteenth century. Each summer, in every rural and

[20] Winslow, C.-E. A., and Hansen, P.: *Reports and Papers of the American Public Health Association,* **29:**141, 1903.

[21] Chapin, Charles V.: *Municipal Sanitation in the United States.* Snow & Farnham, Providence, Rhode Island, 1901.

[22] Chapin, Charles V.: *Sources and Modes of Infection.* John Wiley & Sons, New York, 1912, p. 32.

urban home, there was a tremendous invasion of flies. They bred in the manure heaps of the livery stables of the cities and towns, in the barns of the dairies, and in the stables of each well-to-do householder who kept a driving horse and a family cow. The ceilings of every kitchen, both in restaurants and private houses, were literally black with flies every night in July and August after the sun went down. Screens were invented but were of little avail. All sorts of devices were used to limit the number of flies, such as poison, flytraps, sticky flypaper, and the like. They seemed only to attract flies rather than diminish them.[23]

The investigation of the severe epidemics of typhoid fever among the encampments of the American troops[24] at the time of the Spanish-American War in 1898 suddenly awoke the nation to the fact that flies were not a simple nuisance but a serious hazard to health. This investigation showed that flies were important factors in transmission of enteric infections through badly constructed latrines which were located in close proximity to the kitchens.

The health departments began to make active and extensive efforts to control flies. "Swat the fly" campaigns became the order of the day. Their only value was educational, since "ten flies came to every one fly's funeral." The one way to control flies, of course, was to destroy their breeding places, and this was soon accomplished by an unprecedented application of the invention of the reciprocating gasoline engine. Automobiles began to replace horses about 1900. Within a short time, livery stables disappeared, the farm tractor became popular, and dairy sanitation mechanized manure disposal. The manure pile was no longer seen in the village back alley. By 1950 the fly, together with the English sparrow, had practically disappeared from the face of the land.

In 1913 Rosenau published his famous *Preventive Medicine and Hygiene*.[25] The trend of the times is clearly seen, for this book placed little emphasis on refuse disposal as a public health measure. The

[23] A vivid childhood recollection of the author was the daily morning task of driving the flies out of the kitchen. Mother marshaled her whole family about 9:00 A.M. and armed each with a "shoo-fly"; we then systematically drove the army of houseflies from the kitchen walls to the screened back porch and then out the back door. This was about 1895. Dr. S. J. Krumbine, for many years state health officer of Kansas, coined the term "swat the fly." He died in December, 1954, at the age of 91 years.

[24] Reed, Walter; Vaughan, V. C.; and Shakespeare, E. O.: *Report on the Origin and Spread of Typhoid Fever in United States Military Camps during the Spanish War of 1898*, Vol. 1. Government Printing Office, Washington, D. C., 1904.

[25] Rosenau, M. J.: *Preventive Medicine and Hygiene*. D. Appleton & Co., New York and London, 1913.

chapter on "Refuse Disposal," which was written by George Whipple, encompassed only four pages in a text of over 1,000 pages, whereas in previous texts on hygiene, hundreds of pages were devoted to waste disposal. Within the short space of ten years, garbage and refuse disposal was practically eliminated as a function of the health department. So great was the prestige of Chapin and of Rosenau that their ideas gained ground rapidly. Health departments throughout the nation were reorganized, and within a short time, practically no municipal health department was held responsible for the cleaning of streets and for the removal of garbage.

Burial of the Dead

The custom during the Colonial period was to bury the dead in the center of the village, in a graveyard which surrounded the church; but the advent of the great epidemics and the concepts that arose concerning putrefaction and miasmata as causes of disease led to the obvious conclusion that dead bodies were extremely dangerous.

This subject received great impetus from the report by Edwin Chadwick[26] in 1845 on *The Practice of Interment in Towns*. He was able to demonstrate that the effluvia arising from the decomposition of human bodies was very dangerous. "The occurrence of cases of instant death of gravediggers from accidentally inhaling the concentrated miasma which escapes from coffins is undeniable." Furthermore, corpses polluted the soil, and this in turn resulted in the pollution of ground water which obviously involved the pollution of wells and even public water supplies, leading to such important epidemics as cholera, typhoid fever, and even smallpox.

These observations led to the custom of burying the dead at some distance—at least a mile—from city or town. Quite logically, all questions which related to burial of the dead and to the determination of the location of cemeteries became the responsibility of the health department.

John H. Rauch, who was one of the great public health pioneers of the West and one of the founders of the American Public Health Association, wrote an important pamphlet[27] on this subject in 1866. Dr. Rauch traced, at length, the origin and history of intramural

[26] Chadwick, Edwin: *Report on the Results of a Special Inquiry into the Practice of Interment in Towns.* American Edition printed by C. Sherman, Philadelphia, 1845.
[27] Rauch, J. H.: *Intramural Interments in Populous Cities and Their Influence on Health and Epidemics.* Tribune Co., Chicago, 1866. (The author is in possession of the copy Dr. Rauch presented to Wilson Jewell.)

interments and "proved from chemical, physiological, and pathological standpoints the evil effects of the practice upon the health of the living. We have shown that this custom is universally condemned by the highest medical authorities of both Europe and America, and that in most countries, the authorities have broken it up and compelled the burial of the dead far from the limits of cities and populous towns and at a depth beneath the surface sufficient to prevent the contamination of the air."

Thus, from a false sanitary premise, there was developed our present custom of locating cemeteries in remote rural areas, and also the adoption of laws that require the burial of the dead to a depth of 6 feet. In some communities, even to this day, the health department has the responsibility for the location of cemeteries, for the sealing of coffins for interstate shipment, and for the regulation of the funerals of those who have died from "contagious causes."

Cremation of the dead was initiated in the United States in 1876 at Washington, Pennsylvania, by Dr. J. T. Le Moyne, who built a crematory for the disposal of his own body; but this procedure was not widely adopted for many years. Abbott[28] in 1900 reported a total of only 8,885 cremations in the United States from 1876 to 1900. Between 1900 and 1910,[29] the first ten years of the new century, when the custom had become established, there were 40,000 cremations in this country.

FOOD SANITATION

During pioneer days, the food supply was in the home garden, the wheat field, the barn, the smokehouse, and the cellar bin. Neighbors exchanged food, and there were food markets in the towns, but the food supply was near at hand and did not require special sanitary supervision. Transportation of meat was "on the hoof," and each community had its small slaughterhouse. There were no satisfactory methods of refrigeration nor of mass storage of food. Sanitary food regulations of the towns related only to spoiled food, for there was no concept of transfer of a specific infection through foodstuffs, but only the belief that putrid food is dangerous. Thus we find that the public health ordinances of the City Council of

[28] Abbott, S. W.: *The Past and Present Condition of Public Hygiene and State Medicine in the United States,* Monograph XIX, on American Social Economics. Wright & Potter Printing Co., Boston, 1900.
[29] *Annual Report of the Massachusetts State Board of Health,* 1910.

New Orleans in 1817 contained regulations concerning the seizure and destruction of spoiled food. Furthermore, no oysters could be sold between May 1 and September 1. Sanitary abatement of these health hazards was a function of the police department.

Trichinosis was the earliest known human infection that is due to a specific agent and traceable to food. Tiedemann first noted calcareous cysts in pork tissue in 1822 and James Paget discovered the larvae in pork in 1835. That same year Owen named the parasite *Trichinella spiralis.* Zenker in 1860 discovered that these worms cause disease in man, and gave at that time a good description of the human disease. He demonstrated that the disease is due to the consumption of raw pork. In 1871 Derby reviewed the epidemiology of the disease and reported two outbreaks in Massachusetts.[30] He showed that pickling of pork destroys the larvae and that smoking of pork does not.

Thus, long before the development of bacteriology, a specific infectious disease which was transmitted through food was well understood. The control measures were dependent upon (1) education of the people concerning the necessity of proper cooking of pork and (2) the prohibition of feeding raw pork scraps to hogs. Over a century has passed, yet, down to the present day, no fully protective procedures have evolved, despite many attempts to control this infection. Today trichinosis remains a constant menace. Truly public health moves slowly.

Clark's "Sanitary Code for Cities,"[31] drafted in 1859, contained clauses that related to control of slaughterhouses and to market inspection, but these regulations were concerned largely with abatement of "spoiled" food, such as decayed grain, vegetables, or fruits. There were regulations concerning the weight of a loaf of bread (two pounds) and there also were rules that dealt with adulteration of food, particularly of milk.

In 1872 we find a proposal in a little popular journal called the *Sanitarian*[32] "to establish a national Bureau of Health in the Department of the Interior." One of the purposes of this department would have been to supervise food sanitation.

[30] Derby, George: "Trichinia Disease in Massachusetts," *Reports of State Board of Health of Massachusetts,* p. 46, 1870-1871.
[31] See *Proceedings and Debates of the Third National Quarantine and Sanitary Convention.* Edward Jones & Co., Printers to Board of Education, New York, 1859, p. 647.
[32] *Sanitarian,* 1:1, 1872.

Alsberg,[33] who was to become the great protagonist for our nation's Pure Food and Drug Act, noted, in his review of food sanitation in *A Half Century of Public Health,* that in America there was no serious problem even as late as 1870 in relation to diseases that might be produced by food. Food was raised at home or purchased from neighbors; there was no centralized food processing and no methods for transporting food for long distances.

Adulteration of food was very common and remained the chief problem in food sanitation for over fifty years. Adulteration was not an attempt at fraud, nor designed to damage health, but represented *strained efforts to make money.* This observation was made in 1879 by E. R. Squibb. (This man was to found, at a later date, the great drug supply firm that now bears his name.) He pointed out that watered milk is not harmful, but he also noted that it is not nourishing.[34]

State laws concerning food sanitation were initiated by the state of Illinois in 1874. New York's Food and Drug Law was passed in 1881 and became a model for other states, many of which soon followed the example of the Empire State by passing a state food and drug act. A National Pure Food and Drug Congress was held in Washington in 1899; this Congress urged the establishment of a national department of pure foods. Finally the Federal Pure Food and Drug Act was passed in 1906. President Theodore Roosevelt must be given great credit for his energy in sponsoring this legislation and in driving the bill through Congress.

This act was intended primarily to check the extensive fraudulent practices that had grown up more or less concomitantly with mass processing of foods of all types. The act met with overwhelming popular support which led directly to an improvement in state and local health department regulations concerning cleanliness and more scientific sanitary measures for the preparation and handling of food. As a result of these regulations not only was fraud prevented but a more esthetic quality of food was produced. In the long run there was a great reduction in those diseases that had been so frequently transmitted through contaminated food.

Oysters as a Cause of Epidemics

For a great many years it had been recognized that oysters should not be consumed during the summer months, although shellfish were

---

[33] Alsberg, C. L.: "Progress in Federal Food Control," *A Half Century of Public Health.* American Public Health Association, New York, 1921, p. 209.
[34] Squibb, E. R.: *Tr. New York M. Soc.,* 1879, quoted by Alsberg.

not known until 1894 to be transmitters of typhoid fever or other specific infections. That year Professor H. W. Conn[35] of Wesleyan University traced a severe epidemic of typhoid fever in the student body to a banquet at which raw oysters had been eaten. He was able to trace the epidemiology of the accidental infection and to demonstrate how and when the oysters were infected with typhoid organisms.[36] Out of this simple but clearly delineated example of the dangers of pollution of oysters there developed, in due time, a comprehensive, nationwide program of shellfish sanitation.

Refrigeration of Food

Early attempts at food refrigeration were made during the first half of the nineteenth century with little success. The ammonia absorption process was discovered in 1850, but it was not until 1875 that the first cargo of frozen beef was shipped successfully from the United States to England.

The great development in food sanitation through preservation of food, cold storage of food, and the refrigeration of food during transportation occurred in the early part of the twentieth century. It completely revolutionized the dietary habits and customs of a whole nation in a single generation, and has resulted in a greatly improved nutritional status, with marked reduction in sickness. At the same time there developed standards for purity of food and safeguards against the introduction of infectious agents into foodstuffs to such a degree that by the year 1950 each person in the nation, no matter what his social or economic status, was able to secure at a relatively modest cost, and at any season of the year, a well-balanced diet that was abundant, pure in quality, and safe from infectious agents. This is one of the great public health achievements of the century.

MILK SANITATION

Milk sanitation is a sector of food sanitation that requires special consideration. Charles E. North[37] in *A Half Century of Public Health* gave such a splendid summary of the great struggle for universal pasteurization of milk that we need present in these pages only the high lights of that battle. Universal pasteurization of milk is now

[35] Conn, H. W.: "The Outbreak of Typhoid Fever at Wesleyan University," *Seventeenth Annual Report of the State Board of Health of Connecticut,* p. 243, 1895.
[36] Dr. Gaylord Anderson says that the English had already recognized this danger and that Conn knew of their work.
[37] North, Charles, E.: "Milk and Its Relation to Public Health", *A Half Century of Public Health.* American Public Health Association, New York, 1921, p. 236.

such an accepted procedure that we cannot even imagine the tragedy of those days not so long ago, when as many as 10,000 persons became desperately ill with milk-borne septic sore throat in a single epidemic (Chicago outbreak of 1911). The long, hard fight to introduce milk pasteurization and the bitter opposition to this sanitary measure are now buried in the dusty files of old health department records. But it was a great struggle while it lasted.

Milk was first incriminated as a transmitter of typhoid fever by William Taylor[38] in Penrith, England, in 1857. Seven families were affected. In 1867 the same author recorded an epidemic of scarlet fever in Penrith which he had traced to milk. Ballard[39] in 1870 reported 170 cases of typhoid fever from Islington, England, which were traceable to a single source of milk, and in 1877 E. G. Jacobs reported an epidemic of milk-borne diphtheria in Sutton, England. In 1881, 300 persons taking milk from the same dairy in Aberdeen, Scotland, developed septic sore throat.

Hart[40] read his famous paper on "Collected Reports of Milk Epidemics" at the International Medical Congress in 1881. He described fifty epidemics of typhoid fever, fifteen epidemics of scarlet fever, and four of diphtheria that were traceable to milk.

There must have been many similar epidemics in the United States, but the first reported American milk-borne epidemic of typhoid fever (forty cases) occurred in Allegheny City, Pennsylvania, in 1882. It was not reported until ten years later by Rankin.[41] The first milk-borne diphtheria epidemic in America was reported in Philadelphia by R. L. Pitfield[42] in 1898.

Trask[43] in 1908 gave a summary report on over 250 milk-borne epidemics of typhoid fever, scarlet fever, and diphtheria in the United States. Trask stated that from 1882 to 1892 only fourteen milk-borne epidemics were reported. During the next five years nineteen were noted, and from that time on the milk-borne epidemics increased to twelve or more each year until 1908, when the turning point came.

The great epidemics of septic sore throat in America, with thousands of persons involved, were described during the first decade of the twentieth century. Trask pointed out the reason that milk-borne

[38] Taylor, William: *Edinburgh M. J.*, May 1858.

[39] Ballard, E.: *Brit. M. J.*, 2:589, 1870.

[40] Hart, E.: "Collected Reports of Milk Epidemics," *Tr. Internat. M. Cong.* (London), 4:491, 1881.

[41] Rankin, D. N.: *Pittsburgh M. J.* 3:289, 1893.

[42] Pitfield, R. L.: *University M. Mag.*, 10:669, 1897-1898.

[43] Trask, John W.: "Milk as a Cause of Epidemics of Typhoid Fever, Scarlet Fever, and Diphtheria," *Reports U.S.P.H. Service*, Bulletin 41, 1908.

epidemics of disease were reported so much earlier in England than in the United States:

The degree to which epidemics are reported bears a direct ratio to the number and interest of the personnel of the local health department. One cannot study an epidemic without an epidemiologist.

Dairy inspection was instituted by health departments in America as early as 1882 in Newark, New Jersey. By 1900, standards of dairy sanitation had been well established and a "score card" system of inspection instituted by Woodward of Washington, D. C., in 1904. In 1901 William H. Park of the New York City Bacteriological Laboratory showed that milk, when delivered to the customers in the summer time, might contain over 5,000,000 bacteria per cubic centimeter. Thus it became necessary to establish bacteriological standards for clean milk. This was accomplished early in the twentieth century.

Certified Milk

Dairy inspection and milk sanitation were greatly furthered by the Medical Milk Commission, which was originated by Dr. Henry L. Coit of Newark, New Jersey, in 1890. In order to secure a clean, pure, safe milk supply, a body of physicians organized this commission and made a contract with a dairyman to produce a high-grade milk which was certified by the commission for its purity. The idea spread to all parts of the United States, and "certified milk" was soon available in almost all the larger cities. Certified milk not only provided a very fine raw milk for babies, but the standards that were set by the commission had a profound effect on the improvement of the milk supply for the general market. The great difficulty was that certified milk was very expensive. It was also raw milk and thus, despite all sanitary precautions, it was dangerous.

Theobald Smith demonstrated the presence of living bovine tubercle bacilli in market milk in 1896, and this observation resulted in the testing and exclusion of tuberculous cows from the dairy farms.[44]

Pasteurized Milk

Abraham Jacobi, the foremost early American pediatrician, read a paper before the New York Public Health Association in 1873 in which he recommended the boiling of milk as a sanitary measure.

[44] Kerr, John W.: "Certified Milk and Infant Milk Depots," *Reports U.S.P.H. Service,* Bulletin 41, 1908.

Soxhlet, the great German chemist, suggested in 1886 the boiling of milk as a proper procedure in infant feeding, and when Nathan Strauss opened his infant milk stations in New York in 1892, Jacobi recommended that Strauss utilize the Soxhlet method of heat sterilization at the milk depots. Pasteur, in about 1850, had devised the process of heating wine to 60° C. for a few minutes to destroy certain unfavorable yeasts and molds, but he did not adapt this method to milk sanitation. Denmark developed "flash pasteurization" between 1880 and 1891. The milk was heated rapidly to a boiling temperature and cooled quickly.

Great objection was raised by pediatricians to the boiling of milk.[45] It was claimed that boiling injures the taste, the quality, and the food value of the milk. The Medical Milk Commission believed that cleanliness and good dairy practice could produce safe raw milk and that the boiling of milk would be utilized to cover up poor dairy practice and to disguise dirty milk.

In 1906 Rosenau[46] gave great impetus to the pasteurization of milk by the determination of thermal death points of the more important milk contaminants. He showed that a temperature of 60° C. for twenty minutes destroys all common pathogens that gain access to milk. He also claimed that the heating of milk to 60° C. for twenty minutes produces little or no injury to the quality of milk.

A bitter war now raged between sanitarians and milk producers concerning the public health importance of compulsory milk pasteurization. The matter was settled effectively by the occurrence of very serious epidemics of septic sore throat in Boston in 1910 and in Chicago in 1911. The epidemic in Boston was caused by raw milk of a high quality from a model dairy that had observed cleanly procedures. This dairy had been an outstanding opponent of pasteurization. It capitulated when over 1,000 persons developed a severe infection from consumption of unpasteurized milk from this dairy. For all practical purposes the battle for clean milk, which must be adequately pasteurized, was won. Gradually the dairymen themselves improved their techniques in the handling of milk. Nationwide standards of milk sanitation were established. Pasteurization of milk became an almost universal procedure, and certified milk, which had served such a useful purpose, was largely aban-

[45] North, Charles E.: *op. cit.* p. 271.
[46] Rosenau, M. J.: "Pasteurization of Milk," *Reports U.S.P.H. Service,* Bulletin 41, 1908.

doned. It was a great sanitary victory in a fight which had lasted for nearly thirty years.

DISINFECTION AND FUMIGATION

A disinfectant, according to Sternberg, is "an agent capable of destroying the infective power of infectious material."[47] Disinfection has been employed for centuries on a more or less empirical basis in prevention of spread of disease. We have already noted in our discussion of ship quarantine that Rhode Island in early Colonial days required that the cargo of pestilential ships be aired and exposed to the sun.

During epidemics of yellow fever, and smallpox as well, it will be recalled that it was customary, during the Colonial period, to keep fires burning continually in the streets in order to destroy the infectious agent. Gunpowder, which was exploded between decks of an infected ship, was believed to be a most effective fumigant. Burning tar was also used extensively as a fumigant. Carey,[48] in his discussion of the Philadelphia epidemic of yellow fever in 1793, noted that the citizens burned smudges continuously in the streets to combat the epidemic, but he stated that this procedure had no beneficial effect. One of the most respected and ancient fumigants was sulfur fumes. It was used in periods of plagues and pestilence in medieval days. Chlorine gas was also utilized as a fumigant before the eighteenth century. During the early part of the nineteenth century, chloride of lime was employed as a disinfectant of privies, and slaked lime was generally recognized as an excellent deodorant. Any agent that alleviated odors was believed to prevent infection.

Disinfection was not always included in quarantine procedures. The English Quarantine Act of 1825[49] covered a wide variety of matters relative to ship quarantine, but did not require disinfection of the ship or cargo.

A great deal of confusion occurred, of course, as to just what a disinfectant was. There was no satisfactory method of testing the effectiveness of a disinfectant. Since disease was believed to be due to miasmata that arose from putrescent matter, any simple deodorant

[47] See "Disinfection and Individual Prophylaxis against Infectious Disease," a Lomb Prize Essay by George M. Sternberg in *Prize Essays of the American Public Health Association.* American Public Health Association, New York, 1886, p. 101.

[48] Carey, Mathew: *A Short Account of the Malignant Fever . . . ,* Philadelphia, 1793.

[49] *An Act for Making Provision for the Effectual Performance of Quarantine, etc.* George Eyre & Andrew Strahan, London, 1825.

might well be accepted as an active disinfectant, yet we know now that it might have no power to destroy bacteria.

At the Third National Quarantine and Sanitary Convention in 1859, a report was made upon disinfectants by Dr. Van Bibber.[50] He recognized the natural disinfective power of soil, water, sunlight, heat, and cold. Artificial disinfectants in general use at that time were sulfurous acid gas and chlorine gas. Hypochlorite of lime was recommended as a disinfectant for privies. Metallic salts such as zinc chloride were recognized as effective; and charcoal, which is a good deodorant but has little disinfective power, was considered to be a powerful disinfectant.

At the very first meeting of the American Public Health Association in 1872, a paper on "Disinfection and Disinfectants" was presented by Waller.[51] He pointed out the value of combating infection through destruction of infectious agents by (1) oxidation or by (2) arresting decomposition. For the latter method he suggested (a) carbolic acid,[52] (b) creosote solution, (c) thymol, (d) mineral salts such as bichloride of mercury, and (e) certain common acids and alkalis. He thought that the action of the disinfectant in arresting putrefaction was secured by coagulation of albumen.

In that same volume of the reports,[53] we find an initial discussion on the "Germ Theory of Disease and its Relations to Hygiene" by the president of Columbia University, Dr. Barnard. He pointed out that if infection is propagated by living germs, then "complete disinfection of every spot where pestilence may lift its head" should be a most effective control measure.

Before the development of the germ theory of disease, disinfection had been carried out on a trial-and-failure basis—a purely empirical technique—but now that germs could actually be seen, identified, and cultivated, it was possible to test the effectiveness of disinfectants and to measure their relative value. Koch was one of the first to make these specific tests. Soon it was shown that germs may be dispersed into the air and may remain suspended there. Following this discovery, fumigation became a matter of even greater importance than ever before. But the germ theory of disease was not

[50] Van Bibber, W. C.: "Report on Disinfectants," *Proceedings and Debates of the Third National Quarantine and Sanitary Convention*, Appendix B, pp. 373-85. Edward Jones & Co., Printers to Board of Education, New York, 1859.

[51] Waller, Elwyn: *Reports and Papers of the American Public Health Association*, 1:459-71, 1873.

[52] Carbolic acid was first employed as a disinfectant in 1834 (Chapin).

[53] *Reports and Papers of the American Public Health Association*, 1:70-87, 1873.

widely accepted at the outset and thus disinfection was still in the empirical stage in 1878. In that year A. H. Johnson wrote an article on "Disinfectants for Scarlet Fever" which was published in the *Annual Report of the State Board of Health of Massachusetts*.[54] He suggested the employment of:

1. High temperature (both steam and dry).
2. Nitrous acid.
3. Ozone.
4. Chlorine gas.
5. Sulfur dioxide.

One should hang a cloth saturated with chloride of lime or nitrate of lead at the door of the room of the sick person; chloride of zinc should be used for washing the furnishings of the room, the bed-clothing, and personal clothes. The body of a child who died of scarlet fever should be wrapped in a sheet which was thoroughly dampened with a solution of either carbolic acid or zinc chloride. The body should then be placed in a coffin with a watertight bottom which had been covered with sawdust to a depth of six inches.

In 1885 the awards of the Lomb Prize Essays[55] were announced at the thirteenth annual meeting of the American Public Health Association. Awards were given for the following four essays:

1. "Healthy Homes and Food for the Working Classes" by Victor C. Vaughan of Michigan (prize, $200).
2. "The Sanitary Conditions and Necessities of School-Houses and School-life" by D. F. Lincoln of Boston, Massachusetts (prize, $200).
3. "Preventive Causes of Disease, Injury, and Death in American Manufactories and Workshops, and the Best Means and Appliances for Preventing and Avoiding Them" by George H. Ireland of Springfield, Massachusetts (prize, $200).
4. "Disinfection and Individual Prophylaxis against Infectious Disease" by George M. Sternberg, major and surgeon, United States Army (prize, $500).

These four young men each pioneered in important and uncultivated fields of public health. Each one of them was to distinguish himself in American public health in the years to come.

[54] See *Ninth Annual Report of the State Board of Health of Massachusetts*, pp. 253-327, 1878.
[55] *Prize Essays of the American Public Health Association*. American Public Health Association, New York, 1886.

Sternberg, who won the first prize for his essay on disinfection, utilized tests on bacterial cultures for determining the efficacy of disinfectants, and he showed that many substances that were called disinfectants had little or no power to destroy bacteria. He recommended as the best disinfectants chloride of lime, carbolic acid, and sulfurous acid gas. For the destruction of bacterial spores he suggested steam under pressure, mercuric chloride, chloride of lime, fire, and boiling water. Disinfectants that were effective in the absence of spores were dry heat, carbolic acid, copper sulfate, and chloride of zinc. For fumigation he recommended "time-honored SO_2 gas."

In 1888 disinfection and fumigation really began to thrive. The Committee of Disinfection and Disinfectants of the American Public Health Association wrote a report for the annual meeting. This report was so voluminous that it was published as a separate volume of 265 pages. Dr. Sternberg was chairman of this committee. Large and elaborate devices for disinfecting bedding and clothing were depicted, and the various tests for efficacy of a disinfectant were described.

Knowledge of bacteriology grew tremendously during the last decade of the nineteenth century and, within a few years, the specific causes of most of the common infectious diseases were discovered. This resulted, quite logically, in greatly increased interest in disinfection and fumigation.

Formaldehyde as a Fumigant

This gas was first presented as a possible fumigant by Dr. J. I. Kinyoun of Washington, D. C., at the 1895 meeting of the American Public Health Association in Denver, Colorado. Dr. Kinyoun stated:

I have been carrying on for the last three months some experiments in regard to disinfectants for diphtheria and tuberculosis, and the agent which I recommend to you is known as formaline.[56]

The following year Dr. F. C. Robinson, professor of chemistry at Bowdoin College, Maine, read a paper at the A.P.H.A. meeting entitled "A Formic Aldehyde—Its Practical Use."[57] He had caught Dr. Kinyoun's brief remarks at Denver the year before and had developed a vaporizer for formaldehyde.

[56] Kinyoun, J. I.: "Contribution to the Discussion on Railroad Hygiene," *Reports and Papers of the American Public Health Association,* 21:83, 1896.
[57] Robinson, F. C.: *Reports and Papers of the American Public Health Association,* 21:357, 1896.

From that moment, formaldehyde fumigation swept the country. It was the perfect fumigant. Relatively inexpensive, it had a penetrating and very bad odor. Laboratory tests showed that the gas was a very powerful germicide. It was not destructive to fabrics nor injurious to furniture, silver, brass, or other metals. It was much simpler to use than sulfuric gas. Soon, each home in which a case of infectious disease occured was subjected to terminal fumigation with formaldehyde gas. The people liked it very much. It was so obviously beneficial that the health department was compelled by popular pressure to carry out elaborate fumigation techniques even for the simpler infections. Expensive devices were invented to disseminate the gas.

In Chapin's *Municipal Sanitation in the United States* in 1901,[58] we find an elaborate description of the methods that should be followed in formaldehyde fumigation, and beautiful pictures are given of formaldehyde generators, as well as great autoclaves that were equipped to disinfect the effects of whole households with steam under pressure. A large and expert public health personnel was developed and trained in municipal health departments in order to provide for the intensive demand by the people for terminal fumigation and disinfection of houses where infectious disease had occurred. The peak of absurdity in terminal disinfection was reached about 1905, but, as we have noted before, Chapin, the great municipal health officer of Providence, was his own severest critic.[59] It began to dawn on him that all these expensive and troublesome procedures were futile and of no value. It took great courage to stand all alone at a meeting of the public health section of the American Medical Association in 1906 and to tell his colleagues that formaldehyde fumigation is wasteful, extravagant, and needless. His audience was at first thunderstruck, then angry and vituperative. He was a traitor to public health. He had destroyed at a single blow an idol of great popular appeal and had wrecked the dignity and prestige of the public health department. Nevertheless, so great was Chapin's reputation for intelligence and fearlessness that, within a few years, terminal disinfection was abandoned by the principal cities of the nation. In some areas the use of gaseous fumigation lingered for a long time, for spectacular procedures perish slowly.

When the author went to Sao Paulo, Brazil, in 1918 to study in

[58] Chapin, Charles V.: *Municipal Sanitation in the United States*. Snow & Farnham, Providence, Rhode Island, 1901.
[59] Chapin, Charles V.: "The Fetish of Disinfection," *J.A.M.A.*, 47:574, 1906.

the Instituto de Higiene, he found that great city still employing an elaborate system of terminal disinfection. Disinfectors wore special uniforms, and had special bright red conveyances that drove through the streets pell-mell, like firemen. A great canvas—large enough to cover a house entirely—was expertly drawn over the infected house and fumigation was administered on a lavish scale. All bedding and practically everything in the house that would not be injured by steam was taken to an enormous steam chamber which was large enough to receive a whole truck-body. The great autoclave door on the "infected" side was swung open to receive the material from the household. After sterilization the truck-body was rolled out the other "sterile" side so that there was never any cross-communication between the two sides of the disinfectory.

Soon the whole organization and program were abandoned. Thus the meteoric rise and fall of terminal gaseous fumigation with formaldehyde lasted less than thirty years. Nevertheless it required another twenty-five years to demonstrate the fact that soap, hot water, and scrupulous cleanliness were, after all, the most valuable of all disinfectants.

HOUSING AND HEALTH

Bad housing was not an important health menace in America during the Colonial period. George Wallis,[60] who wrote a book on preventive medicine in 1794, made no allusion to the influence of bad housing upon health. Webster, in his *History of Epidemic and Pestilential Diseases* in 1799, clearly indicated that the location of a house in close proximity to swamps or to other miasmatic situations is an unwise procedure; he emphasized the importance of the proper location of the house, of good ventilation, and the necessity for shutting out the night air by closing the bedroom tightly during the sleeping hours. Franklin was considered a fanatic by his friends, for he insisted that night air is not dangerous, and he actually opened his windows at night in order to secure fresh air. Rush[61] was insistent upon the necessity for community planning. He felt that dwellings should be protected from the bad odors of certain industries, such as tanneries and slaughterhouses; he was a firm believer

[60] Wallis, George: *The Art of Preventing Diseases and Restoring Health, Founded on Rational Principles and Adapted to Persons of Every Capacity.* Samuel Campbell, New York, 1794.

[61] Rush, Benjamin: *Medical Inquiries and Observations.* Fourth Edition, Vol. IV, p. 105, 1815.

in cleanliness of the home and the community at large. He was sure that household and community filth causes epidemics.

In retrospect we realize that the eighteenth century had no serious housing problems, for people lived in individual homes, on the farms or in small villages. Not even the largest cities of America in 1800 exceeded 50,000 population, and the industrial revolution, which was to have such a profound effect on American life, was not yet in its infancy. Bad housing and all its attendant ills have been an integral part of the industrial development of the nation, with the very rapid growth of cities and the production of "slums." The first indication of an interest in housing as a social and health problem was a note by David Hosack in 1810 in which he pointed out that the community has a responsibility for regulating the housing of the poor. In 1837 Dr. McCready[62] made a remarkable statement:

In the rapid growth of our cities the number of buildings has by no means increased in a manner corresponding to the great influx of strangers. The accommodations are insufficient, and the rents, in consequence, extravagantly high.

In our towns the evil is a growing one. Every year adds to its magnitude; unless something be done to check its progress, our cities will ere long present examples of disease and deformity which hitherto could only be found in the overgrown towns of Europe.

This is a very accurate prophecy in which a farsighted man predicted many years in advance the eventual unspeakable slum conditions.

Dr. Griscom, city inspector of health of New York City in 1842,[63] spoke of the dangers of overcrowded dwellings and the habitation of dark damp cellars. He advocated the abolition of pigsties in the city, the removal of slaughterhouses from built-up parts of the town, the necessity for clean streets, and the drainage of marshlands to eliminate malaria.

The Association for Improving the Conditions of the Poor was formed in New York in 1843. Beginning in 1846 this association took up "housing" as one of its important projects. It has maintained this interest down to the present day, for its activities in relation to housing are just as important and pressing today as they were 100 years ago. The association has changed its name to Community

[62] McCready, Benjamin: *Tr. M. Soc. State of New York*, 143:97, 1837.
[63] Griscom, John H.: *Report of the City Inspector of New York*, 1842.

Service Society, but its major unsolved social problems have not changed.

Chadwick's studies on housing of the poor in England which resulted in the passing by Parliament of the Public Health Act of 1848 had a profound influence on the public health in America. Shattuck's report in 1850 gave due credit for the aid and stimulus that he had received from Chadwick's published works. For example, Shattuck's "Recommendation XVII" bears directly on housing:

> In laying out new towns and villages, and in extending those already laid out, ample provision be made for a supply, in purity and abundance, of light, air, and water; for drainage and sewerage, for paving and for cleanliness.

Shattuck referred to Sir John Simon's *Fifth Report of the Registrar-General* concerning the serious effects of bad housing, and in "Recommendation XIX" he suggested the regulation, by the local board of health, of proposed sanitary arrangements in new dwelling houses and factories. His next recommendation was concerned with the mitigation of sanitary evils that arise from overcrowded lodginghouses and cellar-dwellings.

The *Transactions* of the first meeting of the American Medical Association in 1848 recognized the importance of bad housing. The Committee on Sanitary Improvement stated:

> The United States may be considered as a country in which no legislation exists regulating its sanitary condition . . . densely populated cities present the greatest complication of those evils. . . .

Clark[64] in his "Sanitary Code for Cities" in 1859 gave prominence to household sanitation. Under his "Code," the board of health should have the supervision of tenements and of overcrowding, as well as the prevention of nuisances from filth, ashes, rubbish, and the keeping of animals. "Livery stables cannot accumulate more than four cartloads of manure between May and November." Abatement of nuisances under the "Code" were to be at the expense of the property owner. Cesspools could not be constructed *under* any house, and the board had power to enforce construction of "dug privies." A plan for public parks and pleasure grounds was incorporated in the "Sanitary Code" as a public health measure.

---

[64] Clark, Henry: "Sanitary Code for Cities," *Proceedings and Debates of the Third National Quarantine and Sanitary Convention.* Edward Jones & Co., Printers to Board of Education, New York, 1859, pp. 647-72.

Delevan,[65] city inspector of health of New York City in 1862, was much concerned with the worsening sanitary conditions that were due to rapid growth and resultant overcrowding of the city. Healthful districts were becoming unhealthful, with great increase in mortality, particularly infant mortality, because of unwholesome food, impoverished conditions, inattention to cleanliness, intemperance, and large numbers of families occupying apartments in the same house, many with no water closets. Ventilation of many of these tenements was very poor. There were 6,000 families living in underground cellars in New York City. "That life is short and mortality great in these seething places of corruption, is not to be wondered at."

The Metropolitan Health Bill of 1865[66] was intended primarily to improve the very bad housing situation in New York City, but it failed to pass the legislature. Stephen Smith's famous Sanitary Survey of New York City followed in the same year. This survey was basically an exposé of the terrible slum conditions of the dwellings of the poor in the city and resulted in the formation of the Metropolitan Board of Health. Another result of this survey was the passage of the first tenement house law in 1867.

In 1876 Janes[67] wrote a report on the "Health of Tenement Populations." He stated that the number of children that were engaged in factory labor in New York City and environs totaled not far from 100,000.

The degree of aggregation or the dwelling of people in masses must be recognized as a condition which bears very decided relations to the healthy man as well as the future development and sanitary interests of his offspring.

There are certain general causes, such as mode of living, personal habits, and the variety of circumstances . . . which affect health either favorably or unfavorably in proportion to the varying degree of regularity with which well known hygiene laws are observed. For man is largely indebted to his social surroundings for the degree of his physical perfection.

These social influences exert their power, either good or bad, upon all who come within their reach. Hence aggregation of population carries

[65] Delevan, D. E.: *Report of the City Inspector of New York for the Year 1862,* Document 4, p. 8.
[66] *Address of the Committee to Promote the Passage of the Metropolitan Health Bill,* New York, December, 1865.
[67] Janes, E. H.: *Reports and Papers of the American Public Health Association,* 2:115, 1876.

with it an effect like the presence of fluids, tending to reduce to a common level the general mass.

In 1879 Chaillé[68] of New Orleans spoke even more forcefully concerning the dangers of overcrowding:

Every large city has tenements or other crowded houses for the poor, so constructed that it is not possible for the occupants to be either healthy or chaste and in which children from their birth are seized in the remorseless arms of this age's Three Furies—filth, disease, and crime—yet so far are our laws from regulating the healthy construction of dwelling-houses that this is not done even for public edifices, not even for the public schools of our children, thus educating them in anti-hygiene.

Henry Meyer,[69] one of the early sanitary engineers, established a journal, *The Sanitary Engineer,* which later became the *Engineers' Record* in 1877. He became interested in housing and offered a prize for a design of a model tenement. In 1879 this activity resulted in the Model Tenement House Act of New York City.

No city in America grew more rapidly than Chicago, and no health officer was more concerned with the problems of housing than J. H. Rauch.[70] He was one of the first to realize the importance to health of city planning and believed that public parks are a great aid in health promotion. He stated that he considered that it was quite possible, by suitable sanitary procedures, to reduce the death rate of Chicago to *17 per 1,000 per annum.* (The rate has been 10 or below for many years, but a crude mortality rate of 17 was not achieved in Chicago until 1895, twenty years after his prophecy.)

The American Public Health Association at its meeting in St. Louis in 1884 held a symposium on housing.[71] There were three important papers: one by C. W. Chancellor on "The Squalid Dwellings of the Poor—A Social and Sanitary Reproach"; one by S. W. Robinson on "Hygiene of the Habitations of the Poor"; and a third on "The Sanitary Survey of a House" by William K. Newton.

It is quite clear from their reports that public health authorities

[68] Chaillé, Stanford E.: *Annual Address before the Louisiana State Medical Society,* 1879.

[69] Meyer, H. C.: *The Story of the Sanitary Engineer* (by its founder). Monograph, privately printed, 1928.

[70] Rauch, J. H.: "Sanitary Problems of Chicago," *Report Illinois State Board of Health,* p. 94, 1879. See also by same author, *Public Parks: Their Effect upon the Moral, Physical and Sanitary Condition of the Inhabitants of Large Cities with Special Reference to the City of Chicago,* Monograph, 1869.

[71] *Reports and Papers of the American Public Health Association,* 10:145-59, 1884.

of that day realized full well the truth of the statement made by Dr. Biggs[72] many years later:

Disease is a largely removable evil. It continues to afflict humanity not only because of incomplete knowledge of its causes, and lack of individual and public hygiene, but also because it is fostered extensively by harsh

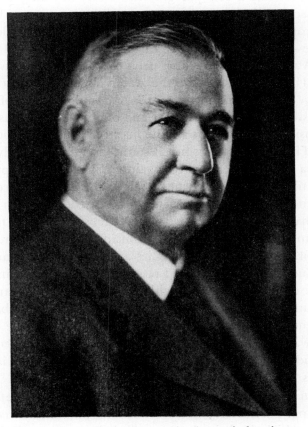

Fig. 29. Victor C. Vaughan, early pioneer in housing.

economic and industrial conditions and by wretched housing in congested communities. These conditions can be removed by better social organization.

The Lomb Prize Essays[73]

In 1885 Henry B. Lomb of Rochester, through the American Public Health Association, offered prizes for the four best essays

[72] Winslow, C.-E. A.: *Life of Hermann Biggs.* Lea & Febiger, Philadelphia, 1929.
[73] *Prize Essays of the American Public Health Association: op. cit.*

on four chosen subjects. One subject was: "Healthy Homes and Food for the Working Classes." The prize was won by V. C. Vaughan, a young professor at the University of Michigan.

Dr. Vaughan, in this prize essay, gave special consideration to the individual house for a workman and his family. Tenement houses he dismissed with a few paragraphs. "Every working man should strive to secure a home, and a tenement house can never be a home in any proper sense." He paid particular attention to location of the house—its construction, drainage, ventilation, and its water supply. Waste disposal by dug privy or water closet was recommended. He emphasized that the water closet is more convenient and "may be made perfectly safe." A double system of sewerage was suggested, one for storm water and one for human wastes. Sewer gas he considered dangerous and he insisted that it must be carefully trapped. The essay contains much sound and practical advice about selecting a house. He warned against "skin" houses put up by "jerry" builders, simply to rent or sell at the highest price.

Following the interest that was created by the Lomb Prize Essays, we find many references, during the latter part of the nineteenth century, to housing, particularly housing for the poor. Most of these reports were by social agencies and not by health authorities. The avalanche of bacteriological research and the absorbing interest in specific causes of infection with resultant efforts toward control of communicable disease absorbed the attention of public health workers during the last years of the old century and the first years of the new. Thus the social aspects of public health faded into the background. But gradually health officers regained an interest in housing as an important factor in promotion of health. There developed an increasing understanding of the unfavorable factors of bad housing, particularly those conditions that influenced the life of families which dwelt in the overcrowded tenements of the rapidly growing cities.

Conditions became so serious that "slum clearance" became a social (and political) password. Unfortunately, however, the social reformers in the field of slum clearance erected great "castles in the air" that were quite beyond the financial resources of the slum dwellers. These unfortunates were displaced when the "model housing projects" were completed, and thus the very measures that were intended for their benefit drove them even deeper into worse overcrowding. As this chapter is written, an examination question for medical students has just crossed the author's desk. It reads as follows:

Housing has been called the most important single unsolved public health problem in America. What evidence can be presented in support of this view?

One hundred years of serious and conscientious public health effort have not succeeded in solving the problem of bad housing and slum conditions in the large industrial cities of America. In fact, in some areas of our large cities, conditions are worse today than they have been during the past century.

CHAPTER 38. *Epidemiology and Communicable Disease Control*

FROM THE CIVIL WAR THROUGH THE END OF THE NINETEENTH CENTURY

> *A great number of cases to observe is in some respects valuable, but confusion and difficulty of study sometimes arise from too great aggregation of disease under the extra artificial conditions of cities, hospitals, etc., and very much is to be learned from a few typical cases occurring under circumstances less complicated.*
>
> *There is often not so much to be learned by observing a very great number of cases as by an exhaustive searching into a few cases, all the facts of which are more within the grasp.*
>
> EZRA M. HUNT, *1872*

The History of American Epidemiology contains a very interesting section by Dr. James Doull,[1] that covers the years from 1876 to 1920. He has called this period the "Bacteriological Era," as indeed it was, since this was the period of the development of the concept of specific agents of infection which produced well-defined disease entities. From this initial concept there grew the idea of individual immunity to specific infection. Furthermore, these hypotheses led to studies relating to the exact mode of transmission of specific infection from the sick to the well.

Up to this time epidemiologists had been greatly puzzled by the sudden appearance of a disease in a community which had had no contact with sick people. Apparently the idea did not occur to these early epidemiologists that a *healthy carrier* might harbor and transmit a specific infectious agent; but the newer bacteriological

[1] Doull, James A.: "The Bacteriological Era (1876-1920)," *The History of American Epidemiology*. C. V. Mosby Co., St. Louis, 1952, p. 74.

techniques proved that this theory was quite correct. This was a new and very important concept in communicable disease transmission. Eventually it revolutionized control measures. The acceptance of this theory was greatly retarded, however, and it did not fully establish itself until the end of the century.

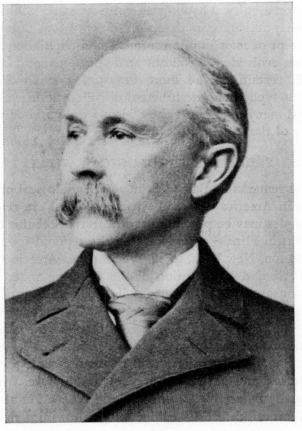

Fig. 30. G. M. Sternberg. Made America's first contribution to bacteriology. (From Watson, Irving A. [editor and compiler]: *Physicians and Surgeons of America.* Republican Press Association, Concord, N.H., 1896.)

The bacteriological era made possible the prevention of infection through direct control of environmental factors. Empirical procedures that had been developed in the sanitation of water supplies and sewage disposal were found to be quite sound, although based on somewhat faulty premises. Thus it was possible to rationalize sanitary procedures for the protection of milk and food and for proper housing, as well as for the development of other environmental measures of health protection. It was feasible also to rationalize the procedures of isolation, of quarantine, and of disinfection. The science of epidemiology became founded soundly on facts rather than on empirical hypotheses, since measures could be undertaken for early and accurate detection of contagious diseases.

The concept of mass immunization of the population by specific measures was evolved, and concentrated and systematic attacks were made upon certain of the more devastating communicable diseases such as typhoid fever, tuberculosis, diphtheria, yellow fever, malaria, and many others. All these ideas were initiated during the last quarter of the nineteenth century.

EARLY EPIDEMIOLOGICAL WORK

It is quite remarkable that such fine epidemiological observations were made in America before the bacteriological era really began. A few examples may be presented as illustrations of this fact. Doull has cited Austin Flint's[2] observation on the typhoid fever epidemic in North Boston, New York, in 1843, as the first American outbreak that was attributed to pollution of the drinking water. Flint did report this outbreak in 1845, but he did not realize until 1873 that it was a water-borne epidemic.[3]

Bigelow,[4] in 1835, gave a bold discourse before the Massachusetts Medical Society on the subject of "Self-Limited Disease." He insisted that treatment is of little avail in cutting short the course of certain diseases, and gave as examples typhoid fever, pneumonia, vaccinia, smallpox, erysipelas, measles, and others. He also brought out an important defect in epidemiological studies that has not been fully corrected even today. He went on to state:

Few authors have published all the cases they have observed, and the greater part have taken only the trouble to present to us the facts which favor their own views. Knowledge has, for its only just and lasting foundation, a rigid, impartial and inflexible requisition of the truth.

[2] Doull, James A.: *op. cit.*, p. 93.
[3] Flint, Austin: "The Relations of Water to the Propagation of Fever," *Reports and Papers of the American Public Health Association*, 1:164, 1873.
[4] Bigelow, Jacob: Lecture at the Annual Meeting of the Massachusetts Medical Society, May 27, 1835.

Bowditch[5] in 1862 obtained data on the prevalence of tuberculosis in various New England towns through a questionnaire to local physicians. His general summary of this correspondence was that:

1. Consumption was not equally distributed throughout New England.
2. The prevalence of consumption depended upon the characteristics of the soil on or near which the affected persons had resided.

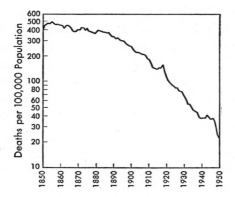

Fig. 31. Tuberculosis in Massachusetts, 1850-1950. (From "A Century of Tuberculosis Control in Massachusetts." Massachusetts Tuberculosis and Health League, Boston, 1953.)

3. The moisture of the soil was the only known characteristic that was connected with consumption-breeding districts.
4. Consumption is not contagious, but may be infectious to some slight extent. "Long attendance on a patient may undermine the constitution of a nurse and produce consumption."

He gave an illustration of two brothers who married sisters. Family *A* remained on the old homestead, a southern slope, dry, warm, and well drained. Family *B* moved to a house subjected to heavy moisture; wet meadow behind, a bog in front, a river nearby. Family *A* had nine children, six of whom grew to adult life in good health. Family *B* had eleven children, of whom the father and two sons survived. The remainder suffered and died of consumption.

[5] Bowditch, Henry I.: "Topographical Distribution and Local Origin of Consumption in Massachusetts," *Communications of Massachusetts M. Soc.* **10:**59, 1862.

Bowditch felt that this was a well-controlled situation on which to base his conclusion, since the only marked variable was the dampness of the housing arrangement.

During the Civil War, excellent epidemiological observations were made by Joseph Jones on contagious disease in the Confederate Army.[6] In 1870 Derby[7] gave a good description of two families in which epidemics of trichinosis occurred in Massachusetts. In each case he discovered the source of infection. That same year Nichols[8] described the prevalence of anthrax in Massachusetts. In all, twenty-six cases were found—fourteen of them fatal. The contamination occurred through animal hair that was imported from Argentina. Nichols discussed the contagious nature of this disease and advanced the theory that anthrax is due to a "living or germinal matter" carried by the animal hair which contained the contagious principle.

Dr. George Derby[9] in 1871 made an extensive study of the causes of typhoid fever in Massachusetts. His information for this study was secured through correspondence with other physicians. He showed that typhoid fever is a rural rather than an urban disease. Polluted water was proved to be an important cause of the disease. He quoted the opinion of Nathan Smith (1787-1822), who believed that typhoid is propagated by contagion. His opinions may be summarized briefly as follows: Typhoid rarely affects the same person twice. It travels from place to place, remains in a village for a longer or shorter period, ceases and appears in another. If communicated from one person to another, it has a specific cause, and cannot be produced without the agency of that çause.

Dr. Derby's correspondents, i.e., physicians who answered his queries, mentioned vacation-typhoid and also recorded a family epidemic involving six persons, in which the family used well water that was contaminated by a privy. A "typhoid house" was cited and a family epidemic of five cases was described, in which the water supply was obtained from a polluted spring. Dr. Derby believed that he had good evidence that typhoid fever could also be trans-

---

[6] Jones, Joseph: *Medical and Surgical Memoirs.* Letter to Surgeon General S. P. Moore, August 6, 1864, Vol. I, p. vi; "Prevalence of Pneumonia and Typhoid Fever," Vol. I, p. 650.

[7] Derby, George: "Trichinia Disease in Massachusetts," *Second Annual Report of the State Board of Health of Massachusetts,* p. 46, 1871.

[8] Nichols, A. H.: "Charbon In Massachusetts," *Second Annual Report of the State Board of Health of Massachusetts,* p. 85, 1871.

[9] Derby, George: "An Inquiry into the Causes of Typhoid Fever in Massachusetts," *Second Annual Report of the State Board of Health of Massachusetts,* p. 110, 1871.

mitted through polluted air from putrid vegetable and animal matter.

Cabell[10] of Virginia also queried his associate practitioners in Virginia in 1877. The correspondents agreed that typhoid fever might be developed in excremental filth, and were willing to accept the water-borne theory of this infectious agent, but they did not believe that this was the only source of typhoid fever, and certainly did not believe that the infection always came from a person with the disease. They stumbled over the "carrier." Apparently this possibility never occurred to anyone, though it was—in retrospect—the simplest and most logical explanation of the varied epidemiological pattern of typhoid fever.

A. N. Bell,[11] in 1877 revived the theory of the infectious nature of bovine tuberculosis. He presented evidence that tuberculosis was transmitted from sick to healthy cows if they were in the same stable, and that the "virus" might be in the milk. He emphasized that this infectious agent was destroyed by cooking. He also pointed out the value of the study of animal diseases in solving human infections, but made no speculations as to the infectiousness of human tuberculosis. In 1879 Noah Cressy held meetings among the farmers in western Massachusetts, explaining to them the infectious nature of bovine tuberculosis and the methods that might be used to combat the disease.[12] In 1889 the Massachusetts Cattle Commission recommended that milk herds be inspected by local boards of health with removal of all milk cows that exhibited the slightest symptoms of tuberculosis. Each of these epidemiological studies was completed without recourse to a bacteriological laboratory and with little knowledge of specific factors in disease production.

Ezra Hunt in 1878 made an important contribution to epidemiology when he formulated a series of principles on "How to Study an Epidemic."[13] Although he had little information concerning specific etiological agents which produce disease, nevertheless his requisites were sound and penetrating. He indicated that the epidemiologist need not be on the spot where the epidemic prevails. It is a requisite in forming a clear, calculated, and impartial judg-

[10] Cabell, James: "Etiology of Enteric Fever," *Tr. Am. M. A.*, 28:141, 1877.

[11] Bell, A. N.: "Tuberculosis in Milk Cows," *Tr. Am. M. A.*, 28:481, 1877.

[12] North, Charles: "Milk and Its Relation to Public Health," *A Half Century of Public Health*. American Public Health Association, New York, 1921, p. 252.

[13] Hunt Ezra M. (secretary, New Jersey State Board of Health): *Tr. Am. Pub. Health A.*, 4:173, 1878.

Table 15

The Great Epidemics of New York City*

1800-1900

YEAR	DISEASE†	TOTAL DEATHS	DEATHS PER 100,000
1832	Cholera	3,513	1,561
1849	Cholera	5,071	1,014
1851	Dysentery	1,173	221
1854	Cholera	2,509	395
1866	Cholera	1,137	113
1872	Smallpox	1,666	118
1875	Smallpox	1,899	125
1881	Diphtheria	4,894	266
1887	Diphtheria	4,509	226

* SOURCE: *Bull. New York City Department of Health*, p. 6, March 1953.
† NOTE: Yellow fever in its highest year (1805) caused only 270 deaths, a rate of 300 per 100,000.

ment that objects shall be placed at a certain distance in order that they may be seen in relative positions and bearings. The following is a synopsis of his seven requisites for proper study of an epidemic:

1. A thorough understanding of the sense in which technical words are used. There may be a confusion of diagnostic terms. For example: "infectious," "contagious," "miasm," "malaria," "fomites," "zymotic," and the like.

2. Specifying the diagnostic character of the disease under investigation. One must be able to recognize the disease. Smallpox causes no confusion—yellow fever causes difficulty. It must be distinguished from other forms of fever.

3. Ascertained and expert methods for collecting facts. The technique should be comparable to the taking of testimony, and should follow legal standards of rules of evidence. "The facts and observations have to be studied inductively, deductively, analogically, numerically, and then grouped rightly for study."

4. Accurate analysis. "It must not make a verdict when possible sources of error have not been eliminated by sufficient massing of cases. . . . The science or art is not in the facts but in logical reasoning thereon." The analysis must follow principles of evidence and methods of logic.

5. Careful collation and consideration of testimony as to former outbreaks and decorous consideration of the opinion of observers thereof.
6. Catechetical method of investigation. The first meaning of "catechetical" is instruction: asking intelligent questions, following the essential as distinct from the incidental, searching into every particular, for we sometimes discover truth where we least expect to find it.
7. Need for material support. One cannot study an epidemic without funds and personnel.

Although three-fourths of a century have passed, a modern instructor in epidemiology might well utilize Hunt's seven requisites as the foundation of his teaching and investigation.

GREAT EPIDEMICS

The first great water-borne outbreak of typhoid fever to be recorded in America occurred in Plymouth, Pennsylvania, in 1885. This outbreak was investigated by L. H. Taylor[14] and has been well described by Sedgwick.[15] In 1890 Sedgwick[16] studied the extensive epidemics of typhoid fever that occurred in Massachusetts at Lawrence and Lowell. These epidemics were due to pollution of the Merrimac River.

Henry P. Walcott[17] made an interesting epidemiological study of the influenza epidemic of 1889-1890. This epidemic lasted from December 1 to February 1. There had been a slow increase all fall, beginning in October and stepping up each week. The rapid increase began the second week in December. The peak of the incidence curve was reached in four weeks, with a rapid decline nearing the base line about the first week in February. There followed scattered cases through March. Then the disease disappeared. In 1895 Professor Conn of Wesleyan University[18] worked out very effectively the epidemiology of an outbreak of typhoid fever that occurred in college students, and which he traced to polluted raw

[14] Taylor, L. H.: *First Annual Report of the Board of Health and Vital Statistics of Pennsylvania*, p. 176, 1886.
[15] Sedgwick, William T.: *Principles of Sanitary Science and the Public Health*. The Macmillan Co., New York, 1902, pp. 200-206.
[16] *Ibid.*, pp. 207-14.
[17] Walcott, Henry P., and Abbott, S. W.: *Annual Report of the State Board of Health of Massachusetts*, p. 747, 1892.
[18] Conn, H. W.: *Annual Report of the State Board of Health of Connecticut*, p. 243, 1895.

oysters. An important outbreak of milk-borne typhoid fever was studied in 1896 by H. E. Smith[19] in Stamford, Connecticut.

In 1898 Reed, Vaughan, and Shakespeare studied the epidemiology of typhoid fever in the United States military camps during the Spanish-American War. This was a truly great pioneer work. The report had an immediate and powerful effect in the development of better methods in typhoid fever control throughout the world.[20]

Milk-borne epidemics of streptococcus infections were reported in England several times during the latter part of the nineteenth century, but the first extensive American outbreak of septic sore throat was reported by Winslow[21] in 1912. It occurred in the suburbs of Boston and was widespread and highly fatal.

One of the great American epidemiologists of the nineteenth century was Henry Carter, who began his field studies in 1887 on the limits of the incubation period of yellow fever, and published his conclusions on the "extrinsic incubation period" of yellow fever in 1900.[22] Reed and his co-workers[23] carried out their work in Havana, Cuba, on the etiology of yellow fever, also in 1900. Their studies proved the theory of Carlos Finlay of Havana that the disease is indeed transmitted through the bite of an Aëdes mosquito.

We have cited these early contributions to the science of epidemiology because they illustrate so well the fact that sound epidemiological work can be carried out without actual knowledge of the specific agents of infection. In very few of the illustrations that we have used did the epidemiologist have at his command exact measures for diagnosis, nor was he able to trace the course of infection by bacteriological techniques. Nevertheless, important results were secured. It is interesting that in no instance did the idea emerge of a normal, healthy *carrier of specific infection.*

Carriers

As Doull[24] has noted, Sternberg was the first to show in 1880 that a normal person might carry a virulent pneumococcus in his

[19] Smith, H. E.: *Annual Report of the State Board of Health of Connecticut,* p. 161, 1896.

[20] Reed, Walter; Vaughan, Victor C.; and Shakespeare, E. O.: *Report on the Origin and Spread of Typhoid Fever in the United States Military Camps during the Spanish War of 1898.* Government Printing Office, Washington, D. C., 1904.

[21] Winslow, C.-E. A.: *J. Infect. Dis.,* 10:73, 1912.

[22] Carter, H. R.: *New Orleans M. & S. J.,* 52:617, 1900.

[23] Reed, W.; Carroll, J.; Agramonte, A.; and Lazear, J. W.: "The Etiology of Yellow Fever," *Philadelphia M. J.,* 6:790, 1900.

[24] Doull, James A.: *op. cit.,* p. 90.

saliva; but the importance of carriers as a source of human infection was first emphasized by Koch in his cholera studies in 1893.

Park and Beebe[25] in 1894 found that 2.4 per cent of 330 healthy persons whom they examined were harboring virulent diphtheria bacilli in their throats. In 1909 Rosenau and his associates[26] found 3 typhoid carriers among 986 normal adults in Washington, D. C. Finally, the dramatic story of the famous cook, "Typhoid Mary,"[27] who left a train of illness and death wherever she went, brought home both to the medical profession and to the laity the danger of healthy carriers in the spread of disease. They soon learned that carriers were important, not only in the transmission of typhoid fever, but in many other diseases as well.

In summary, it may be said that epidemiology, as a science, got a halting start in America and did not get into its stride until after World War I. Chapin's productive studies in Providence, relating to the epidemiology of communicable diseases of childhood, and the work of Lumsden, Frost, Rosenau, and Carter of the United States Public Health Service stand out as oases in a great desert of unproductive efforts. Stiles of the Department of Agriculture did a fine job in his observations on the natural history of hookworm disease, and Ricketts made his brilliant studies on Rocky Mountain spotted fever and typhus fever during the early part of the century. (He died of typhus in 1910.) But by and large, it is only fair to say that most of the productive work in American epidemiology did not get under way until after the era covered by this book had come to an end.

The reader who has a special interest in epidemiology is referred to *The History of American Epidemiology,* edited by Franklin H. Top, C. V. Mosby Company, St. Louis, 1952.

AMERICAN CONTRIBUTION TO THE STUDY OF ETIOLOGICAL FACTORS IN CONTAGION

It must be admitted at the outset that American scientists contributed in a very limited degree to the vast accumulation of bacteriological knowledge that was acquired during the period from 1860 to 1900. Pasteur in 1862 published the results of his critical

25 Park, W. H., and Beebe, A. L.: *M. Rec.* 46:385, 1894.

26 Rosenau, M. J.; Lumsden, L. L.; and Karth, J. H.: *Hygienic Laboratory Bull.,* p. 52, 1909.

27 Soper, George A.: *J.A.M.A.,* 48:2019, 1907.

experiments which terminated the doctrine of spontaneous generation; but Doull has selected the date of initiation of the "Bacteriological Era" as 1876, when Koch demonstrated the essential
role of the anthrax bacillus as a cause of disease. Koch was a pupil
of Henle. He earned his living as a district physician, but somehow
he found the time to carry out his laboratory experiments and to
launch himself on a career in bacteriology. He demonstrated his
results to Conheim in Breslau in 1876, and this great pathologist
recognized at once the importance of Koch's work.

William H. Welch, a young American physician, was a student
in Conheim's laboratory when Koch made his demonstration, and
thus he was precipitated into the very center of this newborn science
of bacteriology. While in Breslau, Welch learned the techniques
of bacterial staining from Weigert, but he did not remain in Germany long enough to absorb much bacteriological knowledge. From
Breslau he hurried to Vienna "where he might more effectively prepare himself for the practice of medicine." Welch's father was a Connecticut physician who wanted his son to practice with him. It was
the fashion of the time for young American physicians to take "graduate courses" of lectures in Munich or Vienna for a three to six
months' period and then to return to the United States as German-
or Austrian-trained specialists. Father Welch felt that it was foolish
for his son to give time to scientific matters "that were visionary
and of no practical importance in the practice of medicine."

Young Welch wanted to be a pathologist and not a practitioner.
Thus on his return from Europe he postponed his entrance into
private practice with his father. Instead he organized a small laboratory at Bellevue Hospital in New York City, and for six years he
taught pathology there. During this period he did no bacteriology,
but he did keep in touch with his German friends who were advancing this science. He was next appointed as pathologist to the new
Johns Hopkins Hospital and Medical School in Baltimore. Before
taking up his task there, he returned to Europe for a short period.
Apparently he was not aware of the importance of Pasteur's work,
for he wrote to his family that he would not stop in Paris "since
there is nothing special of scientific nature to lead me there."[28]
This was in 1884, when Pasteur was just completing his epoch-
making studies on rabies. (Flexner has suggested that Welch may
have been influenced by his German teachers, who underestimated

[28] Flexner, S., and Flexner, J. T.: *Life of William H. Welch.* Viking Press, Inc., New
York, 1941, p. 177.

the importance of Pasteur's work.) So Welch went straight to Germany and took some work under Koch. On his return to Johns Hopkins, he became the leading American scientist in the study and teaching of bacteriology.

We have given this story in some detail, since Welch was one of the great American physicians of his period, and one of the very few Americans who contributed to the field of bacteriology during the entire nineteenth century. The reasons why American scientists did not cultivate this fertile field are quite clear. We had not yet reached the stage of cultural development which provided an opportunity for young men to pursue medical science as a career. Welch, on his return from Germany in 1884, noted that

I was often asked how it is that no scientific work is done in medicine in America. How is it that so many good young men who do well in Germany and show evident talent there are never heard of and never do any good work when they return to their home land? The answer is that there is no opportunity for, no appreciation of, no demand for that type of work here. On the other hand, in Germany every encouragement is held out to the young men with talent for service.[29]

Thus it is that we look in vain for the names of Americans in the long list of contributors to the major discoveries in bacteriology during the great bacteriological era.

Sternberg[30] had discovered the *Micrococcus lanceolatus,* i.e., the pneumococcus, in 1880 by means of inoculating rabbits with his own saliva. Almost simultaneously Pasteur discovered the same organism by inoculating rabbits with the saliva of a child who had died of rabies. Theobald Smith[31] discovered the cause of cattle tick fever, *Piroplasma bigeminum,* in 1889, and this same scientist[32] in 1896 differentiated bovine from human tuberculosis. Welch and Nuttall[33] described the gas bacillus, *Clostridium welchii,* in 1892, and Flexner[34] identified an important cause of bacillary dysentery in 1900. Stiles in 1902 recognized a new species of hookworm which infected the children of our southern states, and demonstrated the great importance of this disease in America. In 1900 Reed and his co-workers determined that the transmission of yellow fever occurs through the bite of an infected Aëdes mosquito.

[29] *Ibid.,* p. 122.
[30] Sternberg, G.: *Nat. Board Health Bull.,* 1:781, 1881.
[31] Smith, Theobald: *M. News,* 50:689, 1889.
[32] Smith, Theobald: *Tr. Am. Physicians,* 11:75, 1896.
[33] Welch, W. H., and Nuttall, G. H. F.: *Bull. Johns Hopkins Hosp.,* 3:81, 1892.
[34] Flexner, S.: *Philadelphia M. J.,* 6:414, 1900.

These contributions were all very important, but they were carried out by a mere handful of young scientists who were working in the Medical Corps of the Army, the United States Department of Agriculture, or the Johns Hopkins Medical School. There was little interest in these matters on the part of medical educators throughout the land. Furthermore, sanitarians did not appreciate the fact that the new science of bacteriology had any direct bearing on preventive medicine or upon the promotion of the public health. Welch, in his lecture on "Public Health in Theory and Practice," has brought out this fact very effectively.

There is some food for thought in the fact that, while a surgeon, Lister, immortalized his name by applying Pasteur's discoveries to the prevention of accidental surgical infections, even before the actual agents of these infections had been recognized, not only did no sanitarian thus early see the bearing of these discoveries upon his field of disease prevention, but the official opinion, as expressed by sanitary authorities at that time, was definitely hostile to the germ theory of disease.

I attach, however, no great importance to this circumstance, for it is not clear what practical use sanitarians would have made of this theory with the knowledge existing at that time. Hypotheses born before their time are often sterile. They must have some relation to the state of knowledge existing at the time, and history affords many instances of the useful purpose served for a time by inadequate and even erroneous theories.

It is doubtful whether any more useful working hypothesis concerning the sources of epidemics could have been framed in 1848 than that which guided most of the sanitary activities at that period and for many subsequent years, erroneous as it was and tenaciously as it was held after it had served its primary purpose. This doctrine, as is well known, was the so-called filth theory of the generation of epidemic diseases, particularly of typhus, typhoid, dysentery, and cholera, which were the most serious scourges to combat.

The acceptance of this theory led to a campaign for the supply of pure water, the proper disposal of sewage and prevention of water pollution, the removal of nuisances, the cleanliness of streets, the inspection of food, the healthfulness of dwellings, ventilation, provision for burial of the dead without injury to the living, in a word, for "general cleaning up." Thus were laid the essential foundations of modern sanitation of the environment, and much of the routine technique of the present-day health officer, particularly of sanitary inspectors, was established in this early period.[35]

[35] Welch, William H.: *Second Sedgwick Memorial Lecture.* Yale University Press, New Haven, 1925, pp. 26-28.

The author of this text has demonstrated that the period of great epidemics in America came to an end before the full development of the bacteriological era.[36] This fact is illustrated by a graph (Figure 32) of the crude death rate of New Orleans from 1820 to 1900. This graph proposes the theory that an attainable base line for deaths in a community is approximately 10 per 1,000 per annum, if reason-

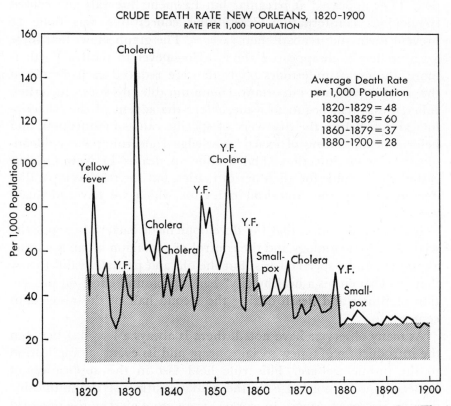

Fig. 32. New Orleans crude death rate, 1820-1900. (From Smillie, W. G.: "The Period of Great Epidemics in the United States," *The History of American Epidemiology.* Ed. by F. H. Top. Copyright 1952 by the C. V. Mosby Co., St. Louis.)

ably adequate general sanitary conditions are provided. This rate was, in fact, the approximate crude death rate in New Orleans in 1950. All deaths above this base line are "excess deaths." The shaded areas of the graph represent the "normal death rate" for each epoch and these areas are made up in great part of the "undertones

[36] Smillie, W. G.: "The Period of Great Epidemics," *The History of American Epidemiology.* C. V. Mosby Co., St. Louis, 1952, p. 52.

of death," e.g., tuberculosis, infantile diarrhea, communicable diseases of childhood, erysipelas, tetanus, typhoid fever, puerperal sepsis, and the like. These diseases were accepted by the people as inevitable, and thus deaths from these causes were to be expected and were considered a normal course of events.

The great epidemics were due to cholera, yellow fever, and smallpox. They appeared at irregular but frequent intervals and caused tremendous consternation. Everything conceivable was done to prevent them and to abate their ravages. The graph shows that these great epidemics disappeared about 1880—never to return. Furthermore, the great undertones of death were reduced each decade of the century. Many important communicable diseases, including tuberculosis, had begun to wane *before* the advent of the bacteriological era, before the discovery of specific causes of infection, and before the unfolding of exact knowledge concerning the epidemiology of acute infection. The decline in deaths in New Orleans is the most graphic for all American cities, but the story is a parallel one in each of the American cities for which we have adequate records.

It is true, of course, that the development of bacteriology put the science of epidemiology and the control of contagion on an accurate, a rational, and a specific basis; but the old and partially valid theory that "a clean city is a healthy city" had a profound effect on prevention of illness and death during the second half of the nineteenth century.

As many observers have noted, there is always a long lag between the introduction of a new social concept and its eventual application to the public welfare. This rule held fast in the application of bacteriological knowledge to the actual control of communicable disease. However, American workers were more alert in the practical application of bacteriology than were their European fellows. American scientists did not discover new etiological factors in disease nor did they develop the concepts of immunology, but one public health technique, namely, the public health diagnostic laboratory, was initiated in the United States and this achievement is worthy of a detailed description.

The Public Health Diagnostic Laboratory

In 1888 the first municipal public health laboratory was established in Providence, Rhode Island, by Dr. Charles Chapin. The director of this laboratory was Dr. G. T. Schwartz. Its primary purpose was the analysis of water and food. That same year, Dr. Victor Vaughan established the Michigan State Hygiene Laboratory for water and food analysis. Dr. George M. Sternberg opened the first privately endowed bacteriological laboratory—the Hoagland Laboratory—in Brooklyn that same year. It is worth noting also that Sternberg employed this laboratory in the teaching of bacteriology at the Long Island Medical College. Each of these three laboratories is still functioning after more than sixty-five years.

The New York City Bacteriological Diagnostic Laboratory was opened in 1892. The story of this very important public health innovation must begin with a brief account of the life of Dr. Hermann M. Biggs.[37]

Hermann M. Biggs was born in the small village of Trumansburg, New York, September 29, 1859. He received his A.B. from Cornell in 1882. He wrote, for a baccalaureate thesis, "Sanitary Regulations and the Duty of the States in Regard to Public Hygiene." For this thesis he demonstrated a fine grasp of the whole philosophy of the responsibility of government in protection of the health of its people; and, although he did not realize it at the time, he had determined his career through the formulation of this thesis, and had constructed the platform that was to become the basis of his life work. During the coming generation Cornell was to train no more valuable man, for the villager from upper New York was to shape the destinies and to promote the health and welfare of uncounted numbers of persons from his own state and from the nation at large.

Dr. Biggs finished his training at Bellevue just at the dawn of the new era in bacteriology and sanitary science. In 1885 he was placed in charge of the bacteriological work at the Carnegie Laboratory. His first job was the study, with Taylor, of a dramatic typhoid epidemic—water-borne—at Plymouth, Pennsylvania (see page 350). The source of this infection was found and the description of the epidemiology of this disaster is now a classic. Biggs was appointed to teach bacteriology at Bellevue, and in 1888 he was made consulting pathologist of the New York City Health Department. As a result of Biggs's activities at Bellevue, he became interested in the bacteriological diagnosis of communicable disease and this interest

[37] For the complete story see *The Life of Hermann M. Biggs* by C.-E. A. Winslow, published by Lea & Febiger, Philadelphia, 1929.

led directly to the formation of a diagnostic bacteriological laboratory.

The New York City Public Health Laboratory

In 1892 New York City was faced with the threat of an epidemic of cholera. In August of that year, Hamburg, Germany, had its first case of cholera and soon an epidemic was raging in that city. Many ships passed continually between the two ports, Hamburg and New York, and the danger of importation of cholera into the latter city was imminent. An advisory committee on cholera, of which Dr. Biggs was made a member, was appointed by the New York City Chamber of Commerce. Dr. J. D. Bryant, then commissioner of health, followed up this move with the establishment of a division of bacteriology and disinfection, and appointed Dr. Biggs chief inspector of this division. A small two-room diagnostic laboratory was opened near the Health Department offices. There were no trained bacteriologists, so a "well-educated chemist" was employed to begin the service. Biggs, who had had bacteriological training, supervised the work and organized the disinfection service. Cholera arrived from Europe on board the "Moravia" on August 31. This vessel was followed in rapid succession by numerous infected ships that had suffered deaths from cholera en route. The barrier that was erected against the disease was effective, for only ten cases of cholera developed in residents of New York City with eight deaths. There were no secondary cases.

The diphtheria diagnostic service of the laboratory was not begun until May 4, 1893, when Dr. W. H. Park entered the laboratory. This story was told to me by Dr. Park in 1937 shortly before his death, and I shall present this interview in full.

Doctors Janeway, Biggs, and Prudden were the Advisory Health Board of the city (New York) in 1891. Dr. Prudden was pathologist in charge of the Pathological Laboratory of Physicians and Surgeons. He became very much interested in the etiology of diphtheria because of the diphtheria epidemic at the Foundling Hospital in 1891 and 1892. Dr. Biggs was pathologist for the city and also Bellevue Hospital. Dr. Dunham did the first diagnostic bacteriological laboratory work for the city. He worked on an outbreak of cholera, the work being done in the pathology laboratory at Bellevue beginning in 1892. Dr. Biggs and Dr. Prudden were great friends and had the confidence of Dr. Bryant, who was Commissioner of Health and also professor of surgery at Bellevue. In 1893

Dr. Biggs opened a small diagnostic laboratory for the city on Mott Street. He rented two rooms in a tenement and fixed them up as a laboratory.

I had returned from a year's study in Europe, where I had gone to specialize in diseases of the nose and throat. I had made no bacteriological

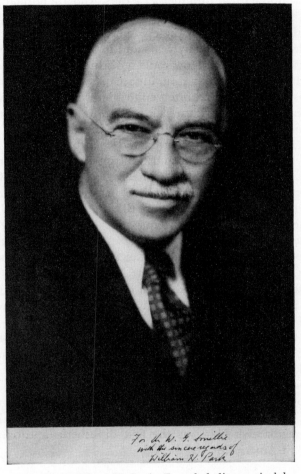

Fig. 33. William H. Park. Founded diagnostic laboratory service.

studies in Europe. Dr. Biggs asked me, as a throat specialist, to see a child at the Foundling Hospital with unquestioned diphtheria, but in whose throat no diphtheria bacilli had been found. I showed him that the case was one of laryngeal diphtheria without the presence of diphtheria bacilli in the nasopharynx. Dr. Biggs was impressed with my understanding of the situation and asked me to take charge of the new City Diagnostic Laboratory when it opened on Mott Street.

Within two years we published the "Report on 5,611 Cases of Suspected Diphtheria."[38] In this report we not only proved the value of the laboratory in the differential diagnosis of diphtheria, but also established the most important fact that diphtheria carriers, who are normal people, with no illness, may be an important source of infection. This phenomenon of the carrier state explained the epidemiological discrepancies that had puzzled physicians for so many years and in so many different diseases.

The question had been: How could a disease be due to a specific agent, transferred from person to person, in face of the well-established fact that isolated cases of disease and often epidemics were initiated without even possible remote contact with a sick person? It was now clear that these puzzling outbreaks were started by normal, healthy carriers.

In 1894 Dr. Hermann Biggs, who was then bacteriologist of the New York City Health Department and director of the infant bacteriological laboratory, was in Europe, where he heard the address of Roux and Behring on the use of antitoxin in the cure of diphtheria. He was so impressed that he cabled me to start the production of diphtheria antitoxin immediately. I and my assistants appealed to the *New York Herald,* and it raised a fund of $8,000. Sixty horses were purchased, and the production of diphtheria antitoxin was begun on a substantial scale in January, 1895. We then asked the New York City Board of Health to appropriate funds for the production of antitoxin. After a great deal of difficulty, $27,000 was secured from the city, and the New York City Serological Laboratory was fully launched.

Late in October, 1894, Dr. Biggs returned from Europe with a small amount of the precious antitoxin. Soon afterward an epidemic of diphtheria broke out in the New York Infant Asylum. I asked Dr. Biggs if he would be willing to spare enough of the antitoxin to give an immunizing injection of 300 units to every child in the institution. He gave me half his supply, and I injected the antitoxin and stopped the epidemic in the asylum immediately. This was the first diphtheria antitoxin to be administered in America.[39]

Other official public health laboratories followed rapidly after the establishment of the New York City Laboratory. Henry P. Walcott, health commissioner of Massachusetts, read Emil Roux's paper on

[38] Park, W. H., and Beebe, A. L.: *New York City Department of Health Scientific Bull.,* No. 1, 1895.

[39] During my interview with Dr. Park, I told him that I hoped to write a history of public health in America. I asked him, on the basis of his more than fifty years of experience, who were the men who had contributed most to the development of the public health in America. He answered without hesitation, "I consider that the great leaders in public health of this nation have been, in order of relative importance, Sedgwick, Welch, Biggs, and Vaughan."

the preventive and therapeutic value of diphtheria antitoxin which was delivered at the International Congress of Hygiene in Budapest in 1894. Dr. Walcott realized the importance of this report and organized a state laboratory for the production of antitoxin in the State House of Massachusetts in November of that same year. This laboratory was under the direction of Dr. J. L. Goodale. In 1896 Theobald Smith came to Boston to assume charge of the antitoxin laboratory and also to become professor of comparative pathology at Harvard. The laboratory was developed to provide to the citizens of the state "free [diphtheria] antitoxins and vaccine lymph."[40]

Philadelphia established a laboratory for the diagnosis, study, and control of diphtheria under the direction of Dr. B. M. Bolton on May 20, 1895.[41] Within a few years each large city and practically each state in the Union had established a diagnostic bacteriological laboratory. Most of the states also provided free biological products to practicing physicians and to health officers for the control of communicable disease. The enormous value of this community service was emphasized by Welch in his Sedgwick Memorial Lecture in 1924.

The two great sanitary contributions of America are:

1. The studies of the fundamental problems of water supply and sewage disposal from the Lawrence Experiment Station.
2. The concept of Biggs that the public health diagnostic laboratory is an essential part of governmental health organization.

[40] Cohn, E. J.: "The University and Biologic Laboratories of the State of Massachusetts," *Harvard M. Alumni Bull.*, 1950.

[41] Laird, John L.: "A Brief History of the Philadelphia Division of Laboratories of the Board of Health upon its Fiftieth Anniversary," radio address, May 19, 1945.

CHAPTER 39. *Health Education*

*In the United States, the permanent value and success of any
method or system of sanitary government will depend upon the
degree in which the people are generally enlightened, concerned and made responsible in regard to sanitary duties.*

ELISHA HARRIS, *1873*

Kendall Emerson once said that "the health standard of a nation
is a fair gauge of its intelligence." But it must be remembered that
the people cannot act intelligently on personal or community matters
unless they are well informed. It is true that sound knowledge does
not always result in wise actions; but it is also true that wisdom
without knowledge is a gift of the very few.

Our leaders who developed the social fields of public health and
preventive medicine in America were slow to realize that the very
foundation of public health in a democratic people must be based
on a firm and broad health education policy for all the people.
This fact was not clearly understood until well into the twentieth
century. One reason was, of course, that public health up to that
time had been developed almost exclusively by physicians. It is
quite clear that the physician is not fitted by training, inclination,
or tradition to plan or to carry out a well-directed program of community-wide health education. The most effective health educators
of this nation have been, for the most part, professional educators
with a crusading spirit. The preachers, college professors, and
schoolteachers, the newspaper publishers and journalists, have been
our great health educators. The best examples perhaps are Cotton
Mather, a preacher, and Benjamin Franklin, an editor.

As we trace the great river of health education from 1950, back
through the last century to the rivulets, brooks, springs, and finally
the headwaters, we find two main tributaries: (1) the teaching
of health practices to school children and (2) presentation of health
information to adults.

In a subsequent chapter (see page 429) we shall discuss in some detail the development of the teaching of school hygiene in the public schools. It is very interesting to note that the early teaching —up to about 1900—was concerned solely with personal hygiene. As the years passed, the students were taught the principles of household sanitation, but only recently have the school children been given instruction in the principles of *community* health organization and community-wide health promotion. Furthermore, the pioneers who were responsible for the teaching of the children were not certain who should teach health matters. J. M. Gregory in the December, 1881, issue of the *American Journal of Education* stated that "the omission of hygiene as a study in the common school is a serious defect in popular education. The same criterion holds true with reference to medical colleges." He suggested further that the training of physicians in sanitation would be of advantage so that "they in turn may instruct the school teachers and the people." At the initial meeting of the American Public Health Association, the Hon. Andrew D. White, president of Cornell University, urged that hygiene and sanitation be taught in all departments of public instruction, in colleges, universities, and medical colleges.[1]

Dr. White had the clear idea that the only way to secure good health education of school children was to give sound public health instruction to the teachers in the teacher-training schools. The difficulty here, however, lay in the fact that there was no one available who was qualified to give this sort of instruction. A solution was not found for this problem until well into the twentieth century and then it came from the educators themselves and not from the health officers or the health departments. The whole question of health education of school children will be discussed at length in Chapter 42, "School Health Services."

Presentation of Health Information

The general subject of health information for all the people may be presented under such varied headings as health pamphlets, health conferences, hygiene museums, crusaders in public health education fields, public health reports both monthly and annual, monthly health journals, and so on. All these modern health education techniques were initiated before the beginning of the present century.

[1] White, Andrew D.: "Sanitary Science in its Relations to Public Instruction," *Reports and Papers of the American Public Health Association,* 1:139, 1873.

Health Pamphlets

The small educational pamphlet which is devoted to a special topic of current interest, and which is intended to reach a large number of people who have a limited insight and interest, was first utilized in America as a public health technique during the Civil War. The United States Sanitary Commission prepared a number of fine leaflets, on a variety of subjects, which were used for promoting the health of the soldiers. This procedure was dropped at the end of the war and was not taken up by health departments or by voluntary health associations for many years to come.

Dr. Prudden in 1890 wrote a small, popular, excellent book on *Dust and Its Dangers*.[2] His purpose was to inform "the people, in simple language, [of] the real danger of acquiring serious disease— especially consumption—by means of dust-laden air, and how this danger may be avoided." Later Dr. Prudden wrote two other small, popular books entitled *The Story of Bacteria* and *Drinking Water and Ice Supplies and Their Relation to Health and Disease*, which were published by Putnam and Sons.

Hermann Biggs, who was a close friend and associate of Prudden, adopted Prudden's idea and carried it much further. In 1889, when Biggs was associated with the New York City Department of Health, he had begun an intensive campaign for the control of tuberculosis. With the aid of Prudden and Loomis, he prepared an educational pamphlet which was intended to be a popular treatise on the prevention of consumption.[3] Although long medical terms were employed in this article rather than simple, popular language, it was well received and it paved the way for more effective pamphlets. The idea caught fire, and from that day on, the popular health education leaflet has been widely and effectively used both by official and voluntary health agencies.

Museums of Hygiene

The Hudson Historical Bureau of New York has, in its collection, a steel engraving which depicts a large building on which appears the name, "Museum of Art, Curiosities, and Relics." The caption

[2] Prudden, T. Mitchell: *Dust and Its Dangers*. G. P. Putnam and Sons, New York, 1890.

[3] Biggs, H. M.; Prudden, T. M.; and Loomis, H. P.: "Report on the Prevention of Pulmonary Tuberculosis." See Appendix II, pp. 393-96, in *The Life of Hermann Biggs* by C.-E. A. Winslow. Lea & Febiger, Philadelphia, 1929.

for this engraving reads as follows: "One of the great events during the Civil War was the great Sanitary Fair held at the corner of Montague and Court Streets by the inimitable P. T. Barnum." A large number of people, particularly women, are seen flocking to this fair. This was in all probability a continuation of the sanitary fairs that were started in Chicago in October, 1863, by Mary Livermore for the purpose of promoting the health of sick Union soldiers.

National Hygiene Museums

Our first intimation of a national museum of hygiene comes from the *Reports of the Annual Meeting of the American Public Health Association* in New Orleans in 1880. Dr. J. N. McCormack introduced a resolution that a committee of five be appointed to consider the advisability of establishing a national museum of hygiene. As a final result of this action a National Museum of Hygiene was established in Washington in 1882 in the Bureau of Medicine of the Navy Department.[4] Surgeon General P. S. Wales signed the order and Congress made a preliminary grant of $7,000 for its housing and staff. The purpose of this museum was to exhibit the history and progress of sanitary science by a collection of publications, models, drawings, and the like, illustrating defects and improvements in food and water supplies, house and hospital construction, heating, illumination, removal of excreta and refuse, for physical culture and "whatever else tends to the preservation of health and prevention of disease."[5]

The Museum Committee of the American Public Health Association presented a report at the annual meeting in 1882 and at each of the annual meetings for several years thereafter. The committee then expired; apparently the museum expired also. It is an interesting observation that the permanent public health museum has never secured an outstanding place in America as a broad health education measure. This is true down to the present time. The Health Museum at Cleveland under Dr. Gerhart's direction has been the chief exception to this rule.

Crusaders in the Public Health Education Field

The initial stage of any social upsurge of a people is marked by the emergence of crusaders, whose work is a religion. These people

---

[4] *Sanitarian*, edited by A. N. Bell, **10**:192, 1882.
[5] *Reports and Papers of the American Public Health Association*, **8**:327, 1882.

are generally considered by their fellows to be fanatics. They are admired by a few and shunned by most. The health education field in America has been enriched by the unselfish, devoted efforts of these most impractical people. We have already described, in some detail, the achievements of one of the greatest of the health educators of America, namely, Dorothea Dix. Her monumental public health achievement was Document 150 of the Thirtieth National Congress of 1849, which provides for a grant of 5,000,000 acres of national land to be set aside for the relief and support of the indigent curable and incurable insane in the United States. This land grant was to be appropriated in such a manner "as shall be of greatest benefit to all who are in circumstances of extreme necessity and who through the providence of God are wards of the nation." This revolutionary bill, which set a precedent in federal aid to the states for medical care, when finally passed by Congress in 1854 but vetoed by President Pierce, provided for 12,225,000 acres.

Another great public health crusader was Edward Jarvis of Concord, Massachusetts (1804-1885). He began his medical practice in Northfield, Massachusetts, but soon developed a great distrust in the therapeutics of his day, and in 1836 gave up his practice because of "medical doubts." He was a friend of Lemuel Shattuck and one of the few medical supporters of Shattuck's work. Jarvis was largely responsible for bridging the gap between 1850, when Shattuck's report was buried in the archives, and 1869, when his theories were finally put into actual practice in the Massachusetts State Department of Health. Jarvis was one of our pioneer statisticians, and the great event of his life was the International Statistical Congress in London in 1860, where he was chosen vice-president. He was a pioneer in the preparation of articles on public health subjects for current journals. His series of three papers on "The Increase of Human Life"[6] in the *Atlantic Monthly* in 1869 were excellent contributions to health education.

The German scientist, Max Pettenkofer, was a man of independent thought and action. He delivered two popular lectures on "The Value of Health to a City"[7] in Munich in 1873. He was a great leader of his day in the field of medical science and thus, through these popular lectures, he set a precedent for distinguished medical

[6] Jarvis, Edward: "The Increase of Human Life," *Atlantic Monthly*, 24:495, 581, 711, 1869. In this same volume is an article on "Inebriates Harbored and Helped," written by an anonymous inmate of the New York State Asylum for the Insane.

[7] *Sanitarian*, 3:248, 1875, and 4:17, 1876.

authorities to come down off their isolated pedestals and talk to the common people in simple language. In 1875 in New York, Jerome Walker wrote a series of popular articles on "Defective Nutrition of Children" which appeared in the *Sanitarian*.[8] But health officials were slow in following these precedents.

The men who organized the American Public Health Association were really public health crusaders, but they had no comprehension of the important place of popular education in public health promotion. It was for this lack of resourcefulness chiefly that the National Board of Health languished and died in 1884. The leaders made an important mistake when they failed to carry the battle for its support to the public at large. It was not until the arrival of Biggs on the horizon of the public health field in 1889 that the modern procedures of public health education were born, for Biggs was, above everything else, a social health educator as well as a great administrator.

There were two great crusaders in the field of public health education, both philanthropic laymen, who deserve special acclaim. The first was Jacob Riis, who came up out of the lower East Side slums of New York to become a potent force in improving the housing conditions of the poor. The second man, Nathan Strauss, is best known for the establishment of milk stations for the babies of the poor. These two men were masters of the techniques of popular health education, and they demonstrated to public health officers that the most effective way to secure advances in community health is to win popular support for these measures by aggressive, businesslike "advertising."

Public Health Reports

One of the very best of all health education methods is the annual report of an official or voluntary health organization. Massachusetts began in 1869 to publish an annual report of the work of the State Health Department, and from the first these reports have been of great educational value. The reports of the annual session of the American Public Health Association have been published continuously since 1873. They are a veritable mine of public health information.[9]

8 *Sanitarian*, 3:108, 172, 205, 1875.

9 Publications of the American Public Health Association: The American Public Health Association published its transactions of meetings in an annual report from 1872 to 1895. The *Journal of the American Public Health Association* began in 1895

Dr. John Woodworth made his first report of the Marine Hospital Service in 1873. These reports were published continuously thereafter for many years, but they contained little public health information. In the later years the *Public Health Reports* of the United States Public Health Service have become one of the most important health educational forces in the nation.

Monthly Health Journals

The annual report of a health organization is a trustee's report, which is intended for a special, discriminating, and interested audience. A much more popular health education tool is the monthly periodical. The monthly health journal put in its appearance in America early in the nineteenth century with the publication of *The Journal of Health*[10] in 1830. It was devoted to discussions of personal hygiene and its motto was, "Health—the poor man's riches, the rich man's bliss." This journal terminated after four volumes because the subscribers "failed to pay their arrearages." *Hall's Journal of Health*[11] was founded in 1854. This lively little journal was concerned for the most part with matters of personal, and to some degree, environmental hygiene.

The *Sanitarian*,[12] a monthly journal which was founded in 1873, was the first real public health journal in America. It had a distinguished group of contributors and has given us a broad yet concise picture of the advances in public health of the nation throughout the formative years. This journal was concerned chiefly with environmental sanitation and it published almost nothing on bacteriology or epidemiology. There were a few discussions on the subjects of child hygiene and nutrition, and there were also a few records of current vital statistics. Dr. A. N. Bell, the editor, lived up to his in-

---

and was published for three years. The association then returned to the annual volume from 1899 to 1908 except for three volumes—two in 1905 and one in 1906. Papers of the Laboratory Section were published in the *Journal of Infectious Diseases*. Beginning in 1908 with Vol. 34, the *American Journal of Public Hygiene* became the official organ of the American Public Health Association. The name was changed to the *Journal of the American Public Health Association* in 1911. See Ravenel, M. P.: "The American Public Health Association, Past, Present, Future," *A Half Century of Public Health*. American Public Health Association, New York, 1921, p. 20.

[10] *Journal of Health,* conducted by an association of physicians, Vol. I. Published in Philadelphia, 1830.

[11] *Hall's Journal of Health,* edited by Dr. W. N. Hall, Vol. I. Published by Henry B. Price, New York, 1854.

[12] *Sanitarian,* edited by A. N. Bell, M.D., Vol. 1. Barnes & Co., New York, 1873.

itial purpose, which he had set forth in the beginning of the first volume as follows:

. . . so to present the results of the various inquiries which have been, and which may hereafter be, made for the preservation of health and the expectations of human life, as to make them most advantageous to the public and to the medical profession.

This monthly journal, which was continued until 1883, was highly successful.

A very interesting official monthly health education journal was initiated by the New Hampshire State Health Department in 1889 by Dr. Irving Watson.[13] He was one of the first to realize the importance of popular health education as a state health department function.

Health Conventions

The very earliest report of the proceedings of a health convention that we have encountered was that of the Second American Health Convention which was held in New York City in 1839.[14] This convention was attended by men from all the New England states, as well as from New Jersey, Pennsylvania, Ohio, Virginia, and by two delegates from the West Indies. The list of names of those registered included over 100 persons, only two or three of whom were physicians. Many of them apparently were ministers.

The statement was made at this convention that the first health convention had been held in Boston the previous year. A Mr. Amasa Walker, vice-president, reported: "It [the convention in Boston the year before] passed off very pleasantly; but what did the Press do about it? Why with few exceptions, the subject was turned into ridicule; but 'bran bread and sawdust pudding' was all their argument."

This second convention was held to discuss the value and importance of the vegetarian diet. The leader was Mr. Graham, and his followers were called Grahamites. They believed that individuals should abstain from "flesh-meat," tea, coffee, and other stimulants, and they recommended the use of whole wheat flour. Thus this flour came to be called "Graham flour."

[13] *Sanitary Volunteer,* edited by Irving A. Watson, Vol. 1, 1889.
[14] *A Report of the Proceedings of the Second American Health Convention;* held in the tabernacle of the Presbyterian Church on Broadway, New York, on the afternoon of Wednesday, May 8, 1839.

The convention was opposed by physicians generally, and one of the doctors who attended is stated to have walked out in disgust. It is apparent from the report of the discussions that many of the members of the group were considered to be fanatics. Simultaneously with this convention another meeting was being held in New York by a group interested in antislavery. Evidently some of the registrants came to New York to attend both meetings. Again it is obvious from the discussions that the members of the antislavery group also were widely regarded as fanatics.

The arguments and statements by various persons who contributed to the program were rather naive, showed little basic physiological knowledge, and were quite religious in tone. There was a great deal of discussion as to whether the Russians, Laplanders, Swedes, and Prussians, who are supposed to eat a great deal of meat, live longer than the Hindustanis, who are vegetarians. Mr. Graham was not willing to concede that North Europeans ate meat to excess. Apparently there was no third annual meeting.

Voluntary Health Organizations

The voluntary health organization, which has played such a tremendous part in the promotion of public health in America, has health education as its essential function and basic purpose. A discussion of the role of these various agencies in the promotion of health in the United States will be the subject of another chapter (No. 45). Suffice it to say at this point that health education as a public health measure has been developed most extensively and effectually by the national voluntary health organizations of America. It has been their major contribution to the field of health promotion.

CHAPTER 40. *Public Health Nursing*[1]

The disease may often be cured by the nurse, but seldom by the physician.

WILLIAM BUCHAN, *1842*

Nursing of the sick in their homes by the neighbors was an essential feature of the mores of our American pioneers. A residual of this tradition is still encountered in certain sections of our rural South, where even today, in the event of serious illness, the neighbors, in whole families, flock to the afflicted home; the women to cook, to do the housework, and assist in the nursing, the men to hang around the barn and discuss farming and politics, the children to play noisily about the yard. Many pioneer women developed a talent for home care of the sick, and some of them made a true profession of nursing—particularly nursing at time of childbirth.

Nurses were required in the hospitals that were first established in America during the latter part of the eighteenth century, but they were recruited from the servant classes and had no special training for their work. They were poorly paid and were often drunken and disreputable. In 1798 Dr. Valentine Seaman[2] organized the first formal training course for nurses at the New York Hospital. This course consisted of twenty-four lectures on anatomy, physiology, care of children, and so on. It was a most elementary form of instruction, but it was at least a beginning and is an important milestone in adequate medical care in America.

[1] Miss Dock has written so extensively and brilliantly on the history of public health nursing that the author feels quite inadequate in presenting this brief summary. He suggests that interested readers turn to the original publications for more comprehensive information:

Dock, Lavinia L.: *A History of Nursing*, 4 vols. G. P. Putnam and Sons, New York, 1907.

————: "The History of Public Health Nursing," *A Half Century of Public Health*. American Public Health Association, New York, 1921, pp. 439-52.

[2] Dock, Lavinia L.: *A History of Nursing*, Vol. II, p. 339.

Charleston, South Carolina, must be given due credit for establishing the first visiting nurse service in America. In 1813 the Ladies' Benevolent Society of that city organized a nursing service for the sick poor. A severe epidemic of yellow fever had devastated the community, and a group of charitably minded ladies assumed the task of providing for home nursing care of the victims. This is the first instance that we have encountered of a benevolent nursing service that was provided to the poor under the auspices of a community agency.

In 1836 Pastor Fliedner and his wife established at Kaiserswerth on the Rhine[3] the system of nursing care in voluntary hospitals which became the forerunner of the present system of nurses' training schools in our modern hospitals. This organization was also a precursor of our present district nursing system, for the ladies provided home nursing care as well as hospital nursing care. The nurses were selected for their piety, industry, and intelligence, and became deaconesses in the church. They made nursing a life career. Miss Dock says, "the Kaiserswerth deaconess was not intended to be a narrow specialist, but was to be prepared for every kind of service that might be needed. She was instructed in nursing, teaching, the management of children and convalescents (this included occupational therapy and organized play and recreation) parish visiting, and religious theory so that she might read and interpret the Scriptures, pray and instruct." In 1849 Pastor Fliedner came to Pittsburgh, bringing with him four of the German deaconesses in an attempt to implant in America a training school for nurses after the Kaiserswerth pattern. The seed that was sown did not flourish.

The Kaiserswerth nursing plan differed from Miss Nightingale's system of bedside nursing in that religious dedication and self-sacrifice were the primary motives of the deaconesses, whereas Miss Nightingale visualized nursing as a profession. It is for this reason that the Nightingale system is practically always referred to as the real initiation of our modern system of nursing education and the establishment of nursing as a professional career.

In 1839 a Nurses' Society of Philadelphia was organized, following an urgent appeal from Dr. Joseph Warrington.[4] Its purpose was to

[3] Waters, Ysabella: "The Rise, Progress, and Extent of Visiting Nursing in the United States," *Charities and the Commons,* 16:17, 1906. This issue was devoted to public health nursing.

[4] Dock, Lavinia L.: *A History of Nursing,* Vol. I, p. 345.

train "pious and prudent" women who would then be paid by the society to give nursing care to the sick poor, particularly in childbirth. Dr. Warrington gave the medical training, and the nurses were supervised by a "lady visitor." By 1850 the society had employed more than fifty nurses, and a "Home" for these nurses had been established where the "pupil nurses" were taught cooking and housekeeping and were given nursing instruction by a physician. A certificate was presented to nurses who completed this course.

The next development in home nursing occurred in 1854. Miss Genevieve Anderson of California has discovered an event in nursing history which has long been forgotten.[5] The Epidemiological Society of London, which was founded in 1850, was the first to promote the concept of a public health nurse. In 1854 the society appointed a committee "for the purpose of determining the feasibility of a plan to secure throughout the country a staff of nurses available for the labouring population when attacked by epidemic disorders, such as fever, cholera, or the like, when at any time overtaken by sickness or during the period of childbirth."[6]

This committee was formed because of a proposal which was submitted to the society by one of its founders, Dr. E. H. Sieveking. This proposal was that suitable inmates of England's workhouses be trained in nursing so that they could go into the community and do nursing among the poor. The plan provided for training of nurses by physicians with subsequent medical supervision of the nurses. There also would be a lay group of advisers. The nurse should be one from the lower class of society, since she would function more satisfactorily as an integral part of the family unit. Furthermore, the plan would stimulate the morale of the trainee from the workhouse and eventually might make her independent. If successful, the plan might encourage respectable women outside the workhouse to enter nursing and thus increase the number of nurses available to all classes of society.

The committee presented the matter to the English Poor Law Board. This resolution stated in part that

. . . if it were possible to provide a staff of nurses easily available throughout the country, and at given points, a material benefit would accrue, perceptible not only by the shorter duration of disease, and the con-

---

[5] Anderson, Genevieve: "An Oversight in Nursing History," *J. Hist. Med.* 3:417, Summer, 1948.
[6] *Ibid.*, p. 417.

sequent diminution of mortality and pauperism among the labouring
classes, but also by the more complete and more speedy arrest of contagious disorders which spread to all classes, and by the diminution of
poor—and country-rates, which are, in a great measure, levied to provide
against direct or indirect effects of suffering preventable by the assistance
contemplated. The committee hold that the sanitary measures which
mark the progress of modern civilization are of vital importance; but
they are also of the opinion that under the most efficient sanitary system,
there will yet always remain a large amount of sickness claiming the aid
of the medical attendant and the nurse.[7]

The Epidemiological Society received little or no encouragement
from the Poor Law Board, so they presented the proposal to the
Medical Relief Committee of the House of Commons, without
avail. Further enlistment of the aid of the Earl of Shaftesbury and
Lord Stanley in a second appeal to the Poor Law Board in 1856
met with further rebuff. The plan failed, but, as Miss Anderson
notes, it did direct the thinking of physicians, and the community
as well, toward the importance and value of trained and supervised
nurses in home care of the sick poor.

In 1862 Florence Nightingale, the patron saint of trained nurses,
aided in the establishment of the first District Nursing Association in
Liverpool, England. The events which led to this important milestone in public health were as follows: Mr. William Rathbone, a
Quaker in Liverpool, England, became interested in the needs of
the poor because of the illness and death of his wife in 1859. His
wife had required prolonged nursing care, and Mr. Rathbone grew
to understand the great value of this service to sick persons. As a
memorial to his wife, he worked out a plan to make nursing care
available to the sick poor in their homes, and with the encouragement and advice of Miss Nightingale, he sent a young woman from
Liverpool to the recently opened Nightingale Training School at
St. Thomas' Hospital in London for training in this new field.
This young woman later returned to take charge of the first nurses'
training school in Liverpool. The school, established through Mr.
Rathbone's efforts, prepared nurses for both hospital and district
nursing. Mr. Rathbone divided the city of Liverpool into eighteen
districts; each district was provided with a nurse and a "lady
visitor." The latter was essentially what we now term a "social
service worker." She gave direct aid, including distribution of
medical supplies and food. Mr. Rathbone himself made rounds to

[7] *Tr. Epidem. Soc.*, 1:10-14, 1855.

homes with the nurses for a year. This effort in district nursing
led directly to reform of the terrible situation in the infirmaries of
the workhouses all over England.

Mr. Rathbone's initial efforts in Liverpool at once attracted the
attention of social leaders in America; but district nursing was not
incorporated in our social structure for years to come, largely because
of the disturbed political conditions of the nation during and after
the war.

The Civil War in America produced an imperative need for
skilled nursing care of the sick and injured soldiers. The need was
met by the organization of the Women's Central Relief Association;
shortly afterward the association became incorporated as an essential
part of the Sanitary Commission. (See page 279.) The commission
turned at once to Miss Nightingale for guidance, and her recent
experiences in the Crimean War proved to be of most timely aid
in the planning of the nursing program for sick and wounded soldiers
in the Civil War. Throughout the war, Miss Nightingale gave valuable suggestions both in the training of nurses and in the outlining
of the functions of nursing in a medical military service.

A serious mistake was made by President Lincoln in the selection
of Dorothea Dix as superintendent of female nurses for the army.
She had great prestige but no training as a nurse. Furthermore, she
was a propagandist and not an administrator. In addition, she was
over sixty years of age and debilitated by tuberculosis as well as
by many previous attacks of malaria (see page 211, Chapter 22,
"Mental Health Promotion"). Miss Dix did not get on well with
the army personnel or with her colleagues. Her standards for the
army nurses were extremely rigid: "No woman under thirty years
need apply to serve in government hospitals. All nurses are required
to be very plain-looking women. Their dresses must be brown or
black with no bows, no curls or jewelry, and no hoopskirts."[8]

Despite these and many other restrictions, a group of able women
served most effectively as nurses during the war. They were not in
any real sense "trained nurses," but were volunteers who were given
a hastily organized short course of intensive training. The nurses
came from all classes of society and included ladies who were
wealthy and socially prominent.[9] The outstanding women to emerge
from the Civil War nursing corps were Mary Livermore, Clara

[8] Civil War recruiting poster for nurses.
[9] Louisa May Alcott, the author of *Little Women,* has written feelingly of her war
nursing experiences.

Barton—who was destined to establish the Red Cross—and Louisa
Lee Schuyler, who later organized the New York State Charities Aid.

A Polish woman physician, Dr. Zakrzewska, in 1862 began the
training of nurses at the New England Hospital for Women in
Boston.[10] During the following ten years she trained some thirty-two
young women in this field. This hospital moved to a new building
in Roxbury in 1872, and here a formal course for the training of

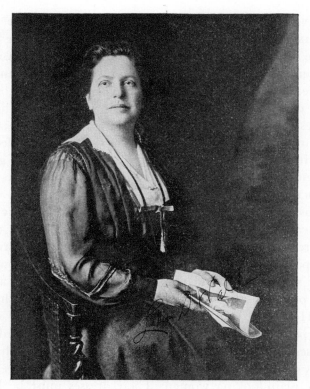

Fig. 34. Lillian Wald. Founded public health nursing in America. (Courtesy of Henry Street Nursing
Service.)

nurses was established. It is generally agreed that the modern school
for trained nurses was initiated with the opening of this school in
Roxbury. Miss Linda Richards was its first graduate.

The American Medical Association appointed a committee on the
training of nurses in 1869, and Dr. Samuel Gross, a very famous
physician, gave the committee's report at the annual meeting of the

[10] Dock, Lavinia L.: *A History of Nursing*, Vol. II, pp. 347-51.

association in New Orleans in that year. Physicians were beginning to be interested officially in the training of nurses as hospital aides.

The next step was the extension of the activities of the trained nurse into the field. In 1877 the New York City Mission, a voluntary philanthropic organization, began the employment of trained nurses for the purpose of giving bedside care to the sick poor in their homes. This action was followed in 1886 by the organization of district nursing associations in Boston and Philadelphia. These philanthropic associations, from the onset, formulated a plan of health instruction as an integral part of home nursing, and thus the modern concept of public health nursing was born. Miss Lillian D. Wald, a young woman of fine family background and good education, was graduated from the Nurses' Training School of the New York Hospital in 1891. Two years later, she and another nurse, Miss Mary Brewster, opened the Henry Street District Nursing Service.[11] From these very simple beginnings, there have developed the splendid concepts and practices of modern public health nursing procedure. The Department of Health gave these young women full encouragement. An official badge was presented to each nurse stating that the Henry Street nurse was sponsored by the Health Department. They were also given authority to vaccinate against smallpox.

Public health nursing now grew rapidly. In 1895 the Procter Marble Company of Procter, Vermont, employed nurses to preserve the health of employees and their families, and in 1897 Wanamaker's Store in Philadelphia initiated an industrial type of nursing service for its employees. Los Angeles in 1898[12] employed a municipal district nurse, whose duty it was to give home nursing care to welfare recipients of the city. Her duties included visits to the public schools. Columbia University established the first collegiate course in nursing in 1899.

In 1902 Miss Wald[13] loaned one of her Henry Street nurses to serve as a school nurse in the New York public school system. It was to be a one month's experiment by one nurse. The name of this nurse was Miss Lina Rogers. Within a short time she was appointed by the Health Department as the first full-time trained school nurse in America. This plan was so successful that twelve more nurses were soon appointed by the commissioner of health to

[11] Wald, Lillian D.: *Windows on Henry Street.* Little, Brown & Co., Boston, 1937.
[12] Waters, Ysabella: *op. cit.,* p. 16.
[13] Wald, Lillian D.: "Development of Public Health Nursing in the United States," *Trained Nurse and Hospital Review,* pp. 689-92, 1893.

serve in the city schools. A few months afterward, Miss Wald loaned a Henry Street nurse to the newly formed Division of Infant Hygiene of the New York City Health Department. This plan also was successful, and the health commissioner began the employment of official public health nurses for the field of infant hygiene.

The New York City Health Department in 1903 initiated instructive home visiting to patients with tuberculosis.[14] Three nurses were appointed at an annual salary of $900 each. During the first year these nurses made 5,028 inspections in homes of persons with tuberculosis. In 1905 this service was increased to fourteen nurses, and these young ladies reported that they made 26,115 home inspections during the year. One can only speculate that the instruction to each patient must have been made by flying leaps from house to house, for each nurse must have averaged 2,000 home visits a year. Since these nurses were appointed to the jurisdiction of the various and separate divisions of the Health Department for special tasks, there developed a system of *specialized nursing* which served a very useful purpose, but which was to cause a great deal of controversy during the years to come. Finally, after many years, the generalized program prevailed over the specialized plan.[15] But that is another story.

It is interesting to note at this point that the first systematic plan of home visits to patients with tuberculosis was organized by William Osler in 1899 when he was professor of medicine at Johns Hopkins Medical College. These visits were not made by trained nurses but by two young women medical students who were assigned by Dr. Osler to give home instruction to tuberculous patients in regard to proper disposal of sputum and other essentials of personal hygiene. The students also gave instruction concerning adequate diet and emphasized the importance of fresh air in the cure of tuberculosis. This is the first instance we have encountered in which the "family health adviser" technique was utilized in the training of medical students.

Public health nursing grew very rapidly from the year 1905 on, and soon was adopted as a community function by local health departments, school boards, state health departments, and eventually by the United States Public Health Service. In 1912 the Na-

[14] Nutting, M. A.: "The Visiting Nurse for Tuberculosis," *Charities and the Commons,* 16:51, 1906.
[15] Dock, Lavinia L.: *A Half Century of Public Health,* pp. 439-52.

tional Organization of Public Health Nursing was formed, and the young and virile profession was established on a solid foundation. The date of birth of public health nursing as a true profession is a little uncertain—probably we should set it at 1886. It came of age in 1912.

CATHOLIC SISTERS OF CHARITY

No review of the history of nursing in America is complete which does not pay suitable tribute to the very important pioneer work of the Catholic Sisters of Charity. These unselfish and devoted women have had a special role in the development of community facilities for medical care throughout the nation. Their primary interest has always been in the considerate care of the destitute, the helpless, and the forgotten. Compassion and complete unselfishness have been the important pillars of their work. Beginning without any funds, often working in an environment of misconception and sometimes hostility, they built slowly but on a firm foundation.

A good illustration of the value of the Catholic order of nurses to the community may be drawn from their pioneer work in Cincinnati, Ohio. This information has been obtained from a book by a Cincinnati physician, Dr. Otto Juettner.[16] The Sisters of Charity first came to this pioneer village on the Mississippi River in 1825. They opened a small school and took six little orphans to live with them. The development of an orphans' home soon became a major responsibility of the Order. This activity grew to include the care and placement of newborn illegitimate children and the rehabilitation of unmarried mothers. The Sisters opened their first hospital in Cincinnati in 1852, the St. John's Hotel for Invalids, with accommodations for twenty patients. It was a tiny place, but it was a good beginning.

During the Civil War the Sisters of Charity served as volunteer nurses for the soldiers who were wounded on the battlefield.

From the group of these heroic women, who worked in the interests of the highest and purest form of humanity, Sister Anthony stands out in bold relief. To the soldiers of both armies her name had a magic ring of wonderful power. To them she was the incarnation of angelic goodness that seemed like a visitation from realms celestial. On the battlefield of Shiloh,

[16] Juettner, Otto: *Daniel Drake and His Followers.* Harvey Publishing Co., Cincinnati, 1909.

amid a veritable ocean of blood, she performed the most revolting duties
to those poor soldiers. Neither the cries of anguish of the dying nor the
unbearable stench from dead bodies could check her in her ministrations.
To the young soldier that lay, fatally wounded, upon that bloody ground
and was thinking of a lone mother at home, Sister Anthony brought the
comfort and peace of a mother's care. In such moments it was the instinct
of the woman in her that enabled her to soothe the aching heart while
relieving the pangs of physical suffering. Then again she stood bravely
and attentively at the side of George Blackman, helping him in his operative work on deck of one of the "floating hospitals" on the Ohio River.
Limbs were quickly amputated and consigned to a watery grave. There
seemed to be no limit to Blackman's endurance. But no matter how hard
the work or how trying the scene, Sister Anthony was always at her post,
her only regret being that she could not do more for her fellowmen, for
her country and for her God.[17]

Following the Civil War in 1866, a wealthy banker in Cincinnati
became interested in the extraordinary work that Sister Anthony
and her associates were doing in the little St. John's Hotel for Invalids. He and his friends raised the funds for the establishment of
the Good Samaritan Hospital and put it in charge of Sister Anthony. One-half the beds were to be reserved for the destitute sick,
preference always being given to women and children. Room must
always be kept for the victims of accidents in shops, on steamboats
and railroads, or from fire or other causes. The nursing care and
the administration of the Good Samaritan Hospital were furnished
by the Sisters. Between the years 1866 and 1891, when the original
hospital was enlarged, over 25,000 patients had received treatment
at the Good Samaritan Hospital. Furthermore, the influence of
the hospital had not only resulted in establishment of other Sister
of Charity hospitals in Cincinnati, but this good example had
spread in ever-widening circles throughout the whole Midwest.

The Sisters of Charity did not, as a rule, develop a program of
public health nursing or home nursing care. Their special health
fields in America have always been hospital administration, hospital nursing care, and the care of orphans, foundlings, cripples,
the destitute, and the abandoned.

[17] Juettner, Otto: *op. cit.,* pp. 418-19.

CHAPTER 41. *Infant Hygiene*

It is not the babies born but those saved that really count.

ANNALS OF THE AMERICAN ACADEMY OF
POLITICAL AND SOCIAL SCIENCE, *1911*

Van Ingen has outlined the chronology of the development of infant hygiene in the United States most succinctly in his contribution to *A Half Century of Public Health*[1] in 1921. In this chronology he has pointed out that in America "the child had hardly been discover'ed before 1872." But there are always pioneers and early discoverers. In 1836 Dr. G. Ackerley wrote a valuable little book called *Management of Children in Sickness and in Health.*[2] He made "careful observation of those measures securing health which clearly fall within the province of the parent to carry into effect . . . omitting long, tedious and unprofitable discussions of the abstrusities of medical science." The book contained excellent suggestions to parents. For example, there was a recommendation for the baby's breakfast of a simple gruel and milk, and a suggestion that the child should not share the family breakfast of "fish, perhaps salted and dried, sausages, hot bread, or buckwheat cakes and hot coffee, such being the diet in general use."

Dr. Ackerley noted that the New York City inspector's report, recently made, gave the following data:

During the past ten years there has been a total of 64,598 interments of children under five years; of these 28,996 were under one year of age. In 1835 alone there were 7,082 deaths in the whole city; over half (3,014) occurred in children under five years of age.[3]

[1] Van Ingen, P.: "The History of Child Welfare Work in the United States," *A Half Century of Public Health*. American Public Health Association, New York, 1921, p. 290.
[2] Ackerley, G.: *Management of Children in Sickness and in Health*. Bancroft & Holley, New York, 1836, 76 pp.
[3] *Ibid.*

New York had a population in 1835 of about 268,000. Thus the death rate for children under five years was higher than the total death rate for all ages in 1935—100 years later.

Van Ingen[4] has told us that a hospital for children was first es-

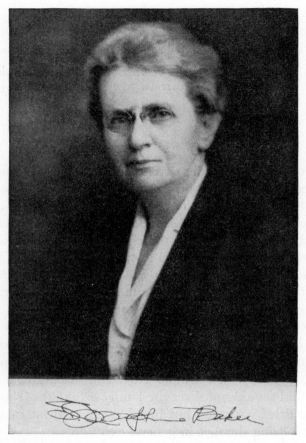

Fig. 35. Josephine Baker. Founded child hygiene in America. (From Baker, S. Josephine: *Fighting for Life*. The Macmillan Co., New York, 1939.)

tablished in Philadelphia in 1855 and that the New York Nursery and Child's Hospital was organized in New York in 1857. Thus pediatrics was definitely initiated in America by the middle of the century.

Teaching of child hygiene to medical students began in 1857.

[4] Van Ingen, P.: *op. cit.*, p. 290.

Dr. Josephine Baker[5] has pointed out that the New York Infirmary Medical College was the first medical college in the United States to establish a chair for the teaching of child hygiene. It also appointed a "sanitary visitor whose duty it was to give simple practical instruction to the poor mothers, on the management of infants and the preservation of the health of their families."

In 1874 the pathetic situation of foundlings was called to public attention by Elisha Harris, who made a report to the Board of Supervisors of Kings County, New York. He stated that in the Infants' Hospital on Randall's Island, New York, in 1868, the mortality of foundlings was 55 per cent. Following better hygienic conditions, this rate was reduced to 36 per cent by 1870. He concluded: "In any alms nursery, if the infant mortality rate exceeds 22 per cent a year there is culpable fault somewhere." He believed that not more than 10 per cent of almshouse children between the ages of one and two should die each year nor more than 3 per cent between the ages of five and ten.[6]

A special committee of the Medical Society of New York State made a report on infant mortality in foundling homes in 1873. Dr. Abraham Jacobi[7] drew up some excellent suggestions for improving the condition of foundlings and abandoned children. He was a great advocate of the utilization of mother's milk. When it was not available he insisted that cow's milk, when fed to infants, should be freshly boiled.

The New York Diet Kitchen began feeding the poor during the great depression that got under way in 1872. As a direct outgrowth of these food stations there developed a new institution in America. When the panic was over in 1878, the food station became a "milk station" for babies and these stations eventually developed into "well baby clinics. This evolution required more than thirty years —as we shall see in our subsequent consideration of these matters.

J. M. Toner in 1873 proposed the adoption of summer camps "for the sick and debilitated children of the poor" as an aid in decreasing the high mortality among children.[8] This idea grew, and in 1875 "fresh air funds" were initiated. Boston people began "country week"—the sending of poor children for a week's outing

[5] Baker, S. Josephine: *Fighting for Life*. The Macmillan Co., New York, 1939, p. 34.
[6] Walker, Jerome: "Causes and Prevention of Infant Mortality," *Reports and Papers of the American Public Health Association*, 15:78-79, 1890.
[7] Jacobi, A.: *Sanitarian*, 1:18, 1873.
[8] *Sanitarian*, 1:71, 1873.

to outlying farm houses in Massachusetts. Seaside excursions for poor children were initiated in 1888. Sarah McNutt, under the auspices of St. John's Guild in New York, hired a barge and fitted it up as a "summer sanitarium" for sick babies. That first year, "of 79 babies under 1 year of age that were admitted, 22 died." Thus the idea of the *floating hospital* was initiated. In *A Handbook for Physicians and Parents,* published in 1952, we find the following account of "The Boston Floating Hospital for Infants and Children":

The Boston Floating Hospital was founded in 1894 by the Reverend Rufus Tobey. His idea was that if sick babies could be taken from the crowded city and given the benefit of the cool sea air during the humid months of July and August, the high infant mortality from diarrheal diseases might be lowered. During the succeeding years the progress from an excursion boat to a well-equipped and well-organized hospital was very rapid. Physicians came from all parts of the world to study pediatrics on the Boston Floating Hospital. During that period important pioneer contributions to the knowledge of artificial infant feeding, diarrhea, metabolic disorders and other pediatric problems emanated from this Hospital.

On June 1, 1927, the hospital ship was destroyed by fire at its dock. By this time the incidence of intestinal diseases of children had greatly decreased and the demand for all-year-round hospital treatment had become evident.

The New York City Health Department employed a summer corps of physicians in 1876 "to search out and treat cases of infant diarrhea."

By the year 1879 Jacobi was professor of diseases of children at the College of Physicians and Surgeons of New York City. He was the first American pediatrician and the greatest, and is now revered as the father and founder of American pediatrics. Thomas Morgan Rotch became instructor of diseases of children at Harvard Medical School in 1879 and gave the first systematic course in pediatrics in that year.

In 1879 Jacobi wrote a chapter in Buck's *Hygiene and Public Health* on "Infant Hygiene."[9] His chief concern was with infant feeding. He noted that "when breast milk was withheld systematically the infant death rate was 499 per 1,000 live births per annum." More than half of those dying in their first year died in the first two months. During the first year 41 per cent of the deaths were

[9] Buck, A. H.: *Treatise on Hygiene and Public Health,* Vol. I, p. 74, 1879.

from digestive disturbances and 21 per cent from respiratory causes. Jacobi insisted upon the proper care and feeding of the mother during the prenatal period. In this article he again stressed the value of breast feeding of the infant, and if this was not possible he insisted that all cow's milk fed to infants be *boiled*. There is not a word in this chapter on community responsibility for the promotion of child health. Apparently the idea had not yet been born, even in the mind of this great and progressive-minded man.

A "milk station" was established by Dr. Koplik at the Good Samaritan Dispensary in New York in 1889. By 1890 it was generally understood that bad milk was an important contributing cause of summer diarrhea and by 1892 most mothers had been informed that cow's milk which was fed to children should be boiled.

Nathan Strauss,[10] the great philanthropist, began the establishment of his milk stations in 1893. He developed this system extensively and effectively, and his methods were widely copied. Nathan Strauss supported these depots for twenty-six years—until 1919. Rochester, New York, established the first *municipal* milk station under health department auspices in 1897. Two types of milk stations were then developed:

1. The Strauss type in which the milk was prepared according to formula, pasteurized and dispensed in nursing bottles from the depot. The mothers were given instruction at the depot.
2. The New York City Health Department type. The milk was distributed from the Center in quart bottles. The nurse was sent to each home and there she instructed the mothers in the proper preparation of the milk, and in the care of the infant in the home.

Both methods were quite effective in reducing infant mortality.

A symposium on infant mortality was held at the meeting of the American Public Health Association in 1889.[11] There were three papers. These were not very informative since the authors had no reliable data on which to base their discussions; births

---

[10] Chapin, Charles: "History of State and Municipal Control of Disease," *A Half Century of Public Health.* American Public Health Association, New York, 1921, p. 150.
[11] Symposium on infant mortality:
White, H. T.: "The Dwellings of the Laboring Classes in Relation to Infant Mortality."
Walker, Jerome: "Causes and Prevention of Infant Mortality."
Beard, R. O.: "The Causes of Infant Mortality."
Reports and Papers of the American Public Health Association, 15:69, 73, 82, 1889.

were not well reported and data from most communities upon deaths of infants were fragmentary. But it was at least a start.

These early efforts were valiant but met with no response. It must be confessed that Van Ingen was right when he said that little real progress was to be made in the health promotion of infants until the new century was well advanced.

Dr. Josephine Baker[12] has given us an excellent description of the vicissitudes of infant hygiene programs during the early part of the present century. During the winter the physicians were busy inspecting the children in the New York schools, and during the summer months they were asked to aid in checking the high infant mortality from summer diarrhea. But these physicians were poorly paid and gave little attention to this work. In 1902 E. J. Lederle was appointed health commissioner and proceeded to have a house-cleaning of the Health Department staff. Dr. Baker was a child health inspector. Her salary was increased from $30 to $100 a month, and she was asked to devote her full time to the care of sick babies. At first these activities were carried out under the Bureau of Contagious Disease. In 1908 Dr. Baker was placed in charge of a new division of child hygiene which was to become of increasing importance, and was to set a pattern for city and state health department administration throughout the land.

That same year J. W. Schereschewsky of the United States Public Health Service published a very important paper on infant mortality.[13] He used as his denominator the census data of 1900 and was able to show that a newborn child in America in 1900 had less chance of surviving a week than did a man of ninety years of age. The chance of a baby surviving a year was less than that of a man of eighty years. He proved that infant deaths were far more prevalent in July, August, and September, and he insisted that this high summer death rate was due to artificial feeding of babies with contaminated milk. His table of infant mortality rates for various cities and states is given in Table 16. Needless to say, this comparative table caused great consternation and was an important factor in the shaping of events that were soon to follow.

In 1909 a conference on the prevention of infant mortality was called by the Academy of Medicine in New Haven, and this meeting

[12] Baker, S. Josephine: *op. cit.*
[13] Schereschewsky, J. W.: "Infant Mortality in Relation to Infant Feeding," *Reports U. S. P. H. Service,* Bulletin 41, p. 631, 1908.

Table 16

Infant Death Rates in America*

1900

STATES	DEATHS PER 1,000 LIVE BIRTHS	CITIES	DEATHS PER 1,000 LIVE BIRTHS
Dist. of Columbia	274	Charleston, S. C.	419.5
Rhode Island	197	Savannah, Ga.	387.5
Maine	194	Atlanta, Ga.	306
Massachusetts	177	Fall River, Mass.	304
New Hampshire	172	Baltimore, Md.	235
New Jersey	167	New Orleans, La.	229
New York	159	Philadelphia, Pa.	197
Connecticut	156	Boston, Mass.	194
Vermont	122	New York, N. Y.	189
Michigan	121		

* SOURCE: Schereschewsky, J. W.: *Reports U. S. P. H. Service*, Bulletin 41, 1908.

resulted in the establishment of the American Child Health Association. The first annual meeting of the American Association for the Study and Prevention of Infant Mortality was held in Baltimore in 1910.[14] J. H. Mason Knox was president. Some of the other distinguished men who participated in this conference were John Fulton, state health officer of Maryland; William H. Welch; Cressy Wilbur, the statistician; Abraham Jacobi; Emmett Holt; and Irving Fisher. Holt had investigated the cause of death in 44,276 infants under one year of age: 28 per cent of these deaths were due to gastrointestinal disease; 75 per cent of the babies who died were bottle-fed.

This conference gave great impetus to the promotion of infant welfare. The following year, 1911, an extensive demonstration in infant welfare was made by the infant health stations of the New York City Department of Health, the New York Milk Committee, and the Diet Kitchen. They showed that 40 per cent of all infant deaths occurred during the first month of life, a fact which led to the establishment of prenatal services. Also in 1911 the American Academy of Political and Social Science published an article on infant mortality in the United States.[15] In 1912 the people of St. Louis and Boston began to interest themselves in prenatal instruction and

[14] *Reports of the First Annual Meeting of The American Association for the Study and Prevention of Infant Mortality*, November 9, 1910. Johns Hopkins University Press, Baltimore.

[15] Newmayer, S. W.: "The Warfare against Infant Mortality," *Ann. Am. Acad. Polit. & Social Sc.*, 37:289, (March) 1911.

postnatal care, although in that same year Holt is quoted as saying that "in maternity hospitals, infants are tolerated as unavoidable incidents of obstetric practice."[16]

The state of Louisiana created a subdivision of child hygiene in the state division of hygiene in 1912, and other states soon followed this example. Finally, in 1912 the Bureau of Maternal and Child Hygiene was established in the federal Department of Labor, with Miss Julia Lathrop as its director. It had an appropriation of only $26,640. With the organization of this service maternal and child health was firmly established in the United States and was to have a brilliant future.

[16] Chapin, Charles: *op. cit.,* p. 310.

CHAPTER 42. *School Health Services*

> *The conditions of health of school children are so commonly overlooked, that it will not be out of place here to lay down a few broad principles which have an application to the matter in hand.*
>
> R. J. O'SULLIVAN
> *First Report as Visiting*
> *Physician of the New York*
> *Board of Education, 1871*

Dr. Samuel Durgin has been lauded as the founder of school health services in America. It is true that he deserves great acclaim, for he was responsible for the establishment of the first permanent system of medical inspection of school children in Boston in 1894. But as we look back through the century we discover that a great deal of time, thought, and effort had been devoted to the protection of the health of the school child before 1894, and that the foundation stones of our school health services were laid about 1875.

American public schools were organized in pioneer days to teach children the three "R's," "reading, 'riting, and 'rithmetic." Any suggestions that new material should be introduced into the curriculum were met with the same solid hostility that we encounter today when it is suggested that medical students should be taught the essentials of preventive medicine or public health.

Physical Training[1]

The first effort to promote the health of school children was the introduction of physical training in Northampton, Massachusetts, in 1825. The following year Dr. Follen introduced the German system of school gymnastics in Boston. The schools had no gymnasia

[1] Sargent, D. A.: "Physical Training," *Reports and Papers of the American Public Health Association*, 9:116, 1883.

or any special equipment, so the children were taught some elementary formal calisthenics. This innovation, however, did not meet with popular approval.

Gymnastic exercises and physical training were developed extensively in the European schools, particularly in Germany, during the nineteenth century. In fact, formal physical training was emphasized to such a degree that the secondary schools were actually called "gymnasia." In America, however, formal, disciplined mass training in gymnastics never gained a vogue, since these exercises did not appeal to the American temperament. It is true that gymnasia were installed in all the larger public schools and physical educators were employed by departments of education to teach physical training to the children, but competitive games proved much more popular than formal calisthenics. By 1885 the public school gymnasium was an accepted institution, and more and more physical training in the schools was emphasized. This trend reached its height about 1900. Gradually, however, calisthenics were abandoned for games and competitive sports.

As an outgrowth of physical training there developed many types of school games, and the physical educator of the school became a coach in each of these different sports. The local schools and colleges entered into competition, first with each other and then with other communities. Eventually these simple sports, which were initiated in the schools and colleges, became professionalized and of nationwide and absorbing interest to large numbers of people. In fact, practically every major American sport today such as baseball, football, all types of track events, basketball, hockey, handball, and, for that matter, almost every kind of popular athletic pastime with the exception of golf and tennis, were introduced initially as a simple form of physical education for school children.

The most unfortunate development of this trend has been the growth of intercommunity school and college athletic contests with overemphasis on community rivalry, obsession with the necessity for victory of one school team over another, and the professionalization of physical educators whose primary function now is to win games. We have completely forgotten that the original purpose of the introduction of physical training into the schools was to promote the health of all the children, and thus we have made an absurd travesty of an initially excellent concept.

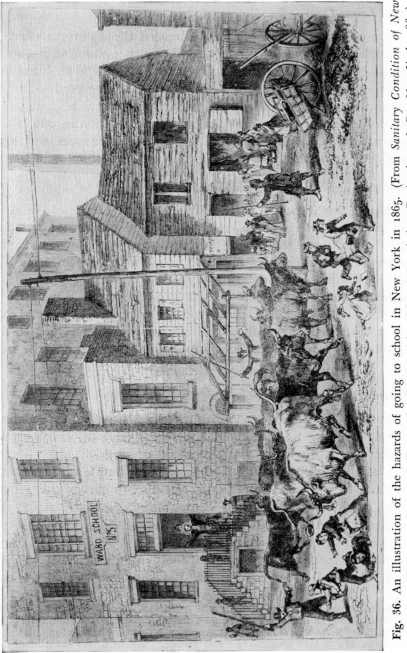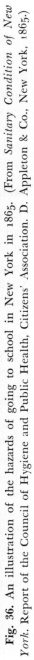

Fig. 36. An illustration of the hazards of going to school in New York in 1865. (From *Sanitary Condition of New York*. Report of the Council of Hygiene and Public Health, Citizens' Association. D. Appleton & Co., New York, 1865.)

425

Child Labor Laws

In a previous chapter we have discussed the disastrous effects of industrial development in America—beginning about 1820—on the health of children of school age. Gradually, laws were introduced into the various states which regulated the working hours of school-age children in cotton mills, coal mines, and factories. Later, compulsory attendance at school, for at least a few months out of each year, was instituted for all the children. All of these measures proved to be very important for promoting the health of school-age children.

Sanitation of Schools and School Buildings

Chapin[2] has informed us that by 1870 local boards of education had assumed definite responsibility for the proper sanitation of school buildings. Dr. R. J. O'Sullivan,[3] who was sanitary superintendent of schools in New York City, read a paper before the New York Academy of Medicine in 1873 in which he set forth the requirements of a good school hygiene program. In this paper he introduced the original idea that not only should the general sanitation of the school buildings be supervised carefully, but also that a system of *medical supervision* of school children should be instituted by the department of education.

Medical Inspection of Schools

Levitan[4] has told us that France was the first nation to undertake school health work. Fulick and Ayers[5] also have informed us that France developed an extensive system of medical inspection of schools in 1842. Physicians there visited every boys' and girls' school not only to inspect the buildings but also to survey the general health of the school children. These authors also have stated that the first medical inspection of schools in a full modern sense was initiated in Brussels, Belgium, in 1874.

The first medical inspector of schools in America that we have been able to discover was Dr. R. J. O'Sullivan,[6] whom we have

[2] Chapin, Charles: "History of State and Municipal Control of Disease," *A Half Century of Public Health*. American Public Health Association, New York, 1921, p. 133.

[3] O'Sullivan, R. J.: *School Hygiene*. D. Appleton & Co., New York, 1873.

[4] Levitan, M.: "School Health—Past and Present." Address before the Annual Conference of School Health Physicians, New York, 1939.

[5] Fulick, L. H., and Ayers, L. P.: *Historical Development of Medical Inspection of Schools*. Russell Sage Foundation, New York, 1908.

[6] O'Sullivan, R. J.: "Sanitary Superintendent of the Public Schools of New York." *Sanitarian*, 1:368-70, 1873.

mentioned earlier in this chapter. He was appointed visiting physician to the Board of Education of New York on January 1, 1871. His initial duty was to report on absences of teachers for more than five days because of illness. Soon after his appointment, an epidemic of smallpox broke out in the city and Dr. O'Sullivan conducted an extensive vaccination campaign among the school children. Some 40,000 children were vaccinated, each with the parents' consent. In 1872 Dr. O'Sullivan's duties were enlarged to include the sanitary supervision of the school buildings. To this task he devoted his entire time during school hours, but apparently his vigorous criticism of the sanitary conditions in the schools aroused opposition. In any case his position was abolished in 1873.

In 1875 there appeared in the *Sanitarian* a report[7] by Dr. D. F. Lincoln, secretary of the Health Department of the American Social Science Association. Earlier in that year, this association had held a symposium in Detroit on "The Health of Pupils in the Public Schools." Subjects that were considered at that session were:

1. Various aspects of school sanitation such as ventilation and lighting of schoolrooms, seating, drinking water, toilets, and the like.
2. Mental hygiene; the title of this discussion was "The Nervous System as Affected by School Life."
3. Gymnastics for schools; this subject was discussed by Dr. S. S. Putnam.
4. Effects of school life upon the eyesight and hearing of school children as revealed by extensive tests.
5. The heights and weights of school children; this was a reference to the study by the famous physiologist, Henry I. Bowditch.
6. Project of a law establishing the office of medical inspection of schools.

The Medico-Legal Society of New York made a report[8] in 1876 on school hygiene. The committee recommended that every school district should have a competent and well-paid medical director who should devote himself thoroughly and conscientiously to the many hygienic duties of the position. The society followed closely the recommendations of the American Social Science Association

[7] Lincoln, D. F.: "School Hygiene," *Sanitarian*, 3:193-202, 1875.
[8] "School Hygiene," Report of a Special Committee of the Medico-Legal Society New York, 1876.
It is interesting to note that Dr. O'Sullivan, who had lost his position as school medical inspector in 1873, was a member of the committee which made this report.

in Detroit in 1875, which we have already cited above. They concluded that the medical inspector should be a physician appointed
by the New York City Board of Education for three years. His
duties should be as follows:

1. To promote the health of teachers and children.
2. To make sanitary investigations of schoolhouses and grounds.
3. To trace the origin and mode of extension of epidemic and
   other diseases in the schools and point out measures for the
   arrest or the prevention of these diseases.
4. To gather and to present such information in respect to the
   interests of the public schools as he might deem proper for
   diffusion among the people.

In the appendix of the report we find that "compulsory measures
have recently been inaugurated relating to vaccination of school
children." These recommendations of the Medico-Legal Society were
excellent, but premature. They were not put into effect for more
than twenty years.

Testing of Eyesight and Hearing in the Schools

In 1876 Clarence J. Blake of Boston published an article[9] in
which he recommended mass methods for testing the hearing of
school children. Among other recommendations he suggested the
following:

. . . some provision should be made for proper determination of the degree of deafness disability. This may be accomplished by instituting competent medical examination in the hands of a medical supervisor of
schools, and the creation of such an office in connection with our public
school system is strongly urged. The frequency of partial deafness in
children, during the period of school life, makes it advisable to make
some definite provision in our public school system for compensatory instruction.

Medical Inspectors

Dr. Lincoln[10] of Boston in 1878 made a report on the sanitation
of public schools in Massachusetts. His major concern was with
the sanitation of the school buildings, but he did suggest a *medical*

[9] Blake, C. J.: "On the Best Methods of Testing the Hearing of School Children
and of Providing for the Instruction of Partially Deaf Children," *Tr. Internat. M.
Cong.*, p. 992, Philadelphia, 1876.
[10] Lincoln, D. F.: "Sanitation in the Public Schools of Massachusetts," *Report
Massachusetts State Board of Health*, 9:227, 1878.

adviser to the board of education whose duties would relate to health policies. One original recommendation by Lincoln was "the certification by a physician before readmitting to school a member of a family in which contagious disease had occurred." He emphasized the importance of isolation in infection and the necessity for disinfection.

An International Congress on Hygiene in Schools was held in Geneva in 1882 and was reported by Dr. Lundy[11] at the American Public Health Association meeting in 1883. He discussed extensively the general sanitation of the schoolrooms and buildings. Physical education was considered, and the subject of mental hygiene was introduced. The first recommendation was that the "cramming process" in education should be avoided. The second recommendation has a familiar sound to educators of medical students—"Reduce the number of subjects and shorten the curriculum." For the first time, one finds the suggestion that the schools should actually give remedial care, for in recommendation No. 7 we find the suggestion that "myopics *be provided* with glasses."

In 1886 Dr. D. F. Lincoln of Boston won the Lomb prize for his essay on "The Sanitary Conditions and Necessities of School Houses and School Life." This essay was concerned chiefly with the details of schoolroom construction. There was a short section on control of contagious disease in schools and the author also presented a tentative suggestion concerning the appointment of a medical inspector of schools. He stated that the extensive program of school medical inspection in Europe, in which medical treatment was given to a large number of children at the school, was a function which goes "beyond what is likely to be thought advisable in America at present." Lincoln felt that the chief duties of the sanitary supervisor of the schools should be (1) the inspection of buildings and (2) the instruction of teachers in the principles of hygiene.

This idea of the formal teaching of hygiene in the schools did not originate with Dr. Lincoln. We possess an old school textbook[12] for the teaching of hygiene in public schools which was published in 1848. This text of over 200 pages is concerned chiefly with anatomy and physiology, but deals to some degree with personal hygiene, and contains much the same material that my brothers and I were taught as fourth grade pupils in a country school in Colorado fifty years

[11] Lundy, C. J.: "School Hygiene," *Reports and Papers of the American Public Health Association,* 9:137, 1883.

[12] Beach, W.: *A Treatise on Anatomy, Physiology and Health,* designed for students, schools, and popular use. Baker & Scribner, New York, 1848.

later. The necessity for taking baths is emphasized, as well as the hygienic requirements of regular hours of rest and recreation and proper attention to clothing. We are instructed in ventilation of houses and suitable illumination to spare the eyesight, and there is a delicate reference to the processes of bodily elimination. In the illustrations of the human torso, all internal organs are outlined in color but the sexual organs are completely omitted from these diagrams, in due respect to the modesty of the schoolteacher.

At the first meeting of the American Public Health Association in 1873, the Hon. Andrew White,[13] president of Cornell University, gave a fine address on health education in the public schools, in which he stated:

Provision should be made for instruction in Human Physiology, Hygiene and Sanitary Science by Departments of Public Instruction in our public schools, also by providing fundamental instruction in Colleges and Universities and in Medical Colleges, by giving more special instruction in matters relating to Public and International Hygiene.

In 1886 Yomans[14] reported to the American Public Health Association on the Geneva International Congress of 1882 on Sanitary Inspection of Schools. He recommended the training of teachers in health and hygiene by the medical inspector of schools.

Yomans also recommended the appointment of a local school physician for each district of not more than 1,000 pupils. The duties of this physician would be to:

1. Inspect the sanitation of schoolrooms.
2. Measure children and place them in suitable seats.
3. Make refractions of the children's eyes.
4. Report communicable disease, and not permit a child who has had a contagious disease to return to school without certification.
5. Act as adviser in the program of students.

Medical Inspector of Schools Finally Appointed

An educator once stated to the author that any sound new idea in education requires a period of twenty-five years between the time

---

[13] White, Andrew: "Sanitary Science in Relation to Public Instruction," *Reports and Papers of the American Public Health Association,* 1:139, 1873.
[14] Yomans, H. P.: "Teaching Hygiene in Public Schools," *Reports and Papers of the American Public Health Association,* 12:99, 1886.

the idea first is evolved and the time that this idea is finally included in the educational schedule. In other words, an educational theory must be incubated twenty-five years before it actually emerges in educational practice. This long gestation period applied in America to the concept of medical inspection of schools, for it was not until 1892 that the first medical inspector of schools was appointed in New York. Fulick[15] has stated that this appointee, Dr. Moreau Morris, was the first medical inspector of schools in America but, as Van Ingen has noted, "he accomplished little." We have met Dr. Morris before in the early organization of the Health Department of New York City. He also accomplished little in his capacity there.

In 1894 medical inspection of schools was finally initiated in America. Dr. Samuel H. Durgin, chairman of the Board of Health of Boston, was faced with an alarming epidemic of diphtheria. He procured an appropriation from the city government and thereby was able to appoint fifty school physicians, one for each district, "to make daily examination of all suspicious cases [of diphtheria] found in the schools, and to see that suitable medical care [is] furnished at home and suitable sanitary precautions taken."[16] As Harrington and Richardson have pointed out, Durgin in 1894 originated medical inspection as a measure for control of contagion. Twenty years later in 1914 they wrote:

To discover incipient cases of communicable diseases, to exclude infected children from school and thereby prevent these diseases from becoming epidemic, is still in the minds of most people the *raison d'etre* of school inspection and the justification for the expenditure of public money upon it.[17]

This concept still holds true in many areas in America to the present day.

Chicago appointed its corps of school physicians in 1895, and New York in 1897 appointed 134 medical inspectors of schools under the direction of the Department of Health in the Division of Communicable Disease. The Division of Child Hygiene was formed in the New York City Health Department in 1908, and school health was then transferred to this division.

---

[15] Fulick and Ayers: *op. cit.*
[16] Harrington, Charles, and Richardson, Mark: *A Manual of Practical Hygiene.* Lea & Febiger, Philadelphia and New York, 1914, p. 680.
[17] *Ibid.,* pp. 680-81.

Compulsory Vaccination

Compulsory vaccination of school children was instituted by the New York City Health Department in 1897. This was not an initial attempt, for, as a matter of fact, compulsory vaccination of school children had been a part of the sanitary code of New York for many years. This law had had a stormy existence. We have encountered a New York State law,[18] passed in 1860, which required compulsory vaccination of school children, but this law almost created a riot and was not enforced effectively at that time or for many years to follow, and for a very good reason. Calf lymph was not generally available until the end of the century; hence vaccination was from arm to arm, with resulting transfer of serious secondary infections, sometimes with fatal outcome. This procedure met with such widespread popular opposition that compulsory vaccination of school children was not well accepted until about 1910.

The School Nurse

The first school nurse in America was appointed in 1902 in New York City. The service was initiated by Miss Lillian Wald of Henry Street at the request of Health Commissioner Lederle. (See Chapter 40, "Public Health Nursing.")

Physical Examination of School Children[19]

In 1903 Vermont passed a state-wide law which required annual eye examinations of all school children. In 1906 the Massachusetts act was passed which required an *annual physical examination of all school children.* Every town and village was required to maintain a system of health inspection, with a competent physician in charge for the following purposes:

1. Exclusion of contagious diseases where possible.
2. Detection of the most obvious physical defects of school children.
3. Correction of these physical defects by the municipality.

This last function aroused great opposition, as might have been expected.

This Massachusetts law of 1906 set an important precedent, since its execution, which included not only the examination of the chil-

[18] Laws of New York State, Chapter 438, Section 1, 1860.
[19] Van Ingen, P.: "The History of Child Welfare Work in the United States," *A Half Century of Public Health.* American Public Health Association, New York, 1921, pp. 296-98.

dren but also specified the functions of the school nurse, was assigned to and became the responsibility of the *Department of Education* and not the Department of Health. Up to this time the medical
aspects of school hygiene had been the responsibility of the local
health department; now the school department assumed these functions. This question of proper responsibility in relation to the health
services for school children was to be debated for fifty years. When
the Massachusetts law was passed in 1906, local health departments
were incompetent, were politically controlled, and were directed and
staffed by untrained, part-time personnel. The departments of education were semiautonomous, well administered, and free from political influence. Thus school health services that were administered by
departments of education were superior to those under health department supervision. As the years went by, local health department
services improved tremendously. Health department personnel became properly trained and well qualified. They insisted that the
health promotion and protection of children of school age is a function of the over-all community health service plan, but the strongly
entrenched vested interests in the school health services of the departments of education have been loath to surrender their well-
established programs. This controversy will not be settled for years
to come.

School lunches were first provided by the schools in New York in
1908. One year later, in 1909, Dr. Haven Emerson initiated the plan
of the education of delicate school children in the elements of nutrition.

School Clinics

In 1912 free clinics were established for school children in New
York City.[20] This service, as well as other school health services in
this city, remained the responsibility of the Health Department and
was not assigned to the Department of Education. These free clinics
which covered various aspects of medical care included:

1. An eye clinic for treatment and correction of eye diseases.
2. A tonsil and adenoid clinic.
3. A general medical clinic.
4. A skin clinic.

[20] *Free Municipal Clinics for School Children,* New York City Health Department
Reprint Series No. 41, 1916.

Here again the establishment of these mass therapeutic activities by the municipality met with active opposition on the part of the medical profession.

In 1918 New York State organized the present plan for school health services. This plan included:

1. The teaching of health practices in the school each day as an incorporated part of the regular school program.
2. Teacher-training in normal schools concerning good health habits for children.
3. Monthly recording of the weight of each child.
4. A comprehensive health examination of each child.
5. An annual physical examination of each child.

The program was the complete responsibility of the respective local *departments of education,* except in New York City, Rochester, and Buffalo. Each of these cities already had a school health service which had been under the supervision of their respective health departments.

SUMMARY

The approximate chronology of school health services began in 1825 with physical training. Sanitation of the school buildings and the teaching of hygiene in the schools developed slowly throughout the nineteenth century as department of education responsibilities.

The concept that the department of education should assume full responsibility for annual physical examinations of all school children, as well as for the school nursing service, the promotion of the nutrition of the school child, and the development of health education in the school curriculum, emerged about the year 1906. Subsequent developments have been promoted jointly by the departments of health and of education, sometimes in friendly co-operation, more often in fiercest rivalry—but always becoming more and more effective. Personal and community rivalry is sometimes an excellent stimulus to efficient public service.

CHAPTER 43. *Health Promotion in Industry*

*Every person in the community is concerned in the conserva-
tion of the health, vitality, energy, and industrial efficiency of
the wage earners.*

JOHN B. ANDREWS, *1916*

Industrial hygiene made no real progress in America during the entire nineteenth century (see Chapter 16, page 178). Legge, in an
analysis of progress in industrial medicine during the first half of the
twentieth century, has noted that in 1900 "only a few hazardous
occupations such as railroading, mining, and lumbering employed
physicians, primarily for the care of traumatic injuries resulting
from accident."[1] Osler's textbook of medicine of that date, 1900,
mentions only two industrial diseases, namely, lead and arsenical
poisoning. The paucity of interest in this field is illustrated by the
fact that Legge found only twenty-two contributions to industrial
hygiene in the entire American medical literature in the two final
decades of the nineteenth century, and those were concerned chiefly
with "the absence of humanizing elements in our industries."

Massachusetts passed a series of regulations in 1877 which gave the
state the right to enter factories in order to determine such simple
matters as proper fire egress, dust removal, and adequate ventilation.
One regulation forbade the employment of small children in factories. Ten years later, in 1887, this same state passed a law which
provided for sanitary supervision of factories and workshops. New
Jersey and Wisconsin passed factory inspection laws in 1883 and 1890.
At about this same time, federal regulations were passed relative to
the inspection of coal mines, particularly with regard to ventilation,
safety cages, measures for promoting accident prevention, and so
forth. One of the federal regulations prohibited children under
twelve years of age from working in the mines.

[1] Legge, R. T.: "Progress of American Industrial Medicine in the First Half of the
Twentieth Century," *Am. J. Pub. Health,* 42:905, 1952.

Federal legislation relating to safety appliances for railroads was enacted in 1893, and a regulation concerning accident prevention on steamboats was passed in 1901. This law also prohibited flogging on board ship and promoted hospital relief for sick and disabled seamen.[2]

One of the subjects that was chosen for the Lomb Prize Essays in 1885 dealt with industrial hygiene. The prize of $500 was won by George H. Ireland[3] of Springfield, Massachusetts, for the best essay on this subject. It was an almost inconceivably ingenuous and juvenile essay, circumscribed in its point of view and with little insight concerning even the major hazards of industry. But it was a start. Ireland discussed fire protection in factories and recommended fire escapes with *flat* treads. Ladders will not do since "women are extremely sensitive about making any seeming exposure of their limbs."

One of Ireland's suggestions for the prevention of inhalation of metal dusts was quite practical. "Persons . . . have been enabled to continue their work by growing a moustache, which caught the particles before they could reach the nostrils." An emergency kit, to be kept in a known place, was recommended, and a mutual relief association was suggested for the purpose of paying hospital fees in case of accident. "Ten cents a week [for each employee] will be sufficient to pay ordinary demands; any excess to be assessed, but not to exceed twenty-five cents in any one week."

What a long road has been traveled since 1886! And that was not so long ago. In fact it was the year the author of this book was born.

Industrial hygiene was first presented to medical students at Georgetown University by George M. Kober in 1890. He did not become deeply interested in this field, however, until 1902, after which time he became a powerful force in the promotion of industrial hygiene in America.

This remarkable man was born in Germany in 1850. He came to America as a seventeen-year-old immigrant boy and got a job in the hospital corps at the United States Army barracks at Carlisle, Pennsylvania. He attracted the attention of the medical officer of the post, who urged him to study medicine. He was appointed hospital

---

[2] For federal labor legislation see George M. Kober in *A Half Century of Public Health*. American Public Health Association, New York, 1921, pp. 368-70.

[3] Ireland, George H.: "The Preventable Causes of Disease, Injury and Death in American Manufactories and Workshops, and the Best Means and Appliances for Preventing and Avoiding Them," *Lomb Prize Essays*. American Public Health Association, New York, 1886.

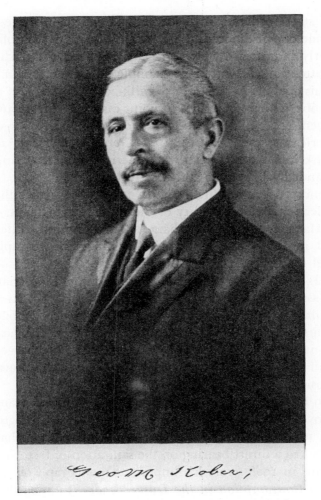

Fig. 37. George M. Kober, great industrial hygien-
ist. (From "Anniversary Tribute to George M. Kober
in Celebration of His Seventieth Birthday," *Am. J.
Phys. Anthropol.*, Vol. III, No. 1, Jan.-March, 1920.)

steward and ordered to Frankfort Arsenal, where he stayed for about
eighteen months. He was then transferred to the surgeon general's
office in Washington, D. C., where he worked in the library. He
studied medicine at night at Georgetown University, graduated in
medicine there, and in 1874 became a medical officer in the United
States Army. He was sent West for active duty in the Indian forays
and there he came under the tutelage of Dr. G. M. Sternberg. He
served in the army for twelve years. Kober was then appointed pro-

fessor of state medicine in Georgetown Medical College in 1889, and became one of the leading physicians of America. Public health, particularly industrial hygiene, became the field to which he gave greatest attention. An excellent example of his interest in epidemiology is his analysis in 1902 of 330 milk-borne epidemics.[4] (Souchon credits Kober as being the first to point out that "flies doubtless are the frequent cause of spreading typhoid.") In 1908 Kober wrote the first American text on *Industrial and Personal Hygiene*.[5] This was a landmark in industrial health in America. From that time on the field expanded very rapidly and effectively.

Massachusetts was the first state, in 1905, to recognize that industrial hygiene is a responsibility of the health department. Dr. William C. Hanson, who was in charge of this division, collected and exhibited in 1907 a splendid series of ninety photographs which illustrated the health hazards of the industry.

Dr. C.-E. A. Winslow had begun the teaching of industrial hygiene at the Massachusetts Institute of Technology in 1905. In 1906 Dr. Frank Fulton, a private practitioner of Providence, Rhode Island, was the first to make a careful effort to supervise the health of a group of industrial workers. He examined, free of charge, a large number of factory employees in order to discover the prevalence of tuberculosis in the typical working man.

In 1909 Dr. Mock[6] introduced the policy of medical examinations for employees of Sears, Roebuck and Company in Chicago. He has informed us that by that year (1909) twenty-one states had passed acts which had a direct bearing on the sanitation of factories.

Hoffman[7] in 1908 wrote his important monograph on *The Mortality from Consumption in the Dusty Trades*. In 1909 the prevention of caisson disease was officially instituted for the first time by an act of the state legislature of New York.

The year 1910 is the eventful year in the development of industrial hygiene in America. Gilman Thompson opened his Occupational Disease Clinic at Cornell University Medical College in New York City; the Illinois State Commission on Industrial Disease was formed

[4] Kober, George M.: "Milk in Relation to Public Health," *Senate Document No. 411*, 1902.

[5] Kober, George M.: *A Report on Industrial and Personal Hygiene*. President's Homes Commission, Washington, D. C., 1908, 175 pp.

[6] Mock, H. E.: "Industrial Medicine and Surgery, a Résumé of Its Development and Scope," *J. Indust. Hyg.* 1:251, 1919.

[7] Hoffman, Frederick: *The Mortality from Consumpton in the Dusty Trades*. Monograph, U.S. Bureau of Labor, 1908.

almost synchronously. The first National Congress on Occupational Disease was also held in 1910 in Chicago. Dr. Alice Hamilton began her industrial hygiene career with a publication on "Lead Poisoning,"[8] and Dr. J. B. Andrews published his studies on "Phosphorous Poisoning."[9] That same year, the United States Bureau of Labor published a list of industrial poisons.[10] A formal course leading to an academic degree in industrial hygiene was established at the Harvard-Massachusetts Institute of Technology School of Public Health in that same momentous year.

The most important single factor in promotion of the health of the worker in America has proved to be workmen's compensation. A tentative Workmen's Compensation Act was passed by New York State in 1910. This was the spark that started the fire burning. Within ten years practically every state in the Union with any industrial problems at all had adopted some form of workmen's compensation for accident, injury, or illness[11] that had been acquired as a result of a man's occupation. In 1911 each of six states passed a uniform law which required the reporting of occupational diseases to the state health department. California had the honor of initiating this law; the other states to adopt it at this time were Connecticut, Illinois, Michigan, New York, and Wisconsin.

The National Safety Conference was first organized in 1911. In 1914 it became the National Safety Congress and it has from that time on played a very important national role in accident prevention, particularly in industrial accidents. The Fifteenth International Congress on Hygiene was held in Washington in 1912. Dr. Kober presided over the deliberations, and made sure that due emphasis was placed on industrial hygiene. This congress was a very important milestone in industrial health promotion in America because of the nationwide publicity that attended these meetings.

In 1914 Gilman Thompson published his classic text on *The Occupational Diseases*.[12] The following year, 1915, the United States Public Health Service created a Division of Industrial Hygiene and Sanitation under the direction of Dr. J. W. Schereschewsky. Drs. A. J. Lanza, David Edsall, Gilman Thompson, George Price, and Otto

[8] Hamilton, Alice: "Lead Poisoning," *Bulletin 95, U.S. Bureau of Labor*, 1910.

[9] Andrews, J. B.: "Phosphorous Poisoning in the Match Industry in America," *Bulletin 86, U.S. Bureau of Labor*, 1910.

[10] "General List of Industrial Poisons," *Bulletin 86, U.S. Bureau of Labor*, 1910.

[11] Compensation for industrial illness was not established until about 1919.

[12] Thompson, Gilman: *The Occupational Diseases*. D. Appleton & Co., New York, 1914.

Geier were selected as consultants. Subsequent events proved that each of these men was to devote a major part of his life to a career in the field of industrial medicine, and each was to take a prominent part in various phases of its advance both in America and throughout the world.

It should be noted that Thompson's text was not the first comprehensive American report on occupational diseases. In 1892 Lloyd wrote "The Diseases of Occupation"[13] for the *Twentieth Century Practice of Medicine*. At that early date he discussed many of the types of poisoning which are due to arsenic, lead, phosphorus, copper, chromium, tin, and other metals, as well as some of the types of chemical poisoning attributed to sulfur and its oxides, carbon and its oxides, aniline, turpentine, nitrobenzene, and quinine. He described the consequences of exposure to dust, heat, compressed air, and constrained attitudes. Writer's cramp and miner's nystagmus were also discussed.

The effects of exposure to silica were not well understood by Lloyd. He considered the predisposing cause of silicosis to be pulmonary tuberculosis, but the relationship of silicosis to many industrial processes was not clear. Caisson's disease was reviewed at length by Lloyd, although he did not understand the cause of the symptoms. He mentioned the animal experiments by Paul Bert, who had worked out the correct solution of the pathology of the disease, but Lloyd did not seem to think much of Bert's theory.

In retrospect it seems almost incredible that industrial hygiene in America should have been held in abeyance for a period of over seventy-five years despite the enormous development of American industry and despite the fact that the European nations had made rapid advances in industrial health promotion for over half a century. Suddenly, in about 1900, the nation became alive to its responsibilities in this field, and within fifteen short years a tremendous growth occurred which was sound in every respect and which has served as a firm foundation for all future development of industrial hygiene in America.[14] This is a concrete and striking illustration of the fact that public health in each and all of its phases is a simple but

[13] Lloyd, J. H.: "The Diseases of Occupation," *Twentieth Century Practice of Medicine*, Philadelphia, 1892.

[14] Andrews, J. B.: "Legislation for the Prevention of Occupational Diseases in the United States," *Diseases of Occupation and Vocational Hygiene* (edited by G. M. Kober and William Hanson). Blakiston Sons & Co., Philadelphia, 1916.

accurate index of the growth of social concepts in the development of a nation.

As a final paragraph in this chapter we have listed those American pioneers of industrial hygiene who have been most effective in promoting this striking social phenomenon.

PIONEER	INITIAL FIELD OF INTEREST	APPROXIMATE DATE OF INITIAL INTEREST
Kober, G. M.	Teaching at Georgetown University	1902
Winslow, C.-E. A.	Teaching at Massachusetts Institute of Technology	1905
Hanson, William	Hazards of factory dusts and fumes (Massachusetts)	1906
Hamilton, Alice	Lead poisoning	1909
Andrews, J. B.	Phosphorus poisoning	1909
Hoffman, Frederick	Hazards of industrial dusts	1909
Hayhurst, E. R.	State Department of Industry and Labor, Ohio	1909
Lanza, A. J.	Health of miners	1910
Schereschewsky, J. W.	Health of garment workers	1911
Thompson, Gilman	Occupational Disease Clinic	1911
Price, George	Garment Workers' Clinic	1912
Edsall, D. L.	Steel Industry of Pittsburgh— its hazards	1912

We have been aided in the selection of this list by Mock, Garrison, and particularly by Kober.[15] The dates are only approximate.

[15] Kober, G. M.: "History of Industrial Hygiene and its Effects on Public Health," *A Half Century of Public Health*. American Public Health Association, New York, 1921, pp. 390-99.

CHAPTER 44. *The Teaching of Public Health and Preventive Medicine*

> *The bulk of the medical profession still looks askance at the invasion of the field of curative medicine by the state. It seems unlikely that the movement is going to be checked and it is a tremendous responsibility for those to whom it is given the opportunity to direct the movement aright.*
>
> CHARLES V. CHAPIN, *1921*

Insofar as we have been able to determine, Dr. Robley Dunglinson was the first professor of hygiene in an American medical college. He gave lectures on this subject in the University of Maryland and published these lectures in book form in 1835.[1] His lectures were devoted almost exclusively to personal hygiene. However, we find in his text a chapter on the influence of climate on health, and discussions of such matters as food and nutrition. We also find a brief mention of mental hygiene and a short section on the draining of malarious soil.

Lemuel Shattuck in his famous report of 1850 made many important recommendations. Not the least of these was Number XLV:

We recommend that persons be specially educated in sanitary science, as preventive advisers as well as curative advisers. . . .

Sanitary professorships should be established in all our colleges and medical schools, and filled by competent teachers. The science of preserving health and preventing disease should be taught as one of the most important sciences.[2]

---

[1] Dunglinson, Robley: *Elements of Hygiene.* Carey, Lea & Blanchard, Philadelphia, 1835, 514 pp.
[2] *Report of the Sanitary Commission of Massachusetts—1849.* Dutton & Wentworth, Boston, 1850, p. 228.

Although Shattuck made this important recommendation more than 100 years ago, it has not yet been carried out in its entirety throughout the United States.

The *Manual of Hygiene* of E. A. Parkes[3] was first published in 1859. Parkes was professor of military hygiene in the Army Medical School of England. The fifth edition was published in 1878 and consisted of 733 pages. Although it was concerned primarily with military hygiene and sanitation, it was also used in America as a medical school text in hygiene. This book contained material on hospital construction, on general sanitation, and on food and nutrition, but it included only scanty discussion of personal hygiene. A few pages were devoted to the control of communicable diseases, notably plague, cholera, malaria, the venereal diseases, and also the enteric diseases. There was a modern touch in a short section on "statistical techniques and calculation of averages." This text was widely read in America. When Dr. Parkes died, a eulogy of his life and works was published in the *Sanitarian*.[4]

A. H. Buck published his great text on *Hygiene and Public Health* in 1879.[5] There were many distinguished contributors to this 791-page book. J. S. Billings wrote the introduction and A. Jacobi, professor of diseases of children at the College of Physicians and Surgeons of New York, wrote on child hygiene. This text deals extensively with environmental sanitation, with housing, and with personal hygiene. Industrial hygiene, food sanitation, quarantine, disinfection, and communicable disease control are included. There is a brief section on infant mortality and vital statistics, as well as a short section on school hygiene by D. F. Lincoln.

As we look back over the years we realize that there was very little effective public health work going on in America in 1879. Yet the extent and depth of knowledge of this subject at this time is clearly attested by Buck's text. This is just one more illustration of a fact that we have noted before; namely, that knowledge precedes accomplishment by more than a generation.

Rohé and Robin[6] presented their "comprehensive treatise on the principles and practice of preventive medicine" from an American standpoint in 1891. Included in this text is a discussion of the *germ*

[3] Parkes, E. A.: *A Manual of Practical Hygiene*, First Edition. London, 1859.
[4] *Sanitarian*, 6:84, 1878.
[5] Buck, A. H.: *Hygiene and Public Health*. William Wood & Co., Philadelphia, 1879.
[6] Roché, G. H., and Robin, Albert: *Text Book of Hygiene*, First Edition. F. A. Davis Co., Philadelphia, 1891, 582 pp.

theory of disease. There is a chapter on the history of epidemic disease and a very short one on vital statistics.

Harrington's enormous *Manual of Practical Hygiene for Students, Physicians and Health Officers*[7] was a book of nearly 1,000 pages (fifth edition, 1914). It contains a chapter on the relation of insects to human disease, and has an excellent section on industrial hygiene.

Rosenau's classical text on *Preventive Medicine and Hygiene*[8] was first published in 1913. This book began a new era in the teaching of public health in America, and was destined to have a profound influence on public health promotion throughout the world.

Although textbooks were available to medical students throughout the nineteenth century, nevertheless hygiene, sanitation, preventive medicine, and public health were taught most casually in medical colleges throughout the entire 100 years. The subjects were assigned to one or more of the professors who were most interested in these fields, and a series of didactic lectures were given to apathetic and uninterested students. Rohé, for example, was professor of therapeutics, hygiene, and mental disease at the College of Physicians and Surgeons in Baltimore when he wrote his text in 1891, and Buck in 1879 was instructor of otology at Bellevue.

Not everyone was uninterested, however, for we note that the need for this type of teaching was frequently emphasized. At the first meeting of the American Public Health Association in 1872, the president of Cornell University, Andrew White,[9] insisted that "fundamental instruction in Colleges, Universities and Medical Colleges should be provided in Physiology, Hygiene, and Sanitation."

In 1881 an educator, J. M. Gregory, writing in the *American Journal of Education,* noted that "the omission of hygiene as a subject for study in medical colleges is a serious defect in the educational system." He believed that, if physicians were given instruction in the elements of hygiene, they in turn could pass on their knowledge to teachers in this field as well as to the general public. But this idea was not well absorbed by medical faculties. The whole trend of the century was to limit the teaching of medical students to the intensely practical fields of diagnosis and treatment.

[7] Harrington, Charles: *A Manual of Practical Hygiene.* Lea & Febiger, Philadelphia. (He was professor of hygiene at the Harvard Medical School before Dr. Rosenau.)
[8] Rosenau, M. J.: *Preventive Medicine and Hygiene.* D. Appleton & Co., New York, 1913.
[9] White, A. D.: "Sanitary Science and Its Relation to Public Instruction," *Reports and Papers of the American Public Health Association,* 1:139, 1873.

Charles W. Eliot, president of Harvard for a great many years, was a clear thinker and farsighted man. He had a vision of the trend of social growth in America and realized that Harvard Medical School was not equipped to train its students to meet these coming needs. Thus in 1910 he decided that a full-time professor of preventive medicine must be placed on his faculty, with the same status as the professor of anatomy, of medicine, or of surgery. Dr. Milton J. Rosenau, then director of the Hygienic Laboratory in Washington, was selected by Eliot to fill this position. Time was to show that Eliot had made a wise choice, for Dr. Rosenau established solidly the principle that the training of medical students in preventive medicine is an integral and essential part of medical education. Dr. Rosenau proved to be a great leader and marvelous teacher.

SCHOOLS OF PUBLIC HEALTH

Victor Vaughan in 1875 was appointed instructor of medical chemistry at the University of Michigan. In 1880 he became interested in the contamination of drinking water, and through this interest he was able to secure a grant from the state of Michigan to build and equip a *hygienic laboratory*. He went to Germany as one of Koch's students in 1888, and at that time he began his career as teacher and research worker in the field of bacteriology and public health. On his return his hygienic laboratory soon became an outstanding bacteriological institute. This laboratory was the first in America to offer systematic teaching in bacteriology, and one of the first to give advanced degrees in the field of sanitary science.[10]

In most medical colleges, public health and sanitation became identified with, and subsidiary to, bacteriology. The reasons are clear. Communicable disease control began to assume more and more importance as a public health responsibility, and obviously the control of contagion was based on a sound knowledge of bacteriology. Welch in 1885 became interested in public health through the field of bacteriology. Ditmars in Ohio entered the field through the same avenue in 1885. E. A. Birge began his teaching in bacteriology at Wisconsin in 1885. H. C. Ernst at Harvard Medical School began his work that same year, and Theobald Smith initiated the teaching of bacteriology at George Washington University in 1886. The influence

[10] *Journal of Laboratory and Clinical Medicine.* Memorial issue to V. C. Vaughan, Vol. XV, No. 9, 1930.

of these men is still felt, for the teaching of preventive medicine and public health is, even today, in some medical colleges allocated to the department of bacteriology.

W. T. Sedgwick, who was destined to become one of the great sanitarians of his generation, began the teaching of sanitary science at the Massachusetts Institute of Technology in 1883. He had had two years of medical school training at Yale, but became interested in the broad science of biology, and transferred to Johns Hopkins. After two years there he began his work in Cambridge, Massachusetts, where he studied the relation of water supplies to public health. A series of epidemics of typhoid fever, which were due to polluted water supplies, occurred in rapid succession. Sedgwick's brilliant epidemiological work on these outbreaks resulted in a "school" of sanitarians at the Massachusetts Institute of Technology which remained a focal point in this field for years to come. In 1902 Sedgwick published *Principles of Sanitary Science and the Public Health*. It was a great book and it did much to enhance his reputation.

Sedgwick believed that there was a career in public health for the *sanitarian*. A medical degree was not a prerequisite in his training, since more of the emphasis in medical school was centered on care of the individual patient, whereas the sanitarian was interested primarily in the community as a unit. Sedgwick carried his ideas into execution and thus, for a time, practically all experts in the field of public health were trained in the Massachusetts Institute of Technology, and most of them did not have a medical degree.

Hermann Biggs[11] had urged the training of physicians for careers in public health as early as 1897. He conceived the idea of a properly organized school of public health, but did not carry this idea into effect.

Shenck[12] has pointed out that the organization of the Army Medical School by Sternberg in 1893 initiated the first school of training in public health and preventive medicine in America. Among the lecturers of this school were Dr. Sternberg, Major John S. Billings, Captain Walter Reed, and C. W. Stiles, the parasitologist. Emphasis in the lectures was upon environmental sanitation and communicable disease control.

[11] Biggs, Hermann: *M. News*, 72:44, 1898.
[12] Shenck, J. M.: "Symposium on Historical Medicine," *M. Rec.*, June, 1944.

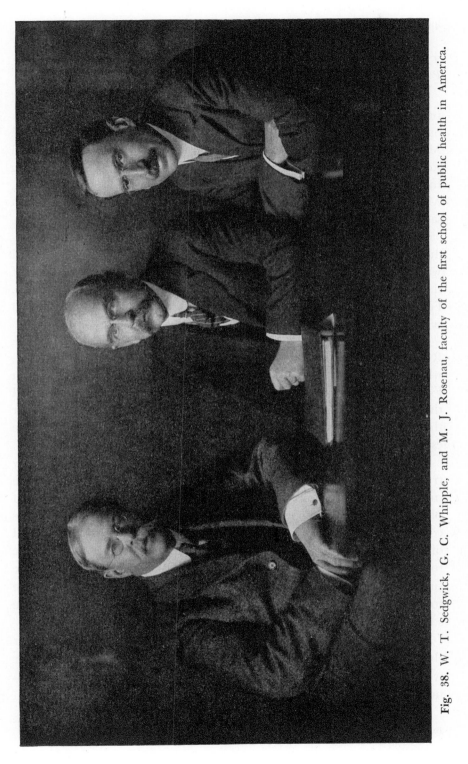

Fig. 38. W. T. Sedgwick, G. C. Whipple, and M. J. Rosenau, faculty of the first school of public health in America.

The Harvard-Massachusetts Institute of Technology School of Public Health

As we have already noted, Dr. M. J. Rosenau had been appointed professor of preventive medicine at Harvard in 1910, and was soon on very friendly terms with his neighbor Sedgwick. In 1913 Harvard Medical School and the Massachusetts Institute of Technology joined together to form the first well-rounded school for graduate training in public health in America. Its three sponsors were W. T. Sedgwick, M. J. Rosenau, and George C. Whipple of Harvard, who was both a sanitary engineer and a statistician. They were a wonderful team, each man complementing the qualities of the other, and they conducted a remarkably effective school for nine years. The joint school was discontinued in 1922 because the courts ruled that the charters of the two institutions did not permit the granting of a joint degree. Following this decision each institution then continued as its own separate school of public health.

On October 16, 1914, an important conference was held by the Rockefeller Foundation,[13] in which Dr. W. H. Welch, Wycliffe Rose, who was director of the International Health Board, Dr. Simon Flexner, Dr. Hermann Biggs, and others participated. It was proposed that a fully endowed institute of hygiene with a full-time staff for the major purpose of training public health personnel should be established as an integral part of a university. Welch felt that the essential feature would be a central institute "which would not only train health officers but would react upon the medical school of the university where it was placed and contribute to the training of physicians going into general practice." On October 1, 1918, this concept was initiated with the opening of the Johns Hopkins School of Hygiene, with Dr. Welch as its director. Subsequent events were to demonstrate that, although the first part of his vision was to be fully realized, the second part was only a mirage. Forty years were to pass before the influence of this great school broke through the solid barrier of a single narrow street.

The founding of these two schools in Baltimore and Boston for the special training of public health personnel set the standard for well-qualified trainees in America, and has resulted in the establishment of other fine schools of the same type. Their influence has been

---

[13] Fosdick, Raymond B.: *The Story of the Rockefeller Foundation.* Harper & Brothers, New York, 1952.

world-wide and has been one of the most important of all stimuli to the promotion of public health in America.

HEALTH SERVICE FOR COLLEGE STUDENTS

A word should be included concerning the instruction of college students in personal hygiene. This idea originated with President Stearns of Amherst College in 1859.[14] He had noted the unnecessary breakdown in student health and, as a result, he established a Department of Physical Education and Hygiene at Amherst. Its principles were:

1. The individual to have charge of the department should be a thoroughly educated physician and should be a member of the college faculty.
2. "Health of the students shall at all times be an object of his special watch, care and council." He should:
   a. Take charge of the gymnasium and give instruction in gymnastics.
   b. Oversee the health of students.
   c. Lecture on hygiene and general knowledge of anatomy and physiology.

President Stearns was an extremely wise man, and his proposed program might well be adopted in its entirety today by all the colleges of our land.

[14] Hitchcock, Edward: "Hygiene at Amherst College," *Reports and Papers of the American Public Health Association,* 4:47, 1877.

CHAPTER 45. *Voluntary Health Agencies*

Agencies of laymen and physicians are formed to promote popular understanding of preventive medicine. The objective is to instill in the people's mind a sense of responsibility for their own health and for that of the communities in which they live.

KENDALL EMERSON, *1942*

The promotion of public health and the prevention of illness in the community is obviously a governmental function. But government, although recognizing this burden, has often been slow to assume it. Socially minded persons, therefore, after unsuccessful efforts to stimulate an official agency to develop a health project in which they are interested, have become impatient and have taken the much more rapid course of initiating this service through voluntary health organizations and activities.

Benevolence, when not disinterested, is not one of the most appealing of human virtues, for it often stems from a desire for personal satisfaction and community esteem. But it has the great advantage that it may be of real assistance to those in dire and immediate need. The author of this text once noted:

The great urge to do something for the welfare of mankind is one of the striking characteristics of our American civilization. It is a characteristic that is easily explainable on the basis of the traditions and historical development of our people. This very quality has been one of the potent forces for the advancement of public health of America. It has accomplished great good. At times it has done real harm. Many of the important health activities that are now incorporated in the standard official public health practice might not have been initiated and certainly would not have been brought to their present state of successful operation were it not for the stimulus of voluntary health organizations. On the other

450

hand, many health services have been over-emphasized and many official programs have been badly planned because of the undue pressure of over-enthusiastic but misguided voluntary health associations.[1]

Types of Voluntary Health Associations

Voluntary health associations may include at least four distinct types of organization, with various subdivisions.

One type of voluntary health organization is epitomized by the American Public Health Association. This type of society may be organized on a local, state, or nationwide basis. It is made up largely of professional workers. Their primary purpose in forming these health associations is the interchange of technical information and the advancement of the quality of public health services, but the organization may also promote community health in a great many effective ways. The historical development of this type of voluntary health organization has already been described (see page 296).

A second type of health organization may be illustrated by the district nursing associations. These benevolent community associations are organized and controlled locally. They render a direct service to the community. These societies stem directly from the ladies' benevolent societies of pioneer days which were planned initially as a Christian service to the sick and deserving poor. We have already described their growth into an effective educational force for health in the community. (See Chapter 40, page 405.) The spread of associations of visiting nurses throughout the country and the gradual assumption of their burdens by the local communities has resulted in the final recognition of public health nursing as an official governmental responsibility.

A third type of voluntary health organization is the national association which is interested in a special health field. Excellent examples are the Red Cross, which is concerned primarily with disaster relief, and the National Tuberculosis Association. These great national associations received their initial impetus from the local community benevolent society, but each has expanded to nationwide scope and all of them have assumed a common pattern of organization.

This third type of health organization, as we have noted, is concerned with a circumscribed public health field. It is essentially edu-

[1] Smillie, W. G.: *Public Health Administration in the United States.* The Macmillan Co., New York, 1936, p. 326.

cational in its character and does not render direct service to local communities, except on a temporary demonstration basis or in emergencies. There is always a national headquarters with state and local subdivisions, and with a bureaucratic and sometimes inflexible type of organization. Funds are raised by a nationwide public appeal.

A fourth type of voluntary health organization is the private foundation for health promotion. This is a unique American institution which required a peculiar combination of social conditions for its inception. Each of these foundations has played a very important role in the development of public health in America. They did not appear until about the beginning of the twentieth century, but they increased almost by geometric proportion during the first half of the century. An illustration of this type of voluntary health organization is the Rockefeller Foundation.

Origin of the Voluntary Health Associations

The initiation and the development of the concept of a local voluntary association for the purpose of promotion of community-wide understanding of health needs is an interesting story. Prior to 1850, the local communities had, for many years, provided facilities for the care of the sick poor. We have already described the general hospitals and the dispensaries that were planned for the care of the needy. For the most part these were supported by benevolent societies and by philanthropy. By the middle of the nineteenth century a few public institutions had been built for the care of the insane and the blind, and for orphaned and needy children. But, for the most part, these health and welfare services were supported through the benevolence of the well-to-do citizens of each community.

In 1854, John Griscom,[2] a distinguished New York physician, proposed: "The establishment of a voluntary association, composed jointly of laymen and physicians, to be called a *Hygiological Society*. Its object of inquiry and action would comprise the entire field of the preservation of public and private health in all its varied and multitudinous relations. . . . It would take under its keeping and guidance the sanitary interests of the whole people in all their aspects and relations, and as a medium of communication between the people and the profession would exert a powerful influence for the good of both."

2 Griscom, John: "Anniversary Discourse," New York Academy of Medicine, November 22, 1854.

In retrospect we realize that the concept of voluntary health organizations was born during the Civil War. This terrible war of 1861-1865 produced an enormous and immediate need for medical, nursing, and sanitary facilities. This need was met by the United States Sanitary Commission (see page 277). The heroic efforts of those pioneer volunteers who organized these services for the soldiers awoke the people throughout the land to the idea that citizens of all ranks could form an association which, by combined effort, would provide the personnel, funds, and material to meet disaster needs. For the first time, the women of the nation found an opportunity to participate effectively in community affairs and to provide those benefits for which they were uniquely fitted.

Two outstanding women came through the tempering fires of this great disaster. Both were voluntary nurses during the Civil War. Both were completely exhausted by their war services and were unable to undertake their true destiny until several years after the war closed. One was Clara Barton, who was to establish the American Red Cross; the other was Louisa Schuyler, who founded the New York State Charities Aid Association.

The New York State Charities Aid Association

We have already discussed in a previous chapter Miss Schuyler's work with the United States Sanitary Commission (see page 282). Miss Louisa Schuyler[3] was only twenty-four years old when the Civil War began. She was a great-granddaughter of Alexander Hamilton, and was "a healthy, vigorous, natural young woman who had been brought up on a Hudson River estate in the security of unpretentious wealth." She was invited by Dr. Elizabeth Blackwell in 1861 to aid in the formation of a "ladies' aid society" for Civil War relief. Miss Schuyler, contrary to the wishes of her family, became actively interested in war service, and when the Women's Central Association for Relief was formed, she became its corresponding secretary. This association then fused its activities with the United States Sanitary Commission, and Miss Schuyler developed a great talent for organization. Her duties covered a large field and she worked strenuously until the end of the war, at which time she was extremely exhausted and required a long rest. Immediately after the war she decided that, when she recovered her strength, she would "form a New York

[3] Greenbie, Marjorie B.: *Lincoln's Daughters of Mercy.* G. P. Putnam's Sons, New York, 1944, 24 pp.

State Association for the betterment of public charitable institutions." She had made a very wide circle of friends through her work in the Sanitary Commission, and furthermore had learned that a voluntary organization could be a great power in the community in the promotion of health and welfare. She also learned that if one is given a good cause to work for, and can secure a well-organized and informed public opinion, then no reform is impossible.

In 1872 Miss Schuyler gathered about her those friends and associates who had been her colleagues in the Sanitary Commission and formed the New York State Charities Aid Association. It was destined to be one of the great voluntary health associations of America, and still serves as a model of intelligent efficiency in social planning.

The American Red Cross

Miss Clara Barton[4] was born in Oxford, Massachusetts. When the Civil War broke out she was forty-one years old. She met Dorothea Dix's severe qualifications for a nurse and served faithfully and well in this capacity throughout the war. At its end she was exhausted and quite ill. In 1869 she went to Europe to rest and recuperate, and by chance she went to Geneva, where she learned for the first time of the International Red Cross.

The International Committee of the Red Cross had been formed in Switzerland in August, 1864. The idea was so splendid that its plans and policies met with almost immediate world-wide recognition. Nine nations adopted the Articles of the Geneva Convention in 1864. Five more joined the following year, and in 1866 six more nations signed the Treaty. In 1868 the president of the Red Cross, Gustave Moynier, wrote to Henry N. Bellows, who was head of war relief in America. In this letter Mr. Bellows was asked to present the International Red Cross Treaty to the federal authorities in Washington for their approval. This was done, but the appeal fell on barren ground.

When Miss Barton arrived in Switzerland in 1869 she was asked why the United States had refused to sign the Treaty of Geneva. European governments felt that the United States, which had just suffered the terrible consequences of war, would be most appreciative of the benefits of the Red Cross. There was no reasonable answer.

Miss Barton, despite her invalidism, entered the service of the

---

[4] Barton, Clara: *The Red Cross: A History of This Remarkable International Movement in the Interest of Humanity.* Washington, D. C., 1898.

Red Cross during the Franco-Prussian War, beginning in 1870. When she returned to the United States in 1873, broken in health, she carried with her a letter from Mr. Moynier, president of the International Committee, to the President of the United States, begging our country to sign the Geneva Treaty. Miss Barton was compelled to spend the next four years in a sanatorium in Danville, New York. In 1877 she carried her official letter from Geneva to President Hayes, but met with no success. In 1881 she succeeded in winning the approval of President Garfield and obtained his assurance that he would refer the matter to Congress. Then Garfield was assassinated. Miss Barton on her own initiative then founded the first Red Cross Society in America while still at the sanatorium in Danville, and made herself its president. With indomitable will she carried on, almost singlehanded, the fight for national recognition. Finally, in July, 1882, President Arthur and the Congress ratified the Geneva Treaty, the thirty-second nation to do so. We signed just after Peru and just before Bulgaria. Miss Barton remained president of the American Red Cross from 1882 until 1904. What a wonderful woman she was, for it must be remembered that she was sixty-one years of age when she first organized the Red Cross in America.

The National Tuberculosis Association

This association has been selected as an example of the national voluntary health associations that are essentially educational in character, are interested in one particular field, and conform most closely to Emerson's definition of a voluntary health organization. The association owes its origin to a Pennsylvania doctor, Laurence F. Flick, who graduated from Jefferson Medical College in 1879. He developed tuberculosis while in college and had repeated relapses. How he ever survived is a miracle. Stumbling over the western plains, without friends and no means of support, with only a few dollars that he had borrowed, he struggled valiantly for bare existence. He attributed his cure to his poverty, for he had to sleep in the open air. He lived largely on milk because it was the only available cheap food. In any event he recovered, and in 1882 he returned to Philadelphia to practice medicine. Here he was soon recognized as a specialist in tuberculosis. He presented a paper on the contagious nature of tuberculosis in 1888, and for years he worked singlehanded in his clinical researches on this disease. As early as 1889 he advocated the reporting and registration of active cases of tuberculosis. In 1892 he organized the Pennsylvania Society for the Prevention of Tuberculosis, the first organized society of its type in the world.[5]

The Pennsylvania Society for the Prevention of Tuberculosis proved to be a great success. In 1898 Dr. Flick began a correspondence with Dr. Otis, Dr. Bowditch, and Dr. Knopf concerning the possibilities of forming a national tuberculosis association. Dr. Knopf organized a conference on tuberculosis in Baltimore in January, 1904, and as a result of this conference, the National Association for Study and Prevention of Tuberculosis[6] was formed in Atlantic City in June, 1904. Its founders were great names all—Drs. Trudeau, Osler, W. H. Welch, Sternberg, Henry B. Jacobs, Charles L. Minor, M. P. Ravenel, Hermann Biggs, S. A. Knopf, and Laurence Flick. The dream of an obscure, local physician who had lived with tuberculosis all his life, and who practiced in the slums of Philadelphia among the destitute and helpless, finally came true. The great National Association for Prevention of Tuberculosis was to be an ever-increasing force in the education of the people throughout the nation, both in the natural history of this disease and in the promotion of technical and administrative procedures for its ultimate eradication. Furthermore, this association set the pattern for other great national voluntary health organizations which were to follow. The American Social Hygiene Association was formed in 1905, the American Child Health Association in 1909, the National Committee for Mental Hygiene was also organized in 1909, and the American Society for the Control of Cancer in 1913. Many others were to follow.

The Rockefeller Foundation[7]

I have chosen the Rockefeller Foundation as an example of the fourth type of voluntary health organization because it is one of the earliest and largest of the privately endowed voluntary health organizations. Also I know it best, as my career in public health began with this organization.

The development of the concept of this foundation is a very human and interesting story. Two men were involved—the silent,

[5] In 1901 Dr. Flick met the philanthropist, Henry Phipps, who became interested in Dr. Flick's little hospital, which was located in the Philadelphia tenements, for the study of tuberculosis. As a direct result, Mr. Phipps established and endowed in 1903 the Henry Phipps Institute for the study of tuberculosis, with Dr. Flick as its director.

[6] Knopf, S. A.: *A History of the National Tuberculosis Association*. National Tuberculosis Association, New York, 1922.

[7] Fosdick, Raymond B.: *The Story of the Rockefeller Foundation*. Harper & Brothers, New York, 1952.

taciturn, cautious, yet bold, financier, John D. Rockefeller, and his spiritual adviser, the eager, fiery, impetuous idealist, Frederick T. Gates. Mr. Gates was a Baptist minister with many of the qualities of a crusading evangelist. Perhaps it might be said that he was a combination of the crusading vision of the prophet Isaiah and the administrative talent of St. Peter. He would thunder at Mr. Rockefeller, "Your fortune is rolling up, rolling up like an avalanche. You must keep up with it! You must distribute it faster than it grows! If you do not, it will crush you and your children and your children's children."

Both men possessed, each in his own way, a religious fervor, a sense of personal destiny, and a deep and sincere feeling for the welfare of his fellow man. Each realized that it is more difficult to spend money in philanthropic efforts than to accumulate money. A careful, well-organized, business-like procedure is essential to philanthropy, with due attendance to efficiency of administration and proper scrutiny of appeals for aid.

Mr. Rockefeller's early benevolences were centered in foreign missions and, out of this interest, the China Medical Board was created. As a young man he had been concerned with the plight of the Negroes and their lack of educational opportunities. From this interest there developed in 1903 the General Education Board. Mr. Gates, in his ubiquitous search for adequate methods to distribute wealth, read Osler's *Practice of Medicine* from front to back covers, and from this careful perusal evolved the idea of a great medical research institution. Thus the Rockefeller Institute was created in 1901. Dr. Simon Flexner was chosen as its director; Wallace Butterick, another Baptist minister, had been chosen by Gates to direct the General Education Board. While canvassing opportunities for the advancement of Negro education, Dr. Butterick met another crusader, Dr. C. W. Stiles, who was a parasitologist in the Department of Agriculture. Dr. Stiles had determined the epidemiology of hookworm disease in our southern states. He knew its cause, its mode of spread, and its method of control. He realized full well the great harm that the disease was causing to the children of a large section of our country, but he had been unable to interest anyone in this great tragedy. Butterick brought his story to Gates, and the Rockefeller Sanitary Commission was formed with a grant of $1,000,000 to be spent in five years to combat hookworm disease in the South. Dr. Wycliffe Rose was chosen as director of this commission.

The stage was set for a great enterprise. Simon Flexner, the son of an itinerant peddler of Louisville, had failed as an apprentice plumber and then clerked in a drugstore. With the self-sacrificing support of his family, he entered Johns Hopkins Medical College, where he came under the eye of William H. Welch and was launched on his career. Butterick started his life career as a brakeman and postal clerk on a railroad in upper New York State. Wycliffe Rose was a modest professor of philosophy in a small women's college (Peabody) in Nashville. These three men, with Gates, were destined to launch a philanthropic organization that had no precedent and no fixed traditions, and which was to have an enormous influence on the promotion of the health and welfare of millions of people throughout the world. Its purpose was, from the outset, "to promote the well-being and to advance the civilization of the peoples of the United States and its territories and possessions and of foreign lands in the acquisition and dissemination of knowledge, in the prevention and relief of suffering, and in the promotion of any and all of the elements of human progress."[8] As Mr. Fosdick has said: "This statement of purpose was obviously the work of Mr. Gates."

The Rockefeller Foundation was conceived in 1909 and was finally incorporated in 1913. During the next fifteen years Mr. Rockefeller was to donate approximately $250,000,000 for the work of this great philanthropy, and its influence was to spread to all parts of the globe. But its chief contribution was not in money given, but in the stimulus and encouragement that it provided for nations and peoples to develop their own resources and to stand on their own feet.

The pattern that was set by the general policy of the Rockefeller Foundation has been followed in detail by the many privately endowed voluntary health and welfare associations that have been chartered since 1910. These organizations have played a very important role in the development of preventive medicine and public health in America and throughout the world.

[8] *Ibid.*, p. 15.

CHAPTER 46. *The Development of*

Federal Health Services

The prevention of preventable disease is the first purpose of a wisely governed state.

ERASTUS BROOKS, *1882*

The major activities of the federal government which relate to promotion of the health of the American people have been assigned to the United States Public Health Service. Dr. R. C. Williams has compiled a comprehensive and beautifully illustrated history of the United States Public Health Service from 1798 to 1950,[1] so that this chapter of our book can be but a short and simple résumé of Williams' compendium.

We are accustomed to consider 1798 as the date that the United States Public Health Service was founded, but, as a matter of fact, the federal government assumed almost no interest in public health affairs until 1872, and it is also a fact that, for the following twenty-five years, the federal health services were extremely limited in scope. The record shows that the increase of concern of the federal government with public health and medical care occurred, for the most part, during the second quarter of the twentieth century, with small beginnings in the early part of the century.

The Constitution of the United States contains no direct reference to national responsibility for health protection or health promotion. All of the existing and most extensive public health and welfare activities of the federal government are based on a single constitutional clause (Article I, Section 8): ". . . provide . . . for the general welfare. . . ." Our forefathers believed firmly and implicitly that

[1] Williams, R. C.: *The United States Public Health Service, 1798-1950.* Commissioned Officers Association of the United States Public Health Service, Bethesda, Md., 1951.

community health protection was a *local responsibility,* and not the responsibility of the Federation of States.

The United States Marine Hospital Service

The origin of the United States Public Health Service may be traced back to a Congressional action of 1792. Alexander Hamilton recommended to the Congress that the federal government establish hospitals "for the relief of sick and disabled seamen." The initial recommendation became a law in 1798. The whole matter was debated with considerable force.[2] Some members of Congress felt that the federal government had no responsibility for matters relating to medical care. They believed that the local communities or perhaps the separate states should be the responsible agents in these matters. The bill as finally passed provided for a deduction of 20 cents a month from each seaman's wages. The local collector of customs was the collector and depositor of these funds. Thus the service was placed administratively in the United States Department of the Treasury and remained there for over 100 years. Each port of the United States was to have a director of marine hospitals. The duty of these directors was to arrange hospitalization and to provide medical care for merchant seamen, and each director was responsible to the local collector of customs. It is difficult to imagine a plan which would provide greater opportunity for political chicanery, with local exploitation of federal funds. During the next seventy-five years there was an occasional amendment to the plan but no major modification. Things worked out exactly as was to be expected. The hospitals were organized and run inefficiently; the service was on a contract basis with little to recommend it. Finally, in 1870 the situation became so bad that the President approved an act "to reorganize the Marine Hospital services and to provide for the relief of sick and disabled seamen." The same act provided for a supervising surgeon whose duty it would be, under the Secretary of the Treasury, to supervise all matters connected with the service. Provision was made also for the disbursement of the central funds that were furnished by the act. Dr. John M. Woodworth was appointed by the President as the first director of the Marine Hospital Service.

The choice was an excellent one. Dr. Woodworth had made a fine record as a medical officer of the army during and after the Civil

2 Mustard, Harry S.: *Government in Public Health.* The Commonwealth Fund, New York, 1945, p. 23.

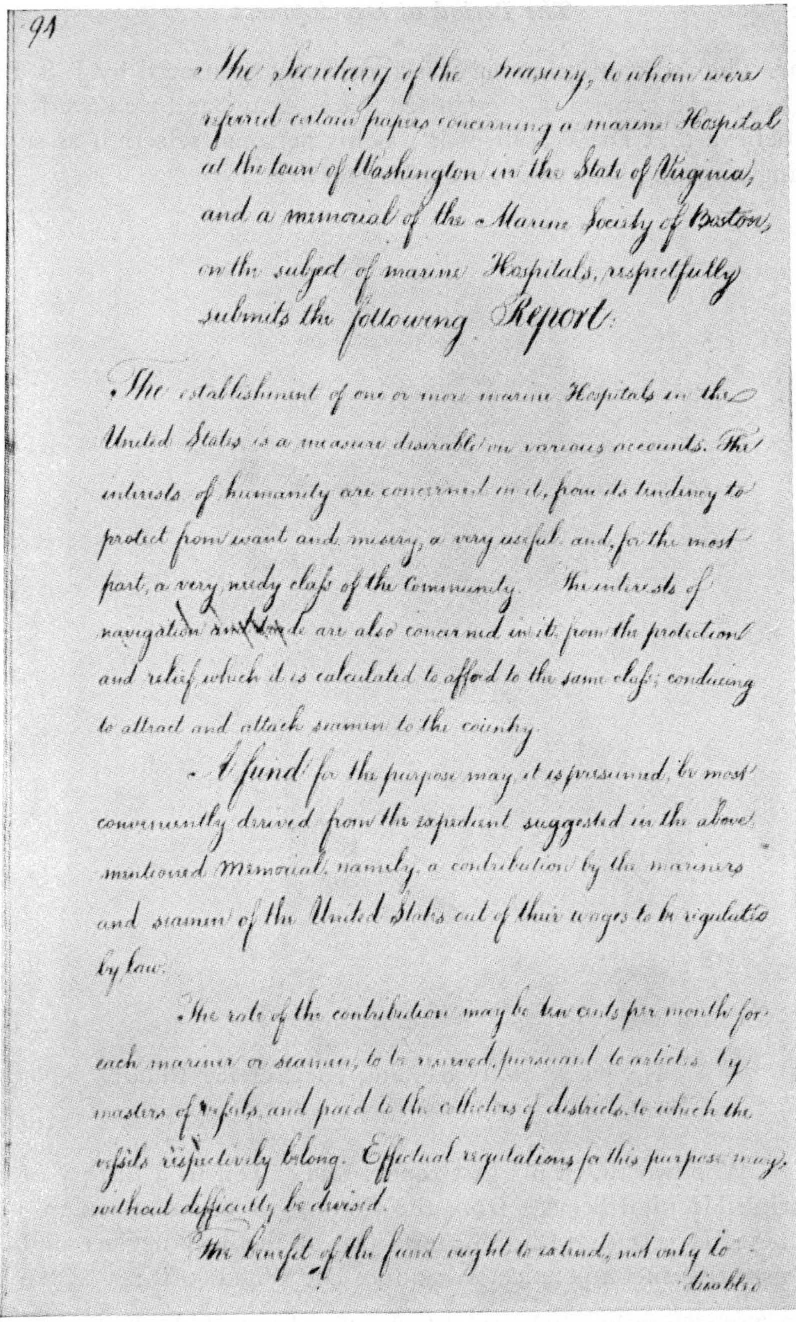

The Secretary of the Treasury, to whom were referred certain papers concerning a marine Hospital at the town of Washington in the State of Virginia, and a memorial of the Marine Society of Boston, on the subject of marine Hospitals, respectfully submits the following Report.

The establishment of one or more marine Hospitals in the United States is a measure desirable on various accounts. The interests of humanity are concerned in it, from its tendency to protect from want and misery, a very useful and, for the most part, a very needy class of the Community. The interests of navigation and trade are also concerned in it, from the protection and relief which it is calculated to afford to the same class; conducing to attract and attach seamen to the country.

A fund for the purpose may, it is presumed, be most conveniently derived from the expedient suggested in the above mentioned Memorial, namely, a contribution by the mariners and seamen of the United States out of their wages to be regulated by law.

The rate of the contribution may be two cents per month for each mariner or seaman, to be reserved, pursuant to articles, by masters of vessels, and paid to the collectors of districts, to which the vessels respectively belong. Effectual regulations for this purpose may, without difficulty, be devised.

The benefit of the fund ought to extend, not only to enable

Fig. 39. Report of Alexander Hamilton, April 17, 1792. (From Mustard, Harry S.: *Government in Public Health.* The Commonwealth Fund, New York, 1945. Reproduced by permission of the Fund and the Harvard University Press.)

War. The reorganization act was apparently sponsored by J. S. Billings, surgeon general of the United States Army, and we have reason to believe that Dr. Woodworth was his personal selection as supervising surgeon of the newly organized service.

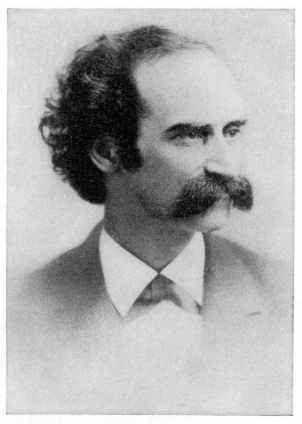

Fig. 40. J. M. Woodworth. Founded the United States Public Health Service.

Dr. Woodworth, in his first report,[3] has given us a history of the Marine Hospital Service from the time of its organization in 1798 to 1872. It is a short but bitter story of medical neglect and administrative incompetence. We quote Dr. Woodworth:

That the marine hospital service had suffered from lack of proper medical supervision, is a fact too apparent to be controverted. Many abuses

[3] Woodworth, J. W.: *First Annual Report of the Supervising Surgeon of the Marine Hospital Service for the Year 1872*. Government Printing Office, Washington, D. C., 1872.

had crept into the service which it was impossible to correct without the aid of a supervising officer versed in sanitary science, and familiar with the management of hospitals.[4]

Dr. Woodworth, following his army traditions, organized the service on a semimilitary basis. Officers were chosen on the basis of competitive examination (beginning in 1876) and were advanced through regular grades that were comparable to military officer rank. His initial reports were concerned almost exclusively with administrative matters relating to hospital management, and there is no mention in these reports of federal assumption of authority in matters relating to public health.

In 1876 Dr. Woodworth read a paper at the International Medical Congress in Philadelphia. He recommended that:

1. The surgeon general of the Marine Hospital Service should draft rules covering quarantine of vessels from foreign ports.
2. Consular officers should inform the United States Government of the sanitary conditions of their ports.
3. The service should publish a weekly report of sanitary information from consular officers.
4. The Marine Hospital Service should be empowered to enforce national quarantine.
5. It should also make investigations of the origin and causes of epidemic diseases, especially yellow fever and cholera.

These five functions were to be the foundation stones upon which the present United States Public Health Service was to stand.

Federal authority in port quarantine had been agitated for many years. In 1796, on May 11, Senator Smith of Maryland proposed to the United States Congress the unprecedented idea of federal regulation of quarantine. There ensued an extensive debate. Senator Lyman of Massachusetts thought that the individual states should have sole control over port quarantine. Senator Heister of Pennsylvania "objected to the principle of the Bill as it proposed to take power from the individual States to regulate what respected the health of their citizens. . . . [It appeared to him] that the governor of each individual State was better calculated to regulate quarantine than the General Government."[5] Since many states were very distant from the seat of government, great havoc might be made among

[4] *Ibid.*, p. 22.
[5] Jones, Joseph: *Medical and Surgical Memoirs*, Vol. 3, Part 1, p. 11, 1887.

citizens before information could be given to the President. Finally, a bill was enacted to the effect that the President of the United States direct revenue officers "to aid in the execution of quarantine."[6]

National Quarantine Act of 1878

This ineffective policy of federal co-operation in regard to port quarantine was continued until 1878, when Dr. Woodworth's five principles were incorporated in a National Quarantine Act. But this act still provided *"that there shall be no interference in any manner with any quarantine laws or regulations as they now exist or may hereafter be adopted under State laws."*[7] Formerly, Massachusetts and Pennsylvania championed state sovereignty; now it was the southern states that were objecting to federal interference in state quarantine procedures.

The doctrine of states' rights had shifted its center of balance from Massachusetts and Pennsylvania in 1796 to Louisiana and South Carolina in 1878, but it was as adamant as ever. This doctrine was to handicap the effective administration of nationwide public health activities for many years to come. Nevertheless, a milestone had been passed, for Dr. Woodworth, as surgeon general of the Marine Hospital Service, had received in 1878, the sanction of the federal government to enforce port quarantine.

A National Bureau of Health

The necessity for a nationwide health service had been discussed from time to time during the entire nineteenth century, although Shattuck in 1850 made no mention of the advantages of a national health department.

A bill for the establishment of a national sanitary bureau was introduced in the United States Congress on December 13, 1872.[8] This bill provided for a commissioner as chief executive officer. Its purpose was:

1. To aid in the establishment of quarantine by the various states.
2. To compile information concerning contagious disease and environmental factors pertaining thereto.
3. To register all deaths.
4. To collect a public health library.

[6] *Ibid.*, p. 14.
[7] "National Quarantine," *Sanitarian*, 6:316, 1878. The act is given in full.
[8] *Sanitarian*, 1:11-13, 1873.

Beside the commissioner, other officers were to be appointed, such as a chief clerk, chemists, and other experts. The bureau was to be attached to the Department of the Interior. Additional functions were suggested, such as a study of medical geography, a study of the sanitary condition of modes of public conveyance, and the sanitary condition of public buildings such as schools, hospitals, and so on. This bill did not pass the Congress.

In 1873 a well-formulated plan for a national sanitary bureau was presented at the first meeting of the American Public Health Association by C. C. Cox,[9] president of the Board of Health, Washington, D. C. He suggested the placing of the bureau in the Department of the Interior.

In 1875 Henry Bowditch discussed "The Future Health of the Nation" in his address to the Section on State Medicine and Public Hygiene of the American Medical Association.[10] He felt that it was premature to establish a national bureau of health before there was a state board of health in every state. He had sent out a questionnaire, and had received twenty-two replies from the various states concerning the establishment of a national health council. He encountered much opposition. Those who favored the plan of a national health council with an official delegate from each state and a central administrator felt that the council should perform the following functions:

1. Investigate epidemiology and prevention of disease.
2. Collect data bearing on health.
3. Help the diffusion of knowledge—"publish real advances in public hygiene, not voluminous documents compiled by scissors."
4. Act in an advisory capacity—suggest to Congress and to the states, laws in relation to quarantine, drainage, immigration, and the like.

The National Board of Health, 1879-1883

We have discussed in a previous chapter (see Chapter 36) the eventual foundation of the National Board of Health in 1879. This board was a logical outgrowth of all the plans and discussions that had been under consideration for years, but it was sure to fail from

[9] Cox, C. C.: "A Report upon the Necessity for a National Sanitary Bureau," *Reports and Papers of American Public Health Association* 1:522, 1873.
[10] Bowditch, Henry I.: *Transactions of the American Medical Association,* 1875. Annual address of the chairman of the Section on State Medicine and Public Hygiene.

the very outset because of an impossible administrative structure. To the National Board of Health was assigned the function of *national quarantine* which Dr. Woodworth of the Marine Hospital Service had worked so hard to create and for which he had just secured the authority to enforce. The loss of this responsibility was a bitter defeat to Dr. Woodworth and probably hastened his death. Dr. John Hamilton succeeded Dr. Woodworth as surgeon general of the Marine Hospital Service. He realized that if the National Board of Health could be discredited and its appropriations curtailed, then the quarantine functions, which had been transferred to it from the Marine Hospital Service, would automatically be returned to him. We have already described the controversy that followed. The National Board of Health knew who its major enemy was, but was unable to cope with him. In 1883 the appropriations for the National Board of Health terminated and the board gradually expired. The actual authority relating to port quarantine was not reconferred upon the Marine Hospital Service until the passage of the Quarantine Act of 1890. This act also provided for the prevention by the Marine Hospital Service of interstate spread of certain infectious diseases. Dr. Hamilton was politically minded and personally ambitious, and he made many enemies, but he must be given due credit, for he did advance the Marine Hospital Service and the national quarantine service as well. In 1891 he resigned from the Marine Hospital Service and left Washington suddenly, for very good personal reasons. He became active in the affairs of the American Medical Association in Chicago where, a few years later (in 1898), he died of typhoid fever.

The federal Quarantine Act of 1893 gave the Marine Hospital Service much more authority in the enforcement of port quarantine than it had had, and made it possible also to erect and to control quarantine stations. The only diseases subject to quarantine by the federal government were plague, cholera, typhus fever, yellow fever, and smallpox. Later anthrax (applying to articles in cargo) and leprosy were added.

The next great step in the development of a federal health service was taken in 1902 when an act was passed providing for the regulation of the interstate sale of viruses, serums, toxins, and similar products. With this act the Hygienic Laboratory was firmly established.

The Hygienic Laboratory

Dr. Joseph I. Kinyoun of the Marine Hospital staff had established a small laboratory in the Staten Island Marine Hospital in 1887. Dr. Walter Wyman was made surgeon general succeeding Hamilton in 1891. Wyman had been Kinyoun's chief in Staten Island, and in 1892 he invited Dr. Kinyoun to move his laboratory from Staten Island to Washington. There Dr. Kinyoun produced diphtheria antitoxin in 1894, and carried out a variety of useful activities, so that his little research laboratory became the nucleus around which the Hygienic Laboratory was formed in 1902. (Dr. Milton Rosenau had succeeded Dr. Kinyoun as director of the Marine Hospital Laboratory in 1899.)

In 1902 also, Congress began to recognize the important place that the federal government must take in public health matters. An act was passed that year creating the United States Public Health and Marine Hospital Service. Finally, in 1912 the present designation of United States Public Health Service was adopted. The great emphasis now was upon public health affairs, but the old functions were continued, for this organization was, and still is, responsible for the medical, hospital, and nursing care of "sick and disabled sailors."

In 1913 funds were provided for field investigations of communicable diseases, particularly those that were of interstate import.

A Committee of One Hundred had been organized in 1906 to promote a National Department of Health. It would absorb the functions of the United States Public Health Service and co-ordinate all the medical and sanitary activities of the federal government that had gradually developed, such as the food and drugs section of the Department of Agriculture, the Indian Affairs and Territorial Health Services in the Department of the Interior, the medical care of federal prisoners, the industrial hygiene studies of the Bureau of Mines, and so forth. Dr. Irving Fisher, famous professor of Yale University, was president of the Committee of One Hundred, and its roster included some very important names. The committee received support from many Congressmen and Senators. It recommended that the director of health should have Cabinet status, but President Taft, whose Committee on Economy and Efficiency had proposed a comprehensive federal health service in 1910, recommended a bureau rather than a department. None of these plans was carried to fruition, and the United States Public Health Service remained under semiautonomous administration within the Department of the Treasury where it had originated in 1798. It was not until 1935 that the Social Security Act was passed, and a comprehensive, co-ordinated plan of the health and welfare functions of the federal government was formulated—in 1939—with a single administrative head, called the Federal Security Agency.

The Children's Bureau

We have discussed in a previous chapter (see Chapter 41) the formation and subsequent activities of the Children's Bureau. Dr. Rosenau once told the author that the original proposal was to organize the Children's Bureau under the direction of the United States Public Health Service. The sponsors of the idea went to interview the surgeon general, Dr. Wyman, about the matter. He was a bachelor of long standing and regarded his staff as his personal family. He was also a gruff, grumpy Marine Hospital officer whose major concern was with the police powers of port quarantine and with the surgical treatment of sailors. At this famous interview he was most emphatic in his refusal to complicate his life with the importunities of a group of sentimental women who were interested solely in the welfare of mothers and infants. Since this activity was not acceptable to the United States Public Health Service, the Children's Bureau was organized in 1912 in the Department of Labor, the rationale being that one of its functions was to administer the maternal and child labor laws. The Children's Bureau became practically autonomous, and developed rapidly under the direction of a group of women who possessed the spirit of crusaders. These women encountered great opposition at first, but they received substantial support when Miss Jeanette Rankin entered Congress as its first woman member. In 1918 she introduced a bill for federal grants-in-aid to states in maternal and child care, and this plan finally was carried into effect through the Shepherd-Towner Act of 1921. To this day the Children's Bureau never has become an integral part of the United States Public Health Service.

Act of 1912

As we have noted at the start of this chapter, the United States Public Health Service has expanded to a greater extent since 1912, which is about the time when this book brings its recital to an end, than during the entire previous century of its existence. But the solid foundation on which it rests and the essential activities which it now carries out were established by the Act of 1912. This act provided for:

1. Investigation and research.
2. Improvement in methods of public health administration.
3. Distribution of federal aid to state and local health departments.
4. Interstate control of sanitation and communicable disease control.

The present United States Public Health Service was really launched at this time.

SURGEONS GENERAL OF THE UNITED STATES PUBLIC HEALTH SERVICE

The list of surgeons general of the United States Public Health Service from the appointment of the first supervising surgeon of the Marine Hospital Service to date have been:

JOHN M. WOODWORTH *(1871-1879)*
  He was only thirty-three years of age when appointed and he died at forty-one years of age.
JOHN B. HAMILTON *(1879-1891)*
  He was thirty-two years of age when appointed. He resigned from this position in 1891 and went to Chicago where he died of typhoid fever at fifty-one years of age.
WALTER WYMAN *(1891-1911)*
  He assumed office at forty-three years of age and served until he died— a long and honorable career.
RUPERT BLUE *(1912-1920)*
  Dr. Blue began his service at forty-five years of age. He served only two terms of four years each and then assumed charge of service operations in Europe. He remained on active duty until 1932.
HUGH S. CUMMING *(1920-1936)*
  Dr. Cumming began his service at fifty-one years of age. Both he and Dr. Blue belonged to the school of dignified southern gentlemen who by tradition dominated the United States Public Health Service staff for many years.
THOMAS PARRAN *(1936-1948)*
  Dr. Parran began his service at forty-four years of age. He was a most able administrator and farsighted statesman.
LEONARD A. SCHEELE *(1948-   )*
  Dr. Scheele was selected at forty-one years of age.

It is interesting to note that all the surgeons general have been appointed while they were young men. The oldest was Dr. Cumming and he was only fifty-one years of age when he took office.

SUMMARY

With this chapter we end our chronology of the growth of public health in America—from the date of the first colony on the Atlantic coast to the great World War in 1914. As we stated at the outset, our interest in public health development was initiated through a request to select the outstanding men of this field. A study of great men required the evaluation of great deeds, and this evaluation led to an understanding of the fact that we were dealing with an important social phenomenon, an irresistible flow of social forces toward the greater happiness and life fulfillment of all the people.

The growth of public health as a social force is, in reality, the growth of an appreciation by the people that each individual has a responsibility to the community; each person, each family, must contribute to the welfare of the whole, and in so doing further his own personal and family welfare.

Thus, public health is an index of the development of knowledge, of idealism, of unselfishness, of self-restraint, and of a greater degree of personal maturity. It is expressed in the responsibility that is aroused in the individual concerning matters that relate to family and communal well-being.

We can say in all truth that the advances in public health in America have been an accurate index of our advancing civilization in all its aspects and connotations. Thus, it becomes an axiom that the degree of the development of public health service, as a well-established and effective community function, is a true measure of the stage of civilization of a nation.

From our observations upon the past, we may now extend our trend lines into the future. Using this long perspective we may rest content with the assurance that a high quality of personal responsibility for the community will continue to develop in America, and that public health will become more widely disseminated and much more effective as the years pass. Our study of the past has given us an understanding of the living present, and the promise for the future is very bright indeed. The author will not live to see the end results of his life efforts—young men must now take up the torch. But he feels quite sure that the future is intrusted to strong hands, alert minds, and devoted hearts.

The Great Pioneers of Public Health in America

APPENDIX. *The Great Pioneers of Public Health in America, 1610-1925*[1]

There were giants in the earth in those days.

GENESIS VI:4

Workers in any field require their heroes. All of us have a need for the great towers of strength to whom we can turn for our inspiration and for spiritual uplift in our periods of weakness, discouragement, and confusion. We may idealize these men and magnify their achievements, but even this exaggeration may enhance the value of their inspiration. Thus, it has been worth while, despite the obvious pitfalls of the task, to seek out the names of those persons whom we may acclaim as the outstanding figures in public health during our whole national history.

The real pioneer in any social field is the man who has the vision to foresee the future; he must possess the perspective, and also the breadth of vision, to understand the unexpressed and often unfelt needs of the people and be able to formulate a plan which will meet these fundamental needs.

The pioneer is often not a leader at all. The effective leader is the man who keeps just a short distance ahead of his followers. In order to be a leader he must maintain close contact with them. Thus, he is seldom the one who has original concepts; rather his function is to carry the pioneer's ideas into execution. Therefore, the leader usually is not the pioneer, in that he does not originate—but develops and promotes—the ideas of others.

However, the originator of a basic concept cannot always be con-

[1] This Appendix was published in its entirety in the *American Journal of Public Health,* **Vol.** 43, No. 9, September, 1953. The author is under great indebtedness to the *Journal* for permission to use this material.

473

sidered a true pioneer. For example, Josiah Nott in 1848[2] suggested that mosquitoes might be an important factor in transmission of malaria, and gave excellent reasons for his unique idea, but he did not follow through with a workable hypothesis and his concept fell on sterile ground.

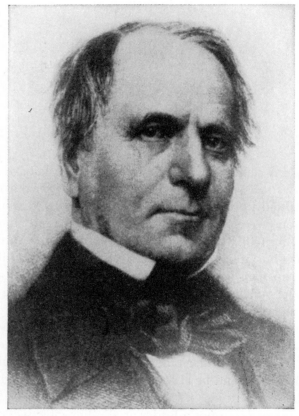

Fig. 41. Lemuel Shattuck. (From Walker, M. E. M.: *Pioneers of Public Health*. The Macmillan Co., New York, 1930.)

The social achievements of a nation may be appraised readily if one utilizes the historical method, and, starting at a given period, measures the advances that have been made, generation by generation. But it is almost impossible to determine just who it was that originated the basic concepts; what individual was chiefly responsible for the initiation of an idea, and who stimulated and fostered its

[2] Nott, Josiah: *New Orleans M. & S. J.*, 4:563, 1848.

growth. For social advancement is a mass phenomenon and is achieved through the activities of numberless undistinguished, but in the aggregate, very important people.

However, there are certain individuals in each generation who have stood out above all the others and who became major instru-

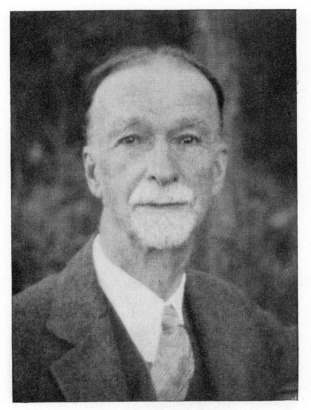

Fig. 42. Theobald Smith.

ments in the promotion of the public health of our country. Who are they?

METHODS OF SELECTION

The whole scope of public health was separated into eleven major categories with appropriate subdivisions, which thus totaled thirty separate divisions of interest. We then compiled a list of names of outstanding men and women who had been active in each of these fields. Each list covered the whole historical range of development of that particular subject as it has been initiated and expanded in America. Some of the lists were short; others, for example, epidemiology and sanitary engineering, each contained fifty or more names. Eventually a total of more than a thousand names were included in the various lists.

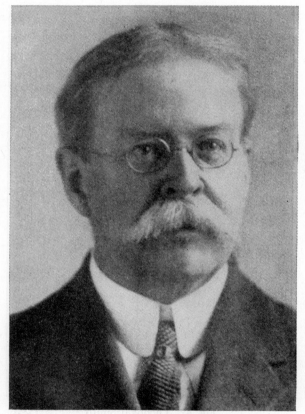

Fig. 43. William T. Sedgwick.

The list of names which was selected for each separate field of activity was then sent to specialists in that particular field. These experts in the special subject were asked to add suitable names and then to select five persons who had made the greatest contributions to their field of public health. From this tabulation, a consolidated list of the thirty categories was prepared with five names in each division. This table was called the "master list" (Table 17). The names in Table 17 do not total 150, since several men, as, for exam-

Table 17

Master List of Pioneers in Public Health in America
1610-1925

FIELD					
I. Communicable Disease Control	Jacob Bigelow	B. Waterhouse	Zabdiel Boylston	W. T. Sedgwick	*V. C. Vaughan*
1. Quarantine	*Wilson Jewell*	J. H. Griscom	Elisha Harris	A. N. Bell	J. M. Woodworth
2. Tuberculosis	Theobald Smith	H. I. Bowditch	*Hermann Biggs*	E. L. Trudeau	M. P. Ravenel
3. Malaria-yellow fever	*Daniel Drake*	G. M. Sternberg	Walter Reed	Henry Carter	W. C. Gorgas
4. Other contagious diseases	*C. W. Stiles*	A. L. Gihon (VD)	William H. Park	Simon Flexner	H. T. Ricketts
5. Diagnostic labs	Hermann Biggs	*William H. Park*	G. T. McCoy	G. M. Sternberg	V. C. Vaughan
6. Immunology	*Theobald Smith*	Simon Flexner	F. F. Russell	V. C. Vaughan	H. T. Ricketts
7. Epidemiology	W. H. Frost	Hibbert W. Hill	L. L. Lumsden	E. O. Jordan	W. T. Sedgwick
II. Sanitation	Noah Webster	*W. T. Sedgwick*	Elisha Harris	George Whipple	A. G. Clark
8. Sanitary engineering	W. R. Nichols	Hiram Mills	J. P. Kirkwood	*Rudolph Hering*	William C. Hazen
9. Food sanitation	E. O. Jordan	H. S. Wiley	H. W. Conn	B. H. Ransom	Samuel Prescott
10. Milk sanitation	M. J. Rosenau	H. W. Conn	William A. Evans	Charles E. North	H. L. Coit
11. Housing	George M. Kober	*Stephen Smith*	Jacob Riis	V. C. Vaughan	Lemuel Shattuck
12. Industrial hygiene and sanitation	George M. Kober	*Alice Hamilton*	Andrew H. Smith	Gilman Thompson	William C. Hanson
III. Health Organization Administration	*Lemuel Shattuck*	H. I. Bowditch	Stephen Smith	*Charles V. Chapin*	J. M. Woodworth
13. Rural health	*Ezra Hunt*	L. L. Lumsden	Wycliffe Rose	W. S. Leathers	C. W. Stiles
14. Municipal health	Stephen Smith	Hermann Biggs	Charles V. Chapin	J. H. Rauch	Edwin Snow
15. State health	Erastus Brooks	R. C. Kedzie	*Lemuel Shattuck*	H. I. Bowditch	Thomas M. Logan
16. National health	*J. M. Woodworth*	Stephen Smith	J. H. Rauch	J. S. Billings	G. M. Sternberg
17. Vital statistics	*Lemuel Shattuck*	E. Wigglesworth	*J. S. Billings*	Cressy Wilbur	Elisha Harris
IV. Maternal-Child Health	Julia Lathrop	*Josephine Baker*	Philip Van Ingen	O. W. Holmes	Henry Koplik
18. Infant care	*A. Jacobi*	Emmett Holt	Lucien Howe	Josephine Baker	J. H. M. Knox
19. School health	D. F. Lincoln	S. H. Durgin	R. J. O'Sullivan	Ellen Richards	Thomas Wood
V. Public Health Nursing	*Lillian Wald*	Mary Gardner	Mary Beard	Alfred Worcester	Lina Rogers
VI. Mental Hygiene	Benjamin Rush	Edward Jarvis	*Dorothea Dix*	Clifford Beers	Thomas W. Salmon
VII. Health Education	Benjamin Franklin	E. Routzahn	A. N. Bell	*Hermann Biggs*	Lemuel Shattuck
VIII. Training for Public Health as a Career	V. C. Vaughan	*W. H. Welch*	W. T. Sedgwick	George Whipple	M. J. Rosenau
IX. Nutrition	*Joseph Goldberger*	Graham Lusk	Nathan Strauss	A. F. Hess	H. C. Sherman
X. Public Health Law	*Dorman B. Eaton*	H. G. Clark	Erastus Brooks	J. Ordronaux	Lemuel Shattuck
XI. Voluntary Organizations	*Clara Barton*	L. F. Flick	Hermann Biggs	L. Schuyler	Fred T. Gates

NOTE: Italicized names are selections for Table 18.

ple, Billings, Shattuck, and Sedgwick, had made major contributions in more than one field.

The master list was then sent to ten distinguished persons who have been active in public health in America. Each of these scientists has manifested a scholarly interest in the historical development of public health. These judges were requested to add appropriate names

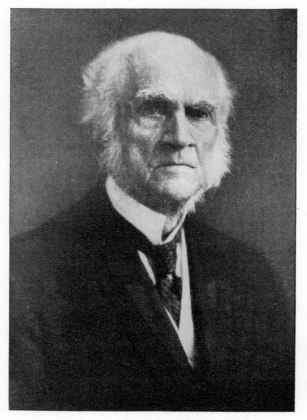

Fig. 44. Stephen Smith.

to the master list and to select the names of twenty-five persons who, in their opinion, had contributed most effectively to the development of public health in America.

The following persons aided in this selection from the master list of the pioneers:

Gaylord Anderson, M.D.
Leona Baumgartner, M.D.

Table 18

Outstanding Pioneers in Each Field of Public Health

1610-1925

FIELD	Name	Principal Contributions
I. Communicable Disease Control		
1. Quarantine	V. C. Vaughan	Epidemiology of Spanish War, typhoid fever, immunology; public health teacher
2. Tuberculosis	Wilson Jewell	Organized Quarantine Convention, 1857
3. Malaria-yellow fever	Hermann Biggs	Began basic services in tuberculosis control
4. Other contagious diseases	Daniel Drake	Diseases of interior valley of North America, 1850
5. Diagnostic labs	C. W. Stiles	Epidemiology of hookworm disease
6. Immunology	William H. Park	Established municipal diagnostic laboratories
7. Epidemiology	Theobald Smith	America's greatest medical scientist
	W. H. Frost	America's greatest epidemiologist
II. Sanitation	W. T. Sedgwick	Outstanding pioneer in general sanitation, brilliant teacher
8. Sanitary engineering	Rudolph Hering	Father of American sanitary engineering
9. Food sanitation	E. O. Jordan	Elucidation of food poisoning
10. Milk sanitation	M. J. Rosenau	Pasteurization of milk
11. Housing	Stephen Smith	Sanitary Survey of New York City, 1866
12. Industrial hygiene and sanitation	Alice Hamilton	Industrial toxicology
III. Health Organization Administration	Lemuel Shattuck	Shattuck report, 1850
13. Rural health	Ezra Hunt	Originated modern concepts of rural health services
14. Municipal health	Charles V. Chapin	America's greatest municipal health officer
15. State health	Lemuel Shattuck	Originated concept of state health department
16. National health	J. M. Woodworth	Founded Marine Hospital Service, which became the U.S. Public Health Service
17. Vital statistics	J. S. Billings	Established vital statistics in America
IV. Maternal-Child Health	Josephine Baker	Developed child health as a municipal function
18. Infant care	A. Jacobi	Father of American pediatrics
19. School health	Samuel Durgin	Established medical school inspection
V. Public Health Nursing	Lillian Wald	Founded "Henry Street Settlement"
VI. Mental Hygiene	Dorothea Dix	Pioneer in provision for care of mental illness
VII. Health Education	Hermann Biggs	Developed modern concepts of health education
VIII. Training for Public Health as a Career	W. H. Welch	Established Johns Hopkins School of Hygiene
IX. Nutrition	Joseph Goldberger	Pellagra studies
X. Public Health Law	Dorman B. Eaton	Basic public health law
XI. Voluntary Organizations	Clara Barton	Founded the Red Cross

Haven Emerson, M.D.
Iago Galdston, M.D.
Hugh R. Leavell, M.D.
Harry S. Mustard, M.D.
George Rosen, M.D.

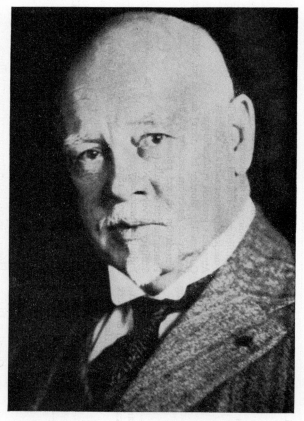

Fig. 45. William H. Welch. (From Bolduan, C. F.: *Illustrious Contributors to Public Health,* privately printed, 1936. Reproduced by permission of the late Dr. Bolduan.)

Richard H. Shryock, Ph.D.
Franklin H. Top, M.D.
C.-E. A. Winslow, Dr.P.H.

From the selections by this group, a solid consensus was obtained and two lists of names compiled: A list which nominates the person who has been judged to have made the greatest contribution to a special field (Table 18); and a final list of twenty-five persons who may be considered as the great pioneers in public health in America (Table 19).

Many students of public health will feel that the names of very important persons have been omitted from the final list. It is obvious, for example, that the names of Haven Emerson and C.-E. A. Winslow

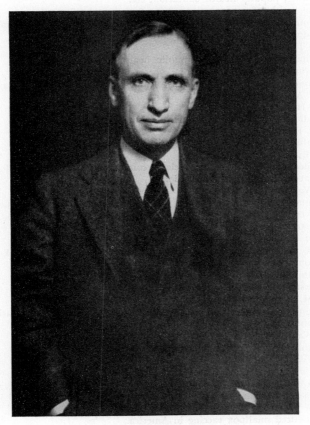

Fig. 46. Wade H. Frost.

belong in any "Temple of Fame" which is erected to public health personnel of America. They have not been included because these men were still active in the field when the selection was made. We considered only those whose major life work was completed by 1925, or at least whose great contributions had been made before that year.

It is apparent that the judgments of any group of men, no matter how thoughtful and judicial they may be, is of transitory import. A

Table 19

Final List of Outstanding Pioneers in the Development of Public Health in America

1610-1925

1. Lemuel Shattuck, 1793-1859
   Founder of public health in America. Recommended state and municipal health organizations on a full-time basis, vital statistics, nurses' training, public health training, popular health education, etc.
2. Theobald Smith, 1859-1934
   Immunologist, bacteriologist, tuberculosis control. Founded state biological products laboratory.
3. William T. Sedgwick, 1855-1921
   Sanitarian, epidemiologist, public health teacher.
4. Stephen Smith, 1823-1923
   Founder municipal health service, also cofounder, National Board of Health and American Public Health Association.
5. William H. Welch, 1850-1934
   Public health statesman, bacteriologist, public health teacher.
6. Wade H. Frost, 1880-1938
   Established epidemiology as a science in America.
7. John S. Billings, 1839-1913
   Epidemiologist, vital statistician, cofounder, National Board of Health; librarian, hospital administration.
8. Charles V. Chapin, 1856-1941
   Communicable disease control, municipal health administration.
9. Walter Reed, 1851-1902
   Determined transmission of yellow fever by a mosquito.
10. Hermann M. Biggs, 1859-1923
    State and municipal health administration, tuberculosis control, health education.
11. Alice Hamilton, 1869-
    Industrial hygienist, particularly toxicology.
12. George M. Sternberg, 1833-1915
    Diagnostic laboratories, bacteriology, malaria, yellow fever, national health administration.
13. Lillian Wald, 1867-1940
    Established public health nursing in America.
14. Oliver Wendell Holmes, 1809-1894
    Epidemiology, "Contagiousness of Puerperal Fever."
15. Dorothea Dix, 1802-1887
    State and national responsibility for care of persons with mental illness.
16. Benjamin Waterhouse, 1753-1846
    Introduced smallpox vaccine in America.
17. John M. Woodworth, 1837-1879
    Organized Marine Hospital Service, 1872, which became U.S. Public Health Service.
18. Josephine Baker, 1874-1945
    Established child health protection as a function of municipal government.
19. Charles W. Stiles, 1867-1941
    Discovered hookworm disease in the South and led development of rural sanitation in America.
20. Howard T. Ricketts, 1871-1910
    Pioneer work in virus disease, etiology, epidemiology, and control of Rocky Mountain spotted fever.
21. Daniel Drake, 1785-1852
    Epidemiology of malaria in America.

Table 19—*Continued*

22. Victor C. Vaughan, 1851-1929
     Pioneer in immunology, epidemiology, sanitation, and teaching of public health.
23. Milton J. Rosenau, 1869-1946
     Teacher of preventive medicine and public health, epidemiologist, milk sanitation.
24. George M. Kober, 1850-1931
     Initiated industrial medicine, exponent of housing, a teacher of public health in medical colleges.
25. William H. Park, 1863-1939
     Communicable disease control, diphtheria immunization, diagnostic laboratories.

NOTE: We have reproduced the photographs of the first ten men on our list.

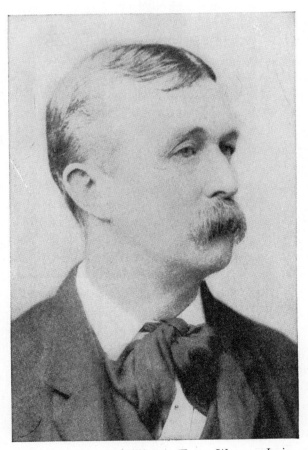

Fig. 47. John S. Billings. (From Watson, Irving A. (editor and compiler): *Physicians and Surgeons of America.* Republican Press Association, Concord, N.H., 1896.)

simple example may be given. Ezra M. Hunt, chairman of the
Section on State Medicine and Public Health of the American
Medical Association in 1877, made an appraisal which was similar
to ours. He selected the great leaders of the public health movement
in America of that generation as follows:

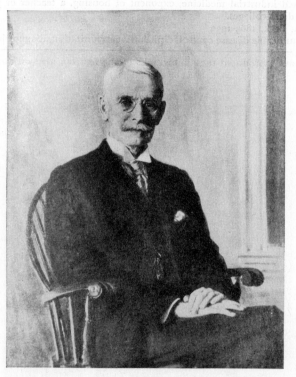

Fig. 48. Charles V. Chapin. (From *Papers of Charles
V. Chapin, M.D.* The Commonwealth Fund, New
York, 1934.)

1. SCIENTIFIC WORK
    Henry I. Bowditch
    C. F. Chandler
    J. S. Billings
2. PRACTICAL WORKERS IN THE FIELD
    E. M. Snow
    J. M. Toner
    Elisha Harris
    H. B. Baker
    Stephen Smith
Only two of these men are on our final list of great pioneers.

As one might anticipate, there was considerable disparity of opinion among the judges in selection of the pioneer group. There was almost complete unanimity in the selection of the first ten names on the list, but considerable diversity of opinion concerning the following fifteen names. For example, I believe that Henry I. Bowditch

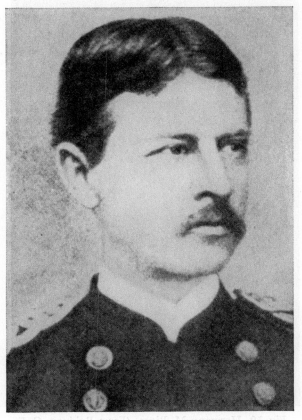

Fig. 49. Walter Reed. (From Bolduan, C. F.: *Illustrious Contributors to Public Health,* privately printed, 1936. Reproduced by permission of the late Dr. Bolduan.)

deserves great acclaim because of his work in the organization of the Massachusetts State Department of Health, for his studies in tuberculosis, and for his advanced social concepts. I also favor the name of Clara Barton, who organized the American Red Cross almost single-handedly, and I included in my pioneer list the name of George Whipple, the great statistician and sanitary engineer. I excluded Benjamin Waterhouse from my list since he simply introduced cowpox vaccine in America and had no part in the initial development of this procedure. As will be noted, I was overruled by my associates. Thus, each judge had his special preferences, but the consensus only is used in the final selection.

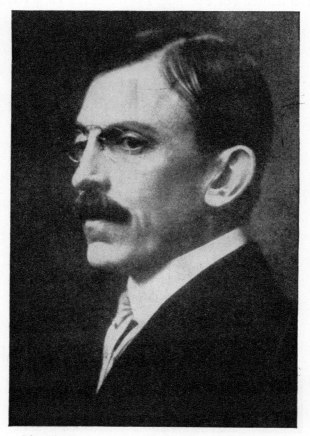

Fig. 50. Hermann M. Biggs. (From Bolduan, C. F.: *Illustrious Contributors to Public Health,* privately printed, 1936. Reproduced by permission of the late Dr. Bolduan.)

Many of the leaders in special public health fields will be in strong disagreement with Table 18, in which one person has been chosen as the greatest single contributor to their specialty. Perhaps they may believe that the most important names have been omitted entirely from their special category in the master table, i.e., Table 17, in which five names are selected to represent each special field.

One of the judges who consented to help in the selection of pioneers in public health emphasized the fact that this type of appraisal is obviously futile, a time-consuming and thankless procedure—but he then pointed out that it would be quite worth while if the effort resulted in an awakened interest in, and a general discussion of, the important milestones in the historical advance of public health in our nation. This in turn would lead to a more solid appreciation of the extraordinary achievements of the founders of public health in America.

PROPER-NAME INDEX

Abbott, S. W., 356, 383
Ackerley, G., 415
Adams, Daniel, 190
Adams, G. W., 273, 277
Adams, James T., 56, 64, 72
Agramonte, A., 384
Alcott, Louisa May, 409
Alsberg, Carl L., 358
Anderson, Gaylord, 478
Anderson, Genevieve, 407, 408
Andrews, John B., 176, 435, 439, 440, 441
Anthony, Sister, 413
Arthur, Chester A., 455
Axon, A. Forest, 314, 319

Bagnal, Anthony, 17, 84
Bailhache, P. H., 333
Baker, H. B., 302, 304, 308, 319, 329, 484
Baker, Josephine, 294, 416, 417, 420, 477, 479, 482
Baldwin, H. D., 314, 319
Bard, John, 71, 79, 86, 98, 103
Bard, Samuel, 52, 86, 90, 91, 98, 102
Bartlett, Elisha, 141, 162, 164, 179
Bartlett, Josiah, 30, 86, 103
Barton, Benjamin S., 86
Barton, Clara, 281, 410, 454-55, 453, 477, 479
Barton, E. H., 259
Baumgartner, Leona, 478
Bayley, Richard, 86
Beach, W., 429
Beard, Mary, 477
Beaumont, William, 185
Beebe, A. L., 385
Beers, Clifford, 477
Bell, A. N., 263, 268, 301, 302, 304, 306, 308, 333, 381, 402-3, 477
Bell, John, 168, 169, 191, 280, 290-91
Bell, William, 85
Bemiss, S. M., 322, 333
Bentham, Jeremy, 238
Bigelow, Jacob, 190, 260, 261, 264, 266, 378, 477
Biggs, Hermann M., 294, 373, 391-92, 398, 446, 448, 456, 477, 479, 482, 486
Billings, J. S., 2, 4-5, 15, 231, 301, 302, 304, 306, 321, 322, 333, 443, 446, 462, 477, 479, 482, 483, 484

Blackwell, Elizabeth, 278, 453
Blackwell, Emily, 305
Blake, Clarence J., 428
Blanton, Wyndham, 57, 88
Blue, Rupert, 469
Boerhaave, Herman, 11, 85, 86, 102
Bolduan, C. F., 113, 201, 294
Bolton, B. M., 395
Bond, Thomas, 86, 89, 101
Booke, T. C., 319
Bowditch, Henry I., 6, 247, 268, 280, 303, 307, 308, 309, 317, 318, 319, 333, 379, 456, 465, 477, 484
Boyd, Mark, 126
Boylston, Zabdiel, 25, 86, 88, 102, 103, 477
Brewster, Mary, 411
Bromwell, W. J., 218
Brooks, Erastus, 329, 459, 477
Buchan, William, 183, 191, 192, 405
Buck, A. H., 344, 443, 444
Budd, William, 164, 342, 344
Butterick, Wallace, 457

Cabell, James L., 301, 305, 306, 309, 322, 333, 335, 381
Carey, Mathew, 34, 37, 69, 363
Carlyle, Thomas, 271
Carroll, J., 384
Carter, H. R., 55, 384, 477
Caulfield, Ernest, 50, 51, 213
Chadwick, Edwin, 237-39, 248, 355, 370
Chaillé, Stanford E., 235, 315, 331, 334, 335, 336, 372
Chambers, J. S., 136, 137, 139
Chandler, C. F., 294, 300, 343, 484
Chapin, Charles V., 6, 75, 77, 213, 286, 353, 367, 390, 419, 422, 426, 442, 477, 479, 482
Cheesborough, E. S., 173, 349
Chesley, A. J., 328, 330
Choppin, Samuel, 36, 314, 322, 327
Clark, A. G., 477
Clark, E. H., 224
Clark, Henry G., 169, 260, 261, 263, 264-65, 267, 280, 303, 352, 357, 370, 477
Clot-Bey, Le Dr., 121
Cochran, Jerome, 300, 308, 319, 323, 333
Cohn, E. J., 395
Coit, Henry L., 361, 477

489

Penn, William, 34, 65
Pepper, William, 90, 177
Pettenkofer, Max, 164, 347, 400
Pfeiffer, Carl, 298-99
Phillips, S. F., 333
Phipps, Henry, 456
Pierce, Franklin, 211, 400
Pintard, John, 228, 287
Plunket, J. D., 321, 322
Pope, Alton S., 154
Prescott, Samuel, 477
Price, George, 439, 441
Prudden, T. Mitchell, 392, 398

Ramazzini, Bernardino, 179
Ramsey, David, 85
Rankin, D. N., 360
Rankin, Jeanette, 468
Ransom, B. H., 477
Ransom, John E., 88
Rathbone, William, 408-9
Rauch, J. H., 122, 298, 300, 301, 302, 303, 305, 306, 319, 321, 322-23, 355-56, 372, 477
Ravenel, Mazyck P., 456, 477
Rawlings, I. D., 154
Redman, John, 98
Reed, Walter, 354, 384, 446, 477, 482, 485
Revere, Paul, 77
Rhazes, 21
Richards, Ellen H., 346, 477
Richards, Linda, 410
Ricketson, Shadrack, 192
Ricketts, Howard T., 477, 482
Riis, Jacob, 401, 477
Rivers, Thomas M., 61
Robin, Albert, 443
Robinson, F. C., 366
Rockefeller, John D., 457, 458
Rogers, Lina, 411, 477
Rogers, Uriah, 28-29, 88
Rohé, G. H., 443, 444
Rolleston, J. D., 21
Roosevelt, Theodore, 358
Rose, Wycliffe, 448, 457, 458, 477
Rosen, George, 294, 480
Rosenau, Milton J., 253, 318, 354, 362, 385, 444, 445, 448, 467, 468, 477, 479, 483
Rotch, Thomas Morgan, 418
Routzahn, E., 477
Rush, Benjamin, 7-12, 37, 46, 53, 57, 58, 59, 73, 74, 77, 79, 85, 86, 96, 98, 99, 101-2, 105, 120-21, 148-49, 170, 222, 271, 351, 368, 477
Russel, Walter, 17, 84
Russell, F. F., 477
Russell, James, 237

Russell, William, 96

Salmon, Thomas W., 477
Sargent, D. A., 423
Scheele, Leonard A., 469
Schereschewsky, J. W., 420, 439, 441
Schuyler, Louisa, 281, 282, 410, 453-54, 477
Schwartz, G. T., 391
Seaman, Valentine, 31, 93, 94-95, 405
Sedgwick, William T., 346, 347, 350-51, 383, 446, 448, 476, 477, 479, 482
Semmelweis, Ignaz Phillip, 156
Shakespeare, E. O., 354, 384
Shattuck, Lemuel, 21, 39, 53, 70, 126, 152, 161, 172, 215, 217, 218, 231, 245, 246-57, 316, 370, 474, 477, 479, 482
Sherman, H. C., 477
Shippen, William, Jr., 94, 98, 101
Shryock, Richard H., 223, 480
Simon, John, 228, 240-41, 248, 343, 370
Smith, A. H., 180, 477
Smith, H. E., 384
Smith, Heber, 299
Smith, Joseph Mather, 245
Smith, Nathan, 216, 380
Smith, Southwood, 178, 226, 239, 241-44, 248
Smith, Stephen, 113, 128, 163, 261, 280, 289, 290, 292, 293, 294, 296-97, 301, 302, 305, 306, 322, 329, 332, 333, 338-39, 352, 477, 478, 479, 482, 484
Smith, Theobald, 361, 387, 395, 445, 475, 477, 479, 482
Snow, Edwin M., 259, 260, 261, 263, 265-66, 280, 286, 297, 301, 302, 303, 304, 306, 477, 484
Snow, John, 342
Soper, George A., 385
Spalding, Lyman, 216
Squibb, E. R., 358
Stearns, Frederick B., 346
Sternberg, George M., 306, 334, 335, 363, 365, 366, 377, 384, 387, 391, 437, 446, 456, 477, 482
Stevens, A. H., 261, 262, 263, 264, 266, 267
Stiles, C. W., 446, 457, 477, 479, 482
Stone, Daniel, 87
Strauss, Nathan, 362, 401, 419, 477
Sydenham, Thomas, 22, 24, 39, 50, 102

Taft, William Howard, 467
Taylor, L. H., 350, 383
Taylor, William, 164, 360
Thacher, James, 46, 48, 86, 87, 91, 152, 192, 221
Thacher, Thomas, 22, 23, 39, 84, 103
Thachrah, Turner C., 179

SUBJECT INDEX[1]

[1] Numbers indicated by *italic type* refer to dates, whereas numbers set in roman type are page references.

Chicago, sanitation during pioneer period, 173
tuberculosis death rate, *1851-1890*, 154
Child health. *See also* School health services
Colonial period, 95
period of development, 415-22
Bureau of Maternal and Child Hygiene, *1912*, 422
death rate, *1900* (table), 421
a division of child hygiene, New York City, *1908*, 420
a state subdivision of child hygiene, Louisiana, *1912*, 422
Strauss milk station, 419
summer camps, *1873*, 417-18
symposium on mortality, *1889*, 419-20
pioneer period, 119, 201-7
deaths, important causes of (table), 206
infant rate (tables), 204, 421
from zymotic diseases (table), 205
intestinal infections of infancy (table), 119
labor laws, 178, 201-3
Children's Bureau, 468
Cholera (Asiatic), 123, 131-40
deaths from, *1850* (table), 118
epidemic of *1832*, 134-36
epidemic of *1849*, 136-38
epidemic of *1866*, 138-39
epidemic of *1873*, 139-40
Cinchona, 57
City health departments. *See* Health departments—city
The City That Was (Stephen Smith), 293
Civilization, essential elements of, 243-44
Cleanliness, community, during Colonial period, 72-75. *See also* Sanitation —environmental
Clostridium welchii, 387
Colonial period, 13-107
communicable disease during, 21-60
industrial hygiene, 176-78
medical care, 83-97
medical education, 98-104
medicine among Indians, 105-7
public health administration during, 61-82
unawareness of public health, 15-20
vital statistics, 213-16
Communicable disease, Colonial period, 21-60
control during latter nineteenth century, 376-95
Consumption. *See* Tuberculosis
Cowpox vaccine, 29-31. *See also* Smallpox
in America, 30-31

"Cyanche trachealis," Colonial period, 53

"Deaconing" of foods, 175
Dental caries, 185
Development, period of, 269-469
American Medical Association, Section on State Medicine and Public Hygiene, 307-10
American Public Health Association, 296-306
Conference of State and Provincial Health Authorities of North America, 321-30
epidemiology and communicable disease control, 376-95
federal health services, development of, 459-69
health departments, city, 284-95
state, 311-20
health education, 396-404
health promotion in industry, 435-41
infant hygiene, 415-22
National Board of Health, 331-39
public health nursing, 405-14
sanitation, environmental, 340-75
military, 271-76
United States Sanitary Commission, 277-83
school health services, 423-34
teaching of public health and preventive medicine, 442-49
voluntary health agencies, 450-58
Diagnostic laboratory. *See* Public health
Diet, of Indians, 105
pioneer period, 181-86. *See also* Food
deficiency diseases during, 183
factory worker, 182
foods, classification of, 184
tomato, legend concerning, 183
Diphtheria, 49 *passim*, 127
antitoxin, *1894*, 394
deaths from, *1850* (table), 118
value of laboratory for diagnosis, 394
Disinfection, 69, 363-68
Dispensaries, Colonial period, 90-92
for Boston, *1796*, 91
for New York, *1790*, 91
for Philadelphia, *1786*, 91
Dysentery, during Civil War, 274
Colonial period, 43-45, 170
pioneer period, deaths in *1850* (table), 118

Employment of male population, *1850* (table), 114
Environmental sanitation. *See* Sanitation —environmental